Healthy ish

**All the goodness
with none of the fuss**

Emma Petersen

PAVILION

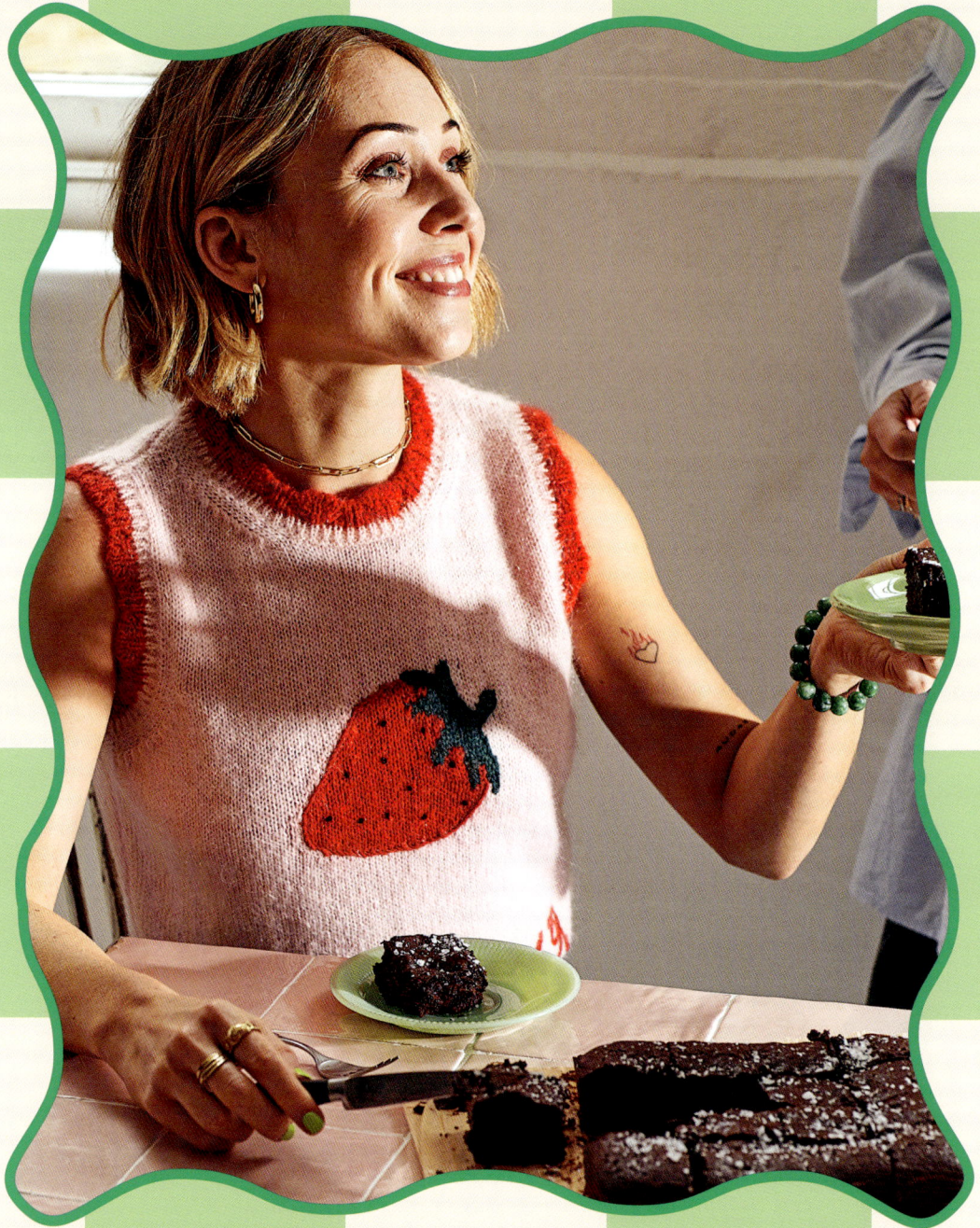

Contents

Describing my cooking style has always been a bit of a challenge. It doesn't neatly fit into any one category – it's not low-carb, not entirely plant-based and certainly not fixated on calorie or macro counts. So, when asked, I often say, 'well, it's healthy-ish'. And that simple, yet perfectly defined, phrase sparked the creation of this book.

So, without further ado, welcome to *Healthy-ish*! My debut cookbook (eeek!) that I have poured my heart and soul into creating, fuelled by my passion for easy and delicious home-cooked food that comforts as much as it nourishes. Whether you follow me on social media, or you've stumbled upon this book simply because you're as fed up as I am with the endlessly confusing narrative around 'healthy eating', I'm so glad and thankful that you're here. Let's begin!

A Little Bit About Me

Why, hello! I'm Emma – a lawyer-turned-food-content-creator, and now I can add turned-cookbook-author (sorry, I will never get over saying that last bit).

Yep, you read that right. Before all of this, I qualified as a solicitor in August 2023. I spent a stressful 6 years chasing my 'dream career' as a corporate lawyer in the City, so when I finally landed a training contract at one of the top firms in London, I thought I had hit the absolute jackpot. But 6 months in, a very different reality hit: I realised I was slowly losing everything else that was important to me – time for cooking, exercising, seeing family, socializing with friends and sharing my love for food online. Burnout became my norm, and so did eating Deliveroo at my desk, alone, at 9pm.

So, on the same day that I qualified, I quit. Scary? Absolutely. Best decision I've ever made? Without a doubt. Everyone else, however, thought I'd lost it.

In hindsight, maybe I should've seen it coming. Although I followed the academic path at school, behind it all I've always been creative. I spent every spare minute of my childhood painting, writing plays, taking hundreds of photos on my mum's digital camera and opening pretend bakeries for my neighbours. Add in the fact that my mum's an avid baker and fantastic cook, and my dad's obsessed with classic cookery, it was no surprise I inherited their passion for food.

University was the first time I really cooked for myself, and I fell in love. That's when I started my secret food page on Instagram. Yes, secret! It was my little hideaway to create and share recipes without anyone knowing. This was back when posting food pics wasn't cool – literally not a food influencer in sight. Safe to say, I never imagined it would grow into what it is now and I have to laugh about it, since over a million people follow me across my platforms. Definitely not a secret anymore!

I tried to keep my food page going while working in the City, but it was just impossible. I felt as though I was doing both things badly, and eventually realised I had to choose: food or the job. That's when I decided to throw myself fully into developing my culinary skills and growing my social media platforms – and I haven't looked back since.

Now, I'm lucky enough to do what I love for a living. I get to inspire people from all walks of life to enjoy simple, delicious food, and that brings me so much joy. But I'll always give credit to my time in the City for teaching me how to get creative in the kitchen with very limited time, and very little energy. It definitely shaped me into the cook I am today, and still allows me to recognise what the regular, busy individual looks for in everyday recipes.

Where I am now is wholly thanks to the incredible support I've received on social media over the past 9 years, and now, from you. If someone had told me a few years ago that I'd be writing a cookbook introduction instead of drafting loan agreements, I would've laughed in their face. But, somehow, here we are! Thank you from the bottom of my heart for being a part of this wild ride and making my dreams come true.

I hope you love *Healthy-ish* as much as I loved creating it.

`Happy cooking, Emma x`

Healthy, But at What Cost?

I think most of us want to eat more healthily and feel our best, but none of us want to sacrifice the joy that food brings, whether that's sharing a meal with loved ones, laughing over a bite out with friends, or enjoying a night in by yourself with something comforting. And we shouldn't have to. For years, I've been preaching that the path to healthy eating shouldn't come at the cost of happiness, or worse, lead to a cycle of restriction and over-control. I've sadly been there myself, and have promised to never go back.

In theory, eating well should be simple, but, in reality, it's a minefield. We have conflicting advice bombarding us from every angle, and labels that leave us with restrictive rules that do more harm than good: cut out carbs; don't eat after 8 p.m.; count every calorie and macronutrient; eliminate fats; avoid sugar in all forms... the list goes on. And it's exhausting! Plus, you don't have to be an expert to realise that trying to follow every piece of dietary advice out there would be impossible (and not to mention miserable), as most of it contradicts itself.

Which is where *Healthy-ish* comes in.

This book is the antithesis of restrictive or puritanical approaches. It focuses on balance, not perfection and embraces the reality of busy lives. I like to think of it as a one-stop solution: easy, everyday recipes that prioritize health and nourishment, but without the labels and without sacrificing on flavour or convenience. My goal is to show as many people as possible that with a little bit of balance – a touch of 'ish' alongside the 'healthy' – it's more than possible to create a lifestyle and way of eating that's totally sustainable, enjoyable and absolutely delicious.

So, while the recipes in this book are all nutritionally diverse and packed with wholesome, unprocessed ingredients (you can read more about my Healthy-ish Principles on pages 8–9), they will also never shy away from comforting touches like melty cheese, a drizzle of melted chocolate or a crispy breadcrumb coating. Because the key to a sustainable diet is all about striking the balance between nourishing our bodies, while leaving space for some comforting indulgences. That's the sweet spot, if you'll pardon the pun.

GOOD FOOD, GOOD MOOD

Before I get too carried away, I'm going to hit pause on talking about nutritionals and move on to the end product, and my favourite part, the food. Because the healthy eating spiel is worth absolutely nothing if it doesn't taste good, right? Right.

I've said it before and I'll say it again: healthy food doesn't have to equal a sacrifice in flavour or excitement. It doesn't have to mean cutting out everything enjoyable and tasty. That's why I've spent many, many months developing these recipes to ensure that they are the most delicious they can be and that they're easy enough to be made, by anyone. There are recipes for those ordinary time-poor weeknights, but there are also impressive dishes that you could serve up with confidence at a dinner party.

So, if you thought that healthy eating meant banishing banging meals like an oozy lasagne (see page 156), creamy ramen (see page 150) or a gooey chocolate cake (see page 184), I'm excited to prove you wrong.

How to Use This Book

To me, an 'everyday' cookbook is one that you could use for every single meal of the day if you wanted to. And that's exactly what we have here: Dinner in Under 30 for when you've had a long day and want to get something on the table quickly; delicious and nutritious Batch Breakfasts that future-you will thank you for when the week's in full swing; tasty One-Pan Winners that are perfect to minimize clean-up and fuss; more indulgent but refined sugar-free Sweet Treats to satisfy any sweet tooth; Weekend Brunch for those long-awaited slower mornings, Simple Lunches that you'll be looking forward to from the moment the day begins; and tasty Snacks to keep any 'hanger' at bay.

DIETARY KEY AND SUBSTITUTIONS

I know how frustrating it can be when a recipe catches your eye, but you're missing an ingredient or have a dietary restriction that prevents you from making it as-is. Or maybe a vegan, vegetarian or gluten-free friend is coming round for dinner and you don't know what to make. Either way, these recipes have you covered. Each one has a variety of dietary substitutions, ensuring that nearly all of the recipes can be adapted to suit various dietary needs.

Just as a general note – whenever you see an ingredient like yogurt, cheese or milk without specifics, it's up to you which variety to use. Go dairy-free or stick with regular – any will work.

These are the dietary labels I've used, with a breakdown of what they mean:

- **(V) Vegetarian:** The recipe contains no meat or fish, but may include dairy and eggs.
- **(V/O) Vegetarian Option:** There are substitutions listed to make the recipe meat-free.
- **(VE) Vegan:** The recipe contains no animal products, including meat, dairy, eggs and honey.
- **(VE/O) Vegan Option:** Choose dairy-free milk, cheese, yogurt, cream, etc., and check the substitutions for other swaps to make the dish plant-based.
- **(DF) Dairy-Free:** The recipe contains no dairy products like milk, butter or cheese.
- **(DF/O) Dairy-Free Option:** This recipe can be made dairy-free by choosing dairy-free milk, cheese, yogurt, cream, etc.
- **(GF) Gluten-Free:** The recipe is free of gluten, a protein found in wheat, barley and rye.
- **(GF/O) Gluten-Free Option:** There are substitutions listed to make the recipe gluten-free.
- **(N) Contains Nuts:** The recipe includes nuts.

A NOTE ON LEFTOVERS

Although I've designed these recipes to minimize leftovers, sometimes you may find yourself with a bit of something extra – like a half-used tub of crème fraîche, for instance. Rather than letting it go to waste, flip to the index. There, you'll find all the other recipes that use that same ingredient, making it easy to incorporate into another dish later in the week. This will not only reduce food waste, but simplify meal planning, as you can build around the ingredients you already have.

Healthy-ish Principles

Every recipe in this book has been developed with 6 key principles in mind. Because I want you to feel confident that whichever recipe you choose, it will be a good one.

1

PROTEIN RICH

Eating a diet rich in protein offers benefits far beyond just muscle growth. It plays a key role in tissue repair and immune function support, and aids the production of essential enzymes and hormones. Protein is also crucial for maintaining healthy skin, hair and nails, making it a cornerstone of overall health (source: NHS UK). On top of that, because we digest protein more slowly than carbohydrates, it helps to stabilize our energy levels, keeping us feeling fuller and more satisfied throughout the day. This means fewer energy dips and a more sustained sense of well-being.

With these benefits in mind, the majority of recipes in this book are designed to deliver high-quality protein in various creative ways. Traditional protein sources like lean meats, eggs and legumes are, of course, included, but I've also integrated less-obvious options, such as blending silken tofu into pasta sauces, dressings and even desserts (trust me, it works).

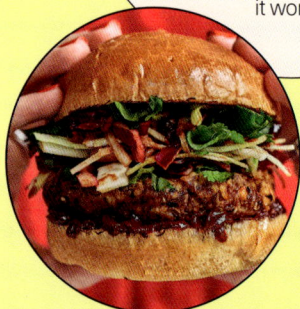

2

FREE FROM REFINED SUGARS

The recipes use natural sweeteners such as maple syrup, dates, honey and coconut sugar.

Sugar is one of those ingredients that tends to spark debate. Personally, I don't think I could live a happy life without it entirely, so that's where my 'ish' comes in. To break it down simply, there are three types of sugar:

• Naturally occurring sugars, found in foods like fruits and vegetables
• Unrefined sugars, like coconut sugar, which undergo less processing and contain more antioxidant compounds
• Refined sugars, such as cane or beet-derived sugars

The last type provides little to no nutritional value, which is why I've excluded it from the recipes in this book. Plus, I do honestly think natural sugars taste way better – but that might just be me!

3

FREE FROM ULTRA-PROCESSED INGREDIENTS

These recipes focus on whole foods. But what are 'ultra-processed' foods? Well, most food is processed to some degree. Even if you're cooking from scratch, ingredients like flour, olive oil and tinned tomatoes are technically 'processed' as they aren't in their raw, whole states. However, UPFs go a step further. They often contain industrial additives used to enhance flavour, texture and shelf life. My general rule is, if I can't pronounce an ingredient on a product's ingredients list, I probably won't buy it.

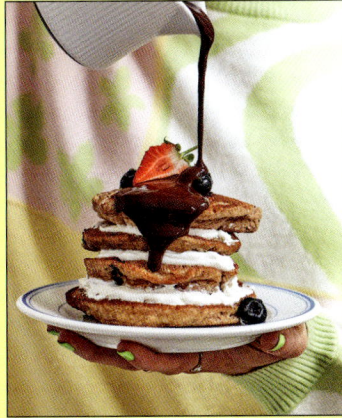

5

PLANT FORWARD

I personally choose to eat a protein-rich diet that limits reliance on animal products, so over 70 per cent of the recipes in this book just so happen to be vegetarian or plant-based. Others, where possible, will include meat and dairy-free substitutions, ensuring as many dietary preferences and restrictions as possible can be catered for. Red meat is absent entirely.

4

CONVENIENCE FOCUSED

'Work smart, not hard' has been my tongue-in-cheek mantra for years. In cooking terms, this means using the right ingredients and techniques, in the right way, to elevate simple dishes quickly and with minimal extra effort – and that is what this book is all about. I want to show you that it's entirely possible to create something innovative that tastes as though you have been sweating over the hob/stove for hours, when in reality you've hardly had to do much at all.

The book's overall structure has been designed to assist the busy home cook. Chapters such as Batch Breakfasts, Simple Lunches, Dinner in Under 30 and One-Pan Winners are solely dedicated to time-saving and/or meal prep. Each recipe also comes with a 'Future You' section, offering information on how to store extra portions in the fridge or freezer, and how to thaw and reheat, if needed.

6

NOURISHING FOR THE MIND AND BODY

This one is possibly the most important, and the principle that can outweigh the others. Because I want to dispel any preconception that eating healthily means losing balance, or having to remove things from your diet completely. Hence Healthy-ish: 'healthy' is for the body, and 'ish' is for the heart and mind.

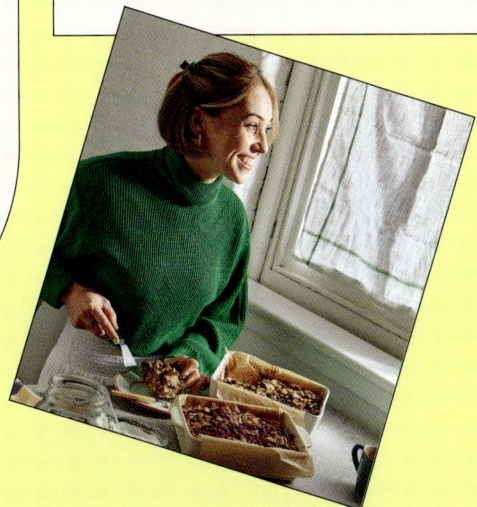

-ish Ingredients

Here are the bits I keep in stock, as well as the tools that are helpful to have to hand.

CHOCOLATE

I don't think I need to go into much detail about why chocolate features in this book. Quite frankly, life is for living, and chocolate (for me) is a big part of that. However, I do choose dark/bittersweet chocolate over milk or white, not just because I think it's the most delicious, but also because it's packed with health benefits. Dark chocolate is rich in antioxidants, flavanols (which support heart health), and polyphenols (great for gut health). You don't have to tell me twice! Ready for some dark chocolate brownies? Jump to 174.

PROTEIN POWDER

I've limited the use of protein powder in this book, since it's a highly processed ingredient and not a pantry staple. That said, I do incorporate it sparingly in my diet because it's a convenient, affordable and tasty way to add plant-based protein to sweet recipes. Whenever it's used in a recipe, there's always a substitution option to leave it out – the choice is yours.

If you do decide to use protein powder, my preferred option is soy protein. Look for one with as few ingredients as possible. My go-to is Myprotein's salted caramel flavour, which simply contains: protein isolate (90 per cent), natural flavouring, salt, apple extract and sweetener (sucralose).

CONVENIENCE OPTIONS

Convenience-focused is one of the key principles of *Healthy-ish*, which sometimes means prioritizing ease over a completely unprocessed option. Again, my general rule is to look at the ingredients list, and if I can't pronounce an ingredient or imagine what it looks like in real life, I'll choose something else.

A few examples of convenience options I use in my kitchen include:

- Microwavable pouches of rice and grains (I opt for unflavoured versions as they tend to be the least processed)
- Store-bought sauces, like pesto
- Bread items, such as flatbreads, bagels and crumpets
- Ready-rolled pastry
- Frozen fruits and veggies, such as peas, spinach and berries

HELPFUL TOOLS TO HAVE ON HAND

All the recipes in this book are simple, and so is the equipment needed to make them. But if I had to list my go-to tools, it would look a little like this:

- 28–30 cm/11–12-in frying pan/skillet with a lid (preferably ovenproof)
- Baking sheet
- Parchment paper
- Medium-sized saucepan
- Microwave-safe bowl with lid and steam escape
- Baking tins (20 cm/8 in square tin, 20 cm/8-in round cake tin, 6- or 12-hole muffin tray)
- Baking dishes (23 x 18 cm/9 x 7-in and 33 x 23 cm/13 x 9-in)
- Microplane grater or cheese grater
- Flat silicone spatula
- A set of mixing bowls
- Sieve/strainer
- Tongs
- Wooden spoons
- Digital food scales

PANTRY SHOPPING LIST

- Oils (mild olive oil for cooking, extra virgin olive oil for dressing, coconut oil for baking, sesame oil for sauces)
- Seasonings (salt, pepper, spices, dried herbs)
- Carbohydrate sources (pasta, noodles, easy-cook rice, oats, potatoes, flour)
- Legumes (tinned beans and lentils)
- Nut butters and tahini
- Harissa paste
- Sun-dried tomatoes
- Sweeteners (maple syrup, honey, agave syrup, coconut sugar)
- Silken tofu
- Soy sauce
- Baking powder and bicarbonate of soda/baking soda
- Nuts and seeds (chia seeds, flaxseeds, hemp seeds, pumpkin seeds, sunflower seeds)
- Dried fruit
- Aromatics (onions, garlic)
- Organic eggs

FRIDGE SHOPPING LIST

- Fresh herbs (parsley, coriander/cilantro, basil, dill)
- Fresh veggies
- Fresh ginger
- Fruit (bananas, stone fruits and berries)
- Lemons and limes
- Milk
- Yogurt
- Cheese
- Extra-firm tofu

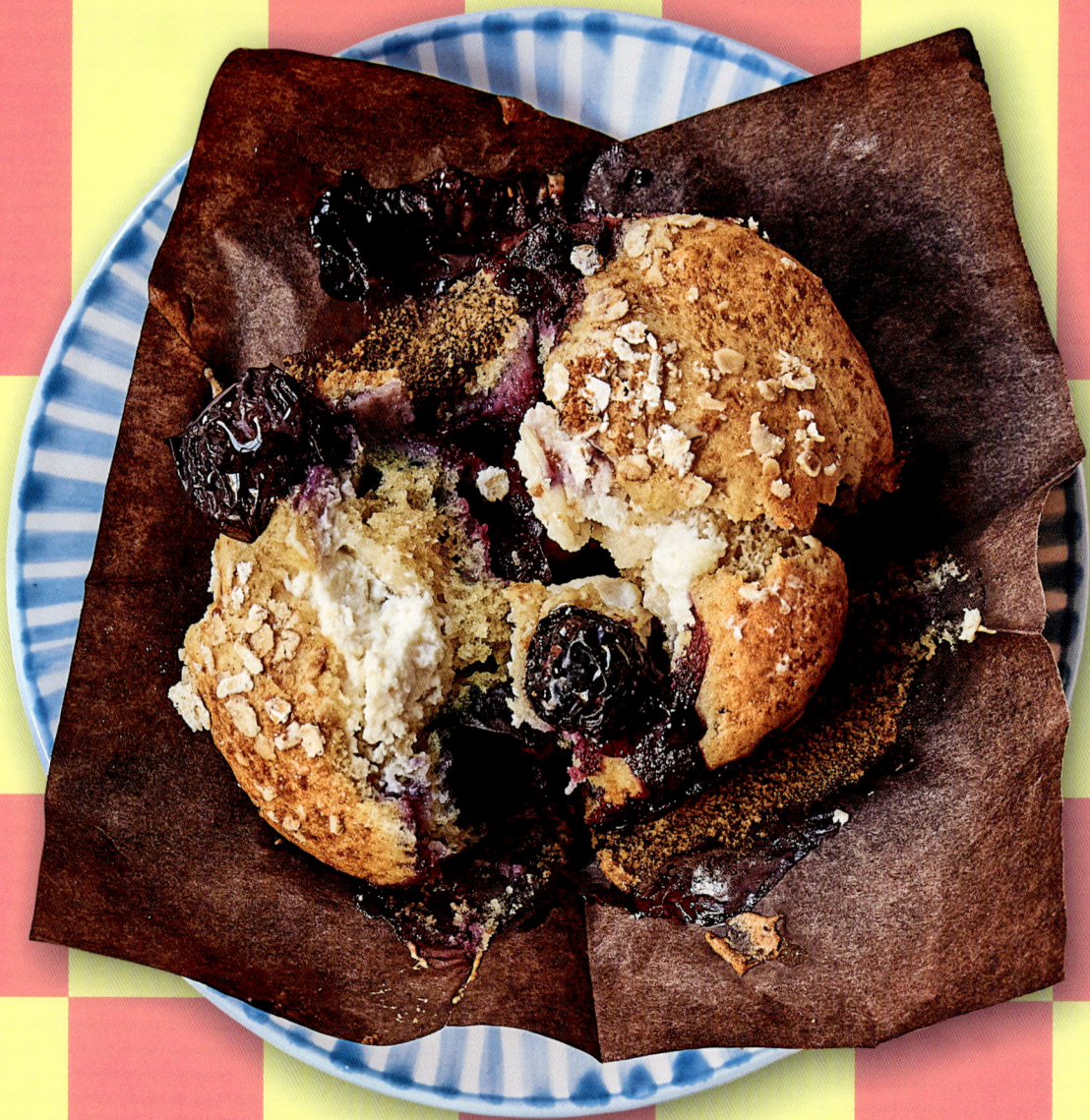

Batch Breakfasts

Make-ahead Breakfasts for Busy Mornings

Meal-prepping breakfast became non-negotiable when I was working in the City. Being a breakfast lover, I refused to settle for mundane, unsatisfying and often overly expensive options when I realised I could cook something delicious once and then enjoy it for the whole week. Even now I work from home and make food for a living, these are still the recipes I lean on the most. Not only do they save so much time, but they are delicious, naturally high in protein and, quite honestly, a reason to get out of bed! My mornings would not be the same without them.

Batch Baked Oats, 2 Ways

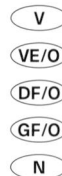

(V)
(VE/O)
(DF/O)
(GF/O)
(N)

Having been unofficially crowned the Oats Queen on social media, it feels safe to say that these are the best baked oats you'll ever make. The flavour possibilities are honestly endless, but to get you started, here are two of my favourite variations that are equally loved by over 10 million viewers across my platforms. All that's needed is 45 minutes of mostly hands-off time, and you'll have grab-and-go breakfasts ready for the whole week.

23 x 15-cm/9 x 6-in baking dish, lined

2 ripe bananas

200 g/7 oz/generous 2 cups rolled/old-fashioned oats

60 g/2 oz/⅔ cup soy protein powder

1 tsp baking powder

420 ml/15 fl oz/1¾ cups milk

yogurt, to serve

For peanut butter and 'jam'

200 g/7 oz/1⅓ cups frozen raspberries

1 tbsp maple syrup

1 tsp chia seeds

60 g/2 oz/4 tbsp natural peanut butter, plus extra to serve (optional)

For chunky monkey

50 g/1¾ oz dark/bittersweet chocolate, roughly chopped

40 g/1½ oz/generous ¼ cup walnut halves, roughly chopped

1 banana, sliced into coins, plus extra to serve (optional)

1   Preheat the oven to 180°C fan/200°C/400°F/gas mark 6.

2   In a large mixing bowl, mash the bananas until smooth, then add the oats, protein powder, baking powder and milk. Stir until everything is fully combined and the mixture has a thick, batter-like consistency.

3   For the peanut butter and 'jam' version, pour the oat mixture into the prepared baking dish, using a silicone spatula to spread it into the corners and smooth the top. Place the frozen raspberries, maple syrup and chia seeds into a microwave-safe bowl and microwave on full power for 1 minute, or until the raspberries are warm and soft. Mash them with the back of a fork until you achieve a jam-like consistency. Dollop alternate tablespoonfuls of the homemade raspberry 'jam' and peanut butter on top of the oats. Using the handle of a teaspoon or a chopstick, swirl them together to create a marbled effect.

4   For the chunky monkey version, fold half of the chopped chocolate and half of the chopped walnuts into the oat mixture, stirring until they are evenly distributed. Pour the mixture into the prepared baking dish, using a flat spatula to spread it into the corners and smooth the top. Arrange the banana coins on top, then sprinkle over the remaining chopped chocolate and walnuts.

5   Place the baking dish onto the middle shelf of the oven and bake for 35 minutes, or until the top is golden and the oats are set in the middle.

6   Once baked, let the oats cool in the dish for 5–10 minutes to allow them to firm up. Slice into 6 portions and serve warm or cold, with your favourite yogurt and extra banana slices or a drizzle of nut butter, if desired.

Substitutions:

● **Gluten-free?** Use gluten-free oats.
● **Nut-free?** Use tahini. ● **No protein powder?** Sub for plain/all-purpose flour and only 300 ml/10 fl oz/1¼ cups of milk.

Future you:

▭ Cool and place in an airtight container, storing in the fridge for up to 5 days.
❄ Cool and freeze for up to 3 months.
💧 Thaw in the fridge overnight, or on low power in the microwave.
🔥 Microwave for 1 minute to warm up, or enjoy cold.

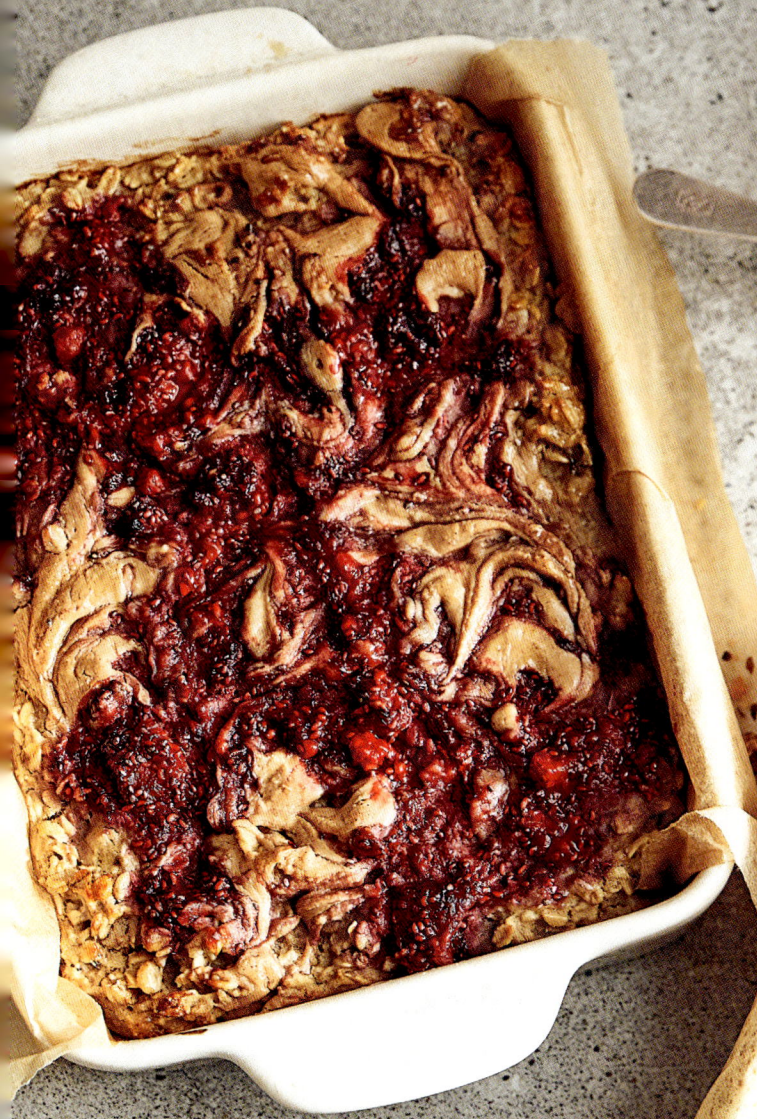

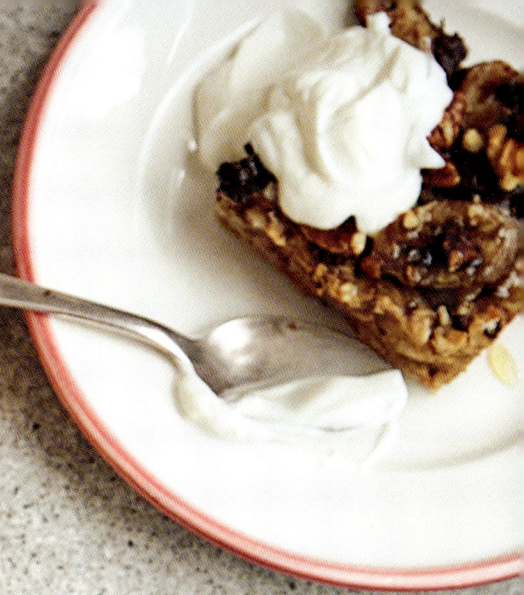

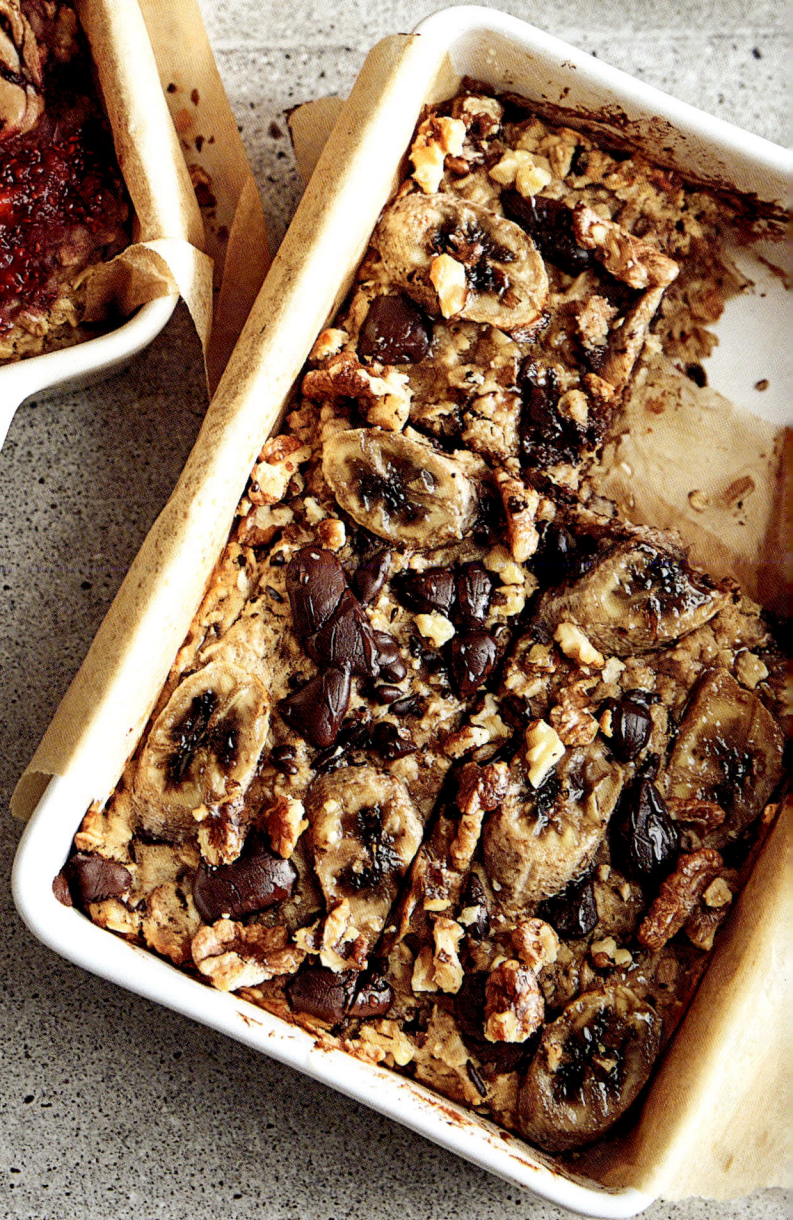

Batch Overnight Oats, 2 Ways

(V)
(VE/O)
(DF/O)
(N)

Every time someone tells me they don't like overnight oats, I sigh – because I just *know* they're doing it wrong. The key is nailing a good, creamy base recipe (luckily I've done that hard work for you) and then focusing on add-ins like nut butters, flavour variations and different textures. I've come to prefer making them in big batches like this, rather than night-by-night, as then all it takes is a couple of minutes each morning to scoop them out and serve with some yogurt, and top with whatever goodies you're craving. So easy, genuinely delicious and totally un-boring.

200 g/7 oz/generous 2 cups rolled/old-fashioned oats

80 g/3 oz/scant 1 cup soy protein powder

15 g/½ oz/1 tbsp chia seeds

600 ml/1 pint/2½ cups milk

yogurt, to serve

almond or peanut butter, to serve

For chocolate cherry

1 tbsp cacao powder

100 g/3½ oz/⅔ cup fresh cherries, halved

25 g/1 oz/2½ tbsp dark/bittersweet chocolate chips

For carrot cake

80 g/3 oz carrot, peeled and finely grated

40 g/1½ oz sultanas/golden raisins or raisins

40 g/1½ oz/generous ¼ cup walnut halves, roughly chopped

2 tsp ground cinnamon

1   In a large mixing bowl, combine the oats, protein powder, chia seeds and milk. Stir well until the mixture forms a thick, batter-like consistency.

2   For the chocolate cherry version, mix the cacao powder into the oat mixture, stirring until fully dissolved with no lumps. Then fold in the cherries and chocolate chips until evenly distributed throughout.

3   For the carrot cake version, fold the grated carrot, sultanas, walnuts and cinnamon into the oat mixture, mixing until evenly distributed throughout.

4   Transfer the mixture to a sealable container, cover with the lid and refrigerate overnight, or for at least 3 hours to allow the oats to set.

5   When you're ready to eat, spoon out a portion and serve alongside a dollop of yogurt, and a drizzle of nut butter.

Substitutions:

● **No protein powder?** Omit entirely and reduce the amount of milk used to 400 ml/14 fl oz/1¾ cups. ● **Nut free?** Omit the walnuts and nut butters.

Future you:

🥡 Cool and place in an airtight container, storing in the fridge for up to 5 days.
❄ Cool and freeze for up to 3 months.
💧 Thaw in the fridge overnight, or room temperature for a few hours.
🔥 Let them come to room temperature before eating, or microwave for 15 seconds.

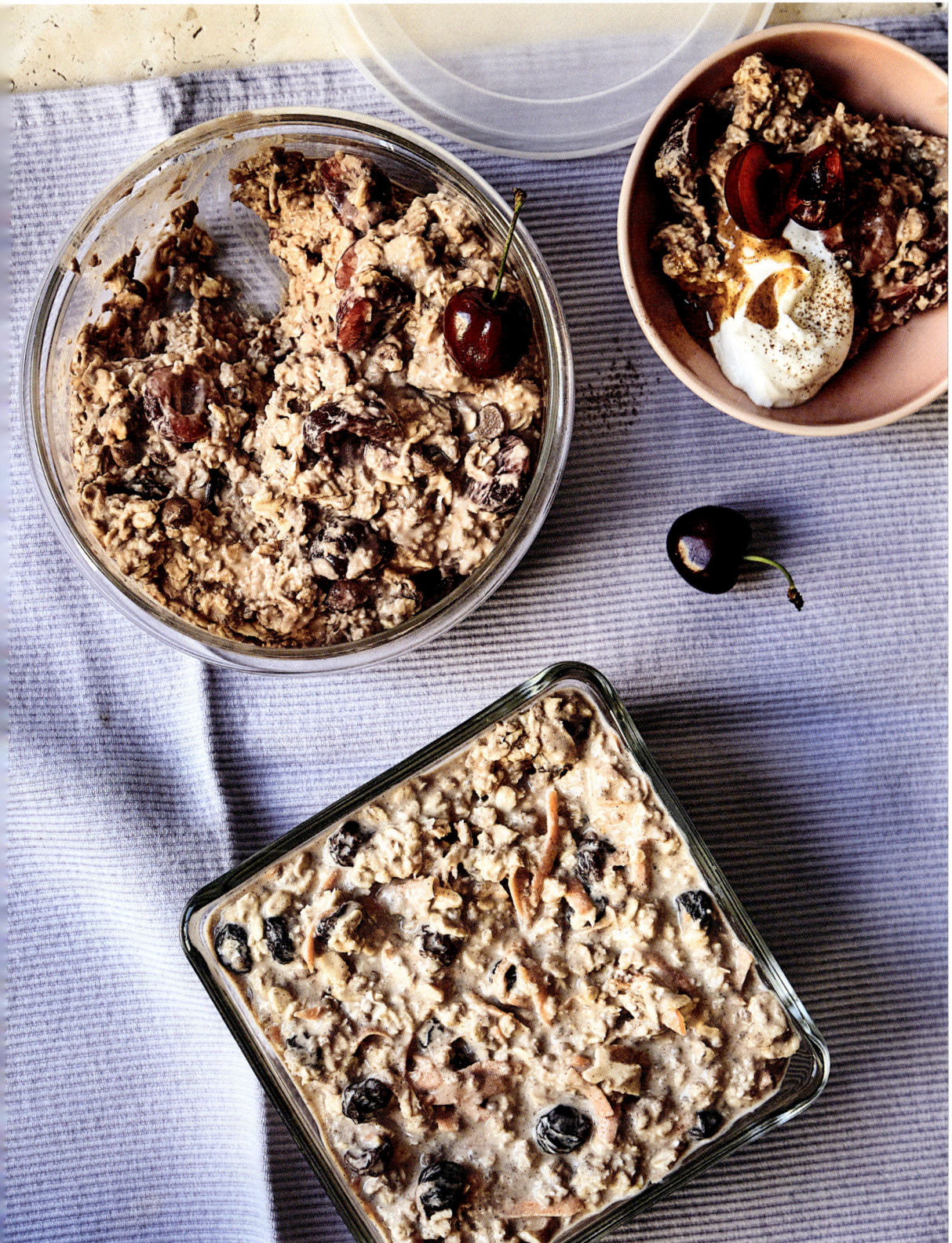

Sweet Potato + Feta Frittata

V

GF

DF/O

Frittatas are a fool-proof way to use up leftover veggies. Try swapping sweet potato for white potato, peppers for broccoli, or parsley for coriander. My only tip: include some bold flavours and a cheese. I've streamlined this into a quick, stovetop-only version. It's a winner.

250 g/9 oz sweet potatoes

8 large/US extra-large eggs

50 ml/1½ fl oz/3½ tbsp milk

1 red onion, finely diced

2 garlic cloves, minced

180 g/6 oz/1 cup roughly chopped jarred roasted red (bell) peppers

50 g/1¾ oz/½ cup sun-dried tomatoes, roughly chopped

1 tsp dried oregano

100 g/3½ oz/scant 2 cups spinach, roughly chopped

100 g/3½ oz/¾ cup crumbled feta

1 tbsp chopped parsley

salt and pepper

olive oil, for cooking

salad leaves, to serve

1   Cooking potatoes in the microwave is my favourite way to save time and washing up. To microwave: pierce the sweet potato(es) with a fork or knife in a few places, then wrap in a damp paper towel. Place in the microwave and cook on full power for 2 minutes. Turn over and microwave for another 2 minutes. The potato(es) should be knife-tender, so continue microwaving in 1-minute intervals if not quite there. Carefully remove, unwrap and set aside to cool.

2   Crack the eggs into a large mixing bowl. Add the milk, with a generous pinch each of salt and pepper, and whisk well until combined.

3   Roughly chop the cooked potato, skin on, into 2.5-cm/1-in chunks. Heat 2 tablespoons of olive oil in a lidded frying pan/skillet over medium heat, cook the onion and garlic for 2 minutes, then add the sweet potato and stir. Increase the heat, cook for 3 minutes until the potato is lightly browned, then add the peppers, sun-dried tomatoes, oregano, and a pinch of salt and pepper. Cook for 1 minute, then stir in the spinach until wilted.

4   Reduce the heat to low. Scoop three-quarters of the potato mixture out of the pan and into a clean bowl. Pour half of the egg mixture into the pan. Return the reserved potato mixture to the pan, a spoonful at a time, then pour the remaining egg mixture over the top. If you're wondering why this step is necessary, creating a layer of egg on the bottom of the pan ensures it cooks through quickly and evenly, without burning.

5   Return the pan to medium heat and sprinkle over the feta and parsley. Cover the pan with the lid and leave everything to cook for around 8 minutes, or until the eggs are set in the middle.

6   Slide the frittata onto a plate, slice it into wedges, and serve with your favourite side salad.

Substitutions:

● **No feta?** Sub for any other cheese.
● **Dairy-free?** Omit the feta or substitute for dairy-free cheese.

Future you:

🗇 Cool and place in an airtight container, storing in the fridge for up to 3 days.
❊ Cool and freeze for up to 1 month.
🌢 Thaw in fridge overnight, or on low power in the microwave.
🔥 Eat cold or microwave each portion for 60–90 seconds to reheat.

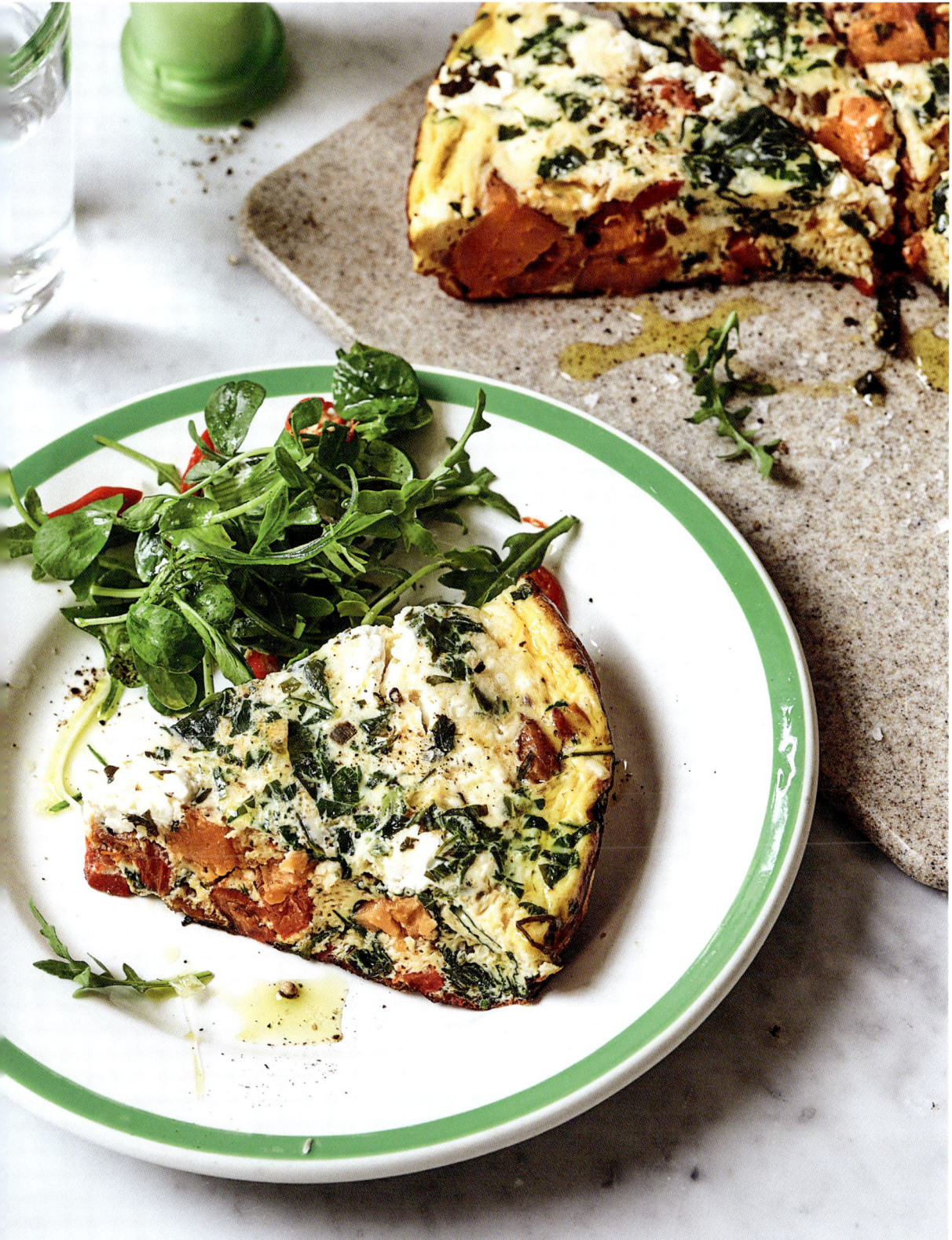

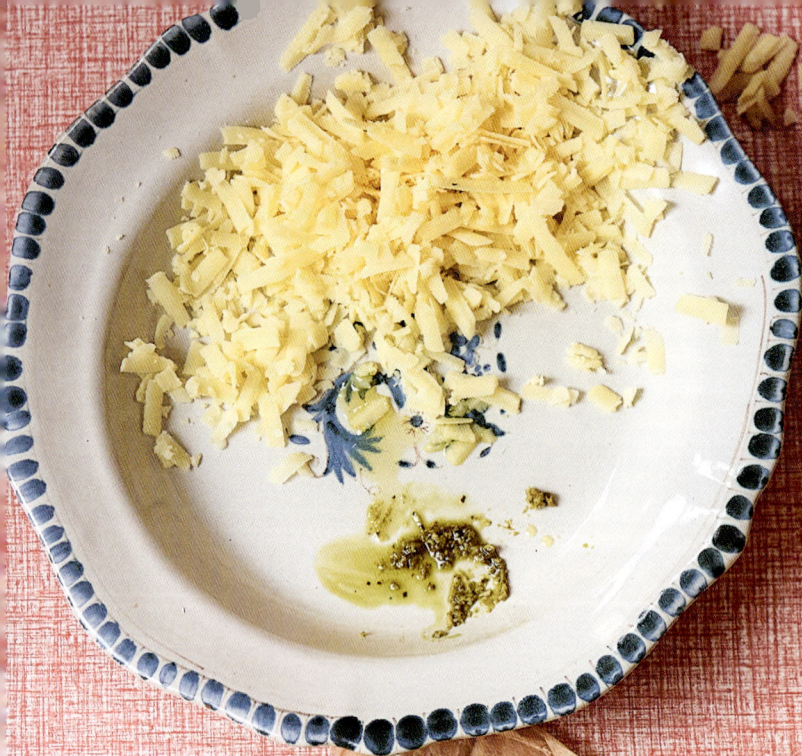

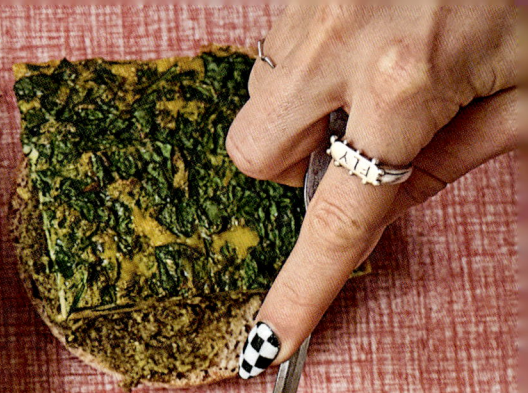

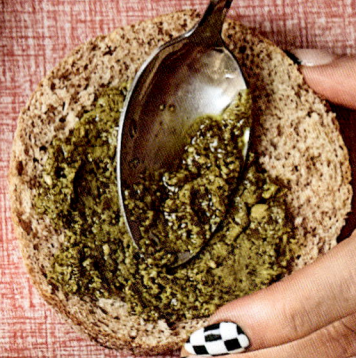

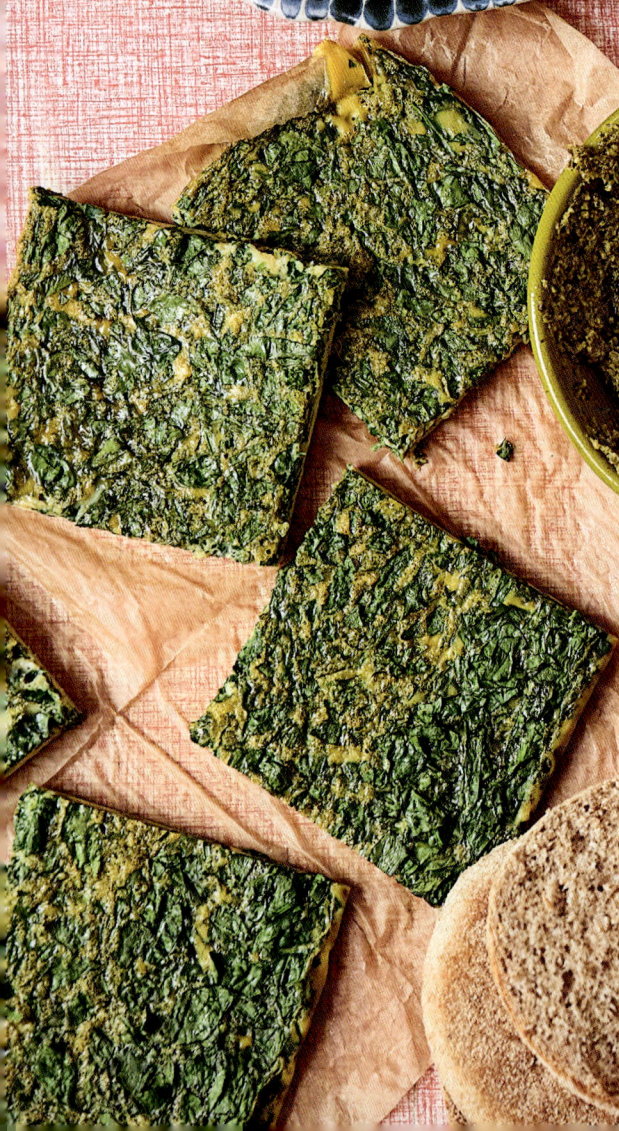

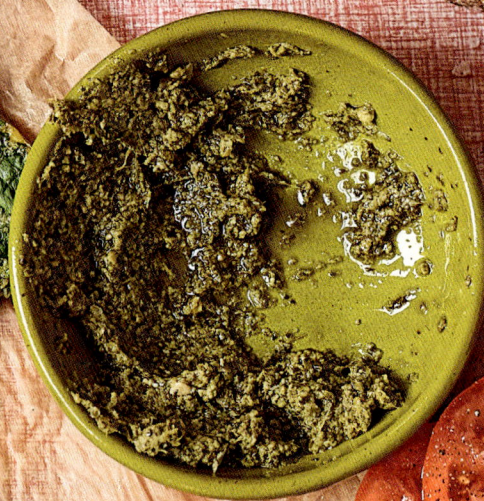

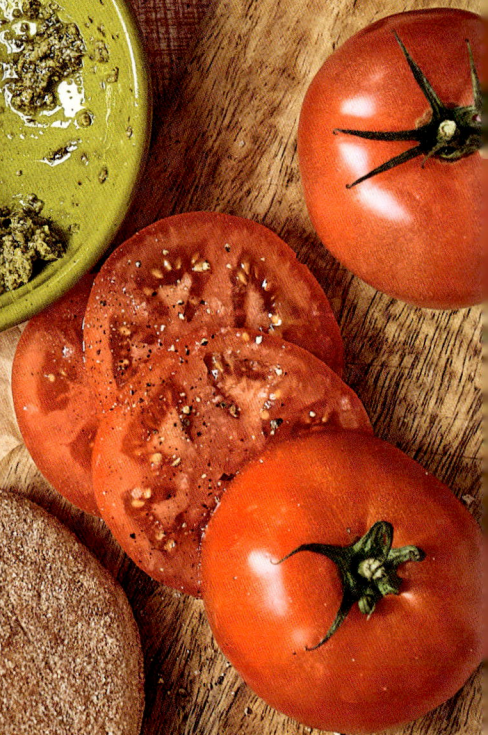

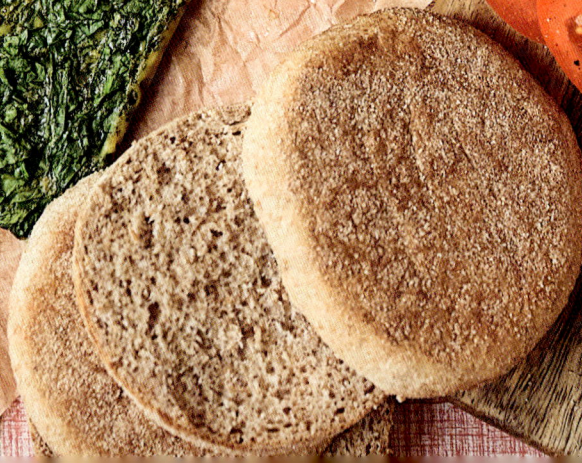

Freezable Egg, Spinach, Pesto + Cheese Sandwiches

(V) (DF/O) (GF/O)

These are a gift to your future self. They can be reheated straight from frozen – so when you're racing out of the door in the morning, you'll thank yourself for having a stash ready to go. They use my easy homemade pesto recipe to kick things up a notch, but if time's not on your side, I'll look the other way if you go for store-bought.

23 x 18-cm/9 x 7-in baking dish, lined (make sure it fits in your air fryer, if using one)

6 large/US extra-large eggs

100 g/3½ oz/scant 2 cups spinach, roughly chopped

6 wholemeal/whole-wheat English muffins

60 g/2 oz/½ cup grated cheddar or mozzarella

salt and pepper

tomato slices, to serve

For the pesto

30 g/1 oz fresh basil

1 garlic clove

15 g/½ oz/scant 2 tbsp pine nuts

20 g/¾ oz/¼ cup grated Italian hard cheese

3 tbsp extra virgin olive oil

salt and pepper

1 Preheat the air fryer or oven to 180°C fan/200°C/400°F/gas mark 6.

2 Crack the eggs into a mixing bowl and whisk them until the yolks and whites are completely combined. Stir in the spinach and season generously with salt and pepper. Pour the egg mixture into the prepared dish and place it into the air fryer or oven. Cook for about 10 minutes, or until the eggs are fully set and firm in the centre.

3 While the eggs are cooking, prepare the pesto. In a food processor, combine the basil, garlic, pine nuts and Italian hard cheese. With the lid on (and the cap removed), slowly drizzle in the olive oil while blending, and keep blending until the mixture emulsifies into a smooth pesto. Taste and adjust the seasoning with salt and pepper, if desired.

4 Once the eggs are cooked, remove them from the oven or air fryer and let them cool slightly before cutting into 6 even slices.

5 With everything now ready, it's time to assemble the sandwiches. Slice each muffin in half and spread a generous spoonful of pesto on each half. Place a slice of cooked egg on each of the bottom halves, sprinkle over the grated cheese and add the top of the muffin.

6 If you plan to eat them immediately, arrange the filled muffins on a baking tray and return them to the oven or air fryer for about 5 minutes, or until the cheese is melted and the muffin is slightly crispy. Once warmed through, insert the slices of tomato and serve. If you're saving them for later, follow the storage instructions below.

Substitutions:

● **Dairy-free?** Use dairy-free cheese (in both the muffin and the pesto).
● **Gluten-free?** Use a gluten-free English muffin.

Future you:

🗄 Cool and wrap in parchment paper, then in foil. Refrigerate for up to 3 days.
❄ Cool and wrap in parchment paper, then in foil. Freeze for up to 2 months.
🔥 To reheat from frozen, remove the wrapping and place muffin on a paper towel then microwave for 90 seconds, turning halfway. To reheat from chilled, remove the wrapping and follow step 6 again, or microwave for 30 seconds.

Breakfast Cookies

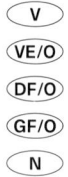

V

VE/O

DF/O

GF/O

N

Because who doesn't want cookies for breakfast?! Of course, these ones are different from your typical bakery treat, but that's what makes them so great. They're sweetened only with bananas, and packed with oats and other wholesome goodies that not only satisfy your sweet tooth but also sneak in a hefty dose of protein, fibre and heart-healthy fats to fuel your morning. A glorious grab-and-go breakfast option for busy days.

2 baking sheets, lined

2 ripe bananas

40 g/1½ oz/2½ tbsp natural peanut butter

½ tbsp cacao powder

40 ml/1⅓ fl oz/2½ tbsp milk

180 g/6 oz/scant 2 cups rolled/old-fashioned oats

15 g/½ oz/1 tbsp hemp seeds

15 g/½ oz/1 tbsp chia seeds

15 g/½ oz/1½ tbsp dark/bittersweet chocolate chips, plus extra to decorate

yogurt, to serve

fruit, to serve

1　Preheat the oven to 180°C fan/200°C/400°F/gas mark 6.

2　In a large mixing bowl, mash the bananas until smooth. Add in the peanut butter, cacao powder and milk, mixing until you have a chocolatey batter. Fold in the oats, hemp seeds, chia seeds and chocolate chips, mixing until everything comes together.

3　Using an ice-cream scoop or spoon, divide the mixture into 8 roughly equal portions and space them out on the prepared baking sheets. They won't spread much, or at all, in the oven, so shape them into your desired cookie shape and thickness now. I also like to press in a few extra chocolate chips on the cookie tops to decorate.

4　Slide the baking sheets into the oven and bake for 10–12 minutes, or until the edges are crisp and the centres are still a little soft to the touch.

5　Allow the cookies to cool on the baking sheets undisturbed for 10 minutes, to ensure they set and hold their shape.

6　If eating right away, serve 2 cookies with a portion of yogurt and some fruit of your choice.

Substitutions:

● **Gluten-free?** Ensure your oats are gluten-free. ● **Nut free?** Use tahini instead of peanut butter.

Future you:

🍱 Cool and place in an airtight container, storing at room temperature for up to 4 days, or in the fridge for up to 7 days.
❄ Cool and insert a piece of parchment paper between each. Stack and freeze for up to 3 months.
💧 Thaw in the fridge overnight, or at room temperature for a few hours.
🔥 Enjoy at room temperature or warm by microwaving for 20 seconds.

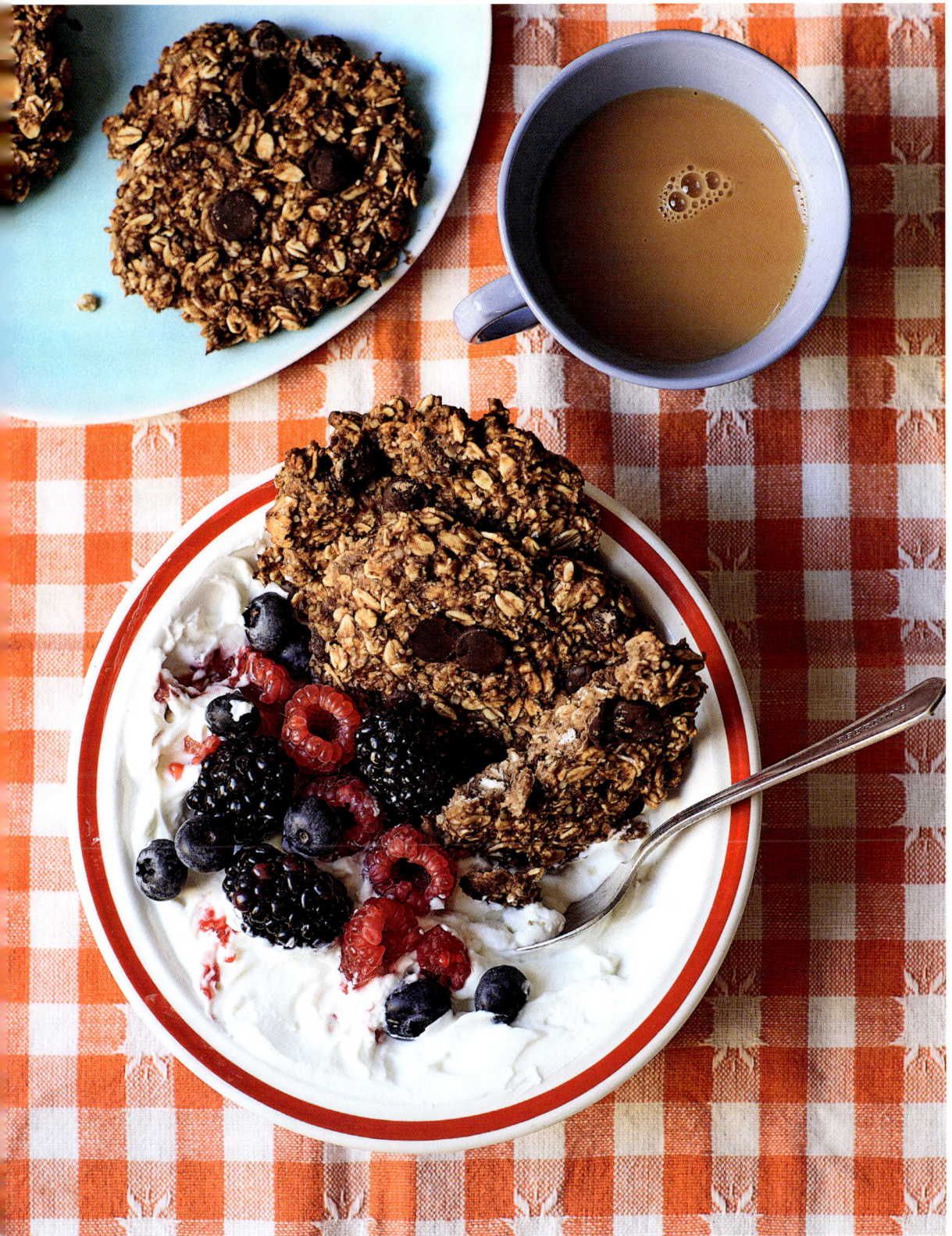

Freezable Breakfast Burritos

(V)
(VE/O)
(DF/O)
(GF/O)

Like the delicious breakfast sandwiches on page 21, these nutritious, freezer-friendly breakfast burritos are perfect for batch cooking and making sure you always have a grab-and-go meal ready for breakfast (or lunch, or dinner – because who am I to judge when you eat them?!). They're filled with a flavoursome tofu scramble and a spiced bean mix, then to seal the deal – quite literally – they're crisped in a hot pan to ensure none of those precious fillings make an escape.

4 wholemeal tortilla wraps

100 g/3½ oz/generous ½ cup jarred roasted red peppers, roughly chopped

sriracha, to taste (optional)

For the spiced beans

½ red onion, finely diced

1 garlic clove, minced

1 x 400-g/14-oz can black beans, drained

1 tsp chipotle paste

1 tsp ground cumin

1 tsp hot smoked paprika

50 g/1¾ oz/scant 1 cup spinach

salt and pepper

olive oil, for cooking

For the tofu

1 x 300-g/10½-oz block extra-firm smoked tofu

½ tsp ground turmeric

½ tsp garlic granules

½ tsp onion granules

1 tbsp nutritional yeast

1 tbsp milk

1 First up, the spiced bean mix. Heat a tablespoon of olive oil in a frying pan/skillet over medium heat. Add the onion and garlic and cook for about 3 minutes until soft. Stir in the drained beans, chipotle paste, cumin, paprika and a good pinch each of salt and pepper. Let everything cook for another 3 minutes. Grab a masher, or fork, and lightly mash the beans to break some down for texture, but leave most whole. Add the spinach and stir until it wilts. Once done, remove the mixture from the pan and set it aside to cool.

2 Next, the scrambled tofu. Add a little more oil to the same pan and return to medium heat. Press out any water from the block of tofu (this will vary depending on the brand you use), crumble it into the pan with your hands, and stir in the turmeric, garlic granules, onion granules and nutritional yeast. Season with salt and pepper, add a splash of milk to loosen the mixture, and cook for 2–3 minutes.

3 With all the components ready, it's time to assemble the burritos. Spread the bean mixture onto the tortillas, followed by the tofu and chopped jarred red peppers. Give them a drizzle of sriracha (if using), then fold in the opposite sides of each tortilla and roll up tightly.

4 If you're eating the burrito(s) right away, heat a clean frying pan over medium–high heat and drizzle lightly with oil. Place the burrito seam-side down and cook for about 1 minute, then flip it over and cook the other side for another minute – this will seal and crisp up the edges, ensuring no filling falls out.

Substitutions:

● **No tofu?** If you are not vegan, substitute the scrambled tofu for scrambled eggs. ● **Gluten-free?** Use gluten-free tortilla wraps.

Future you:

☗ Cool and wrap in parchment paper, then in foil. Refrigerate for up to 3 days.
❋ Cool and wrap in parchment paper, then in foil. Freeze for up to 2 months.
💧 Thaw in the fridge overnight before reheating.
🔥 Microwave in just the parchment paper for 3 minutes, flipping halfway. Flash the burrito in the pan (see step 4) to make it crispy again.

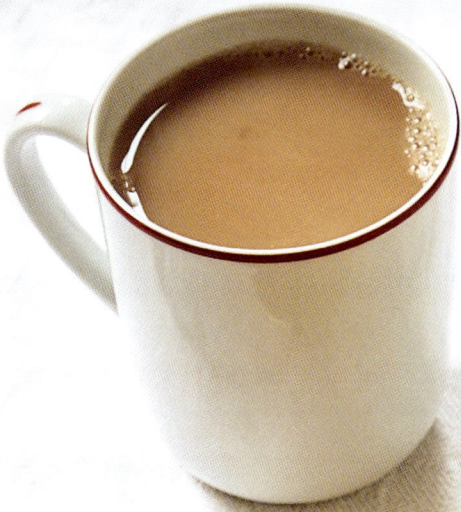

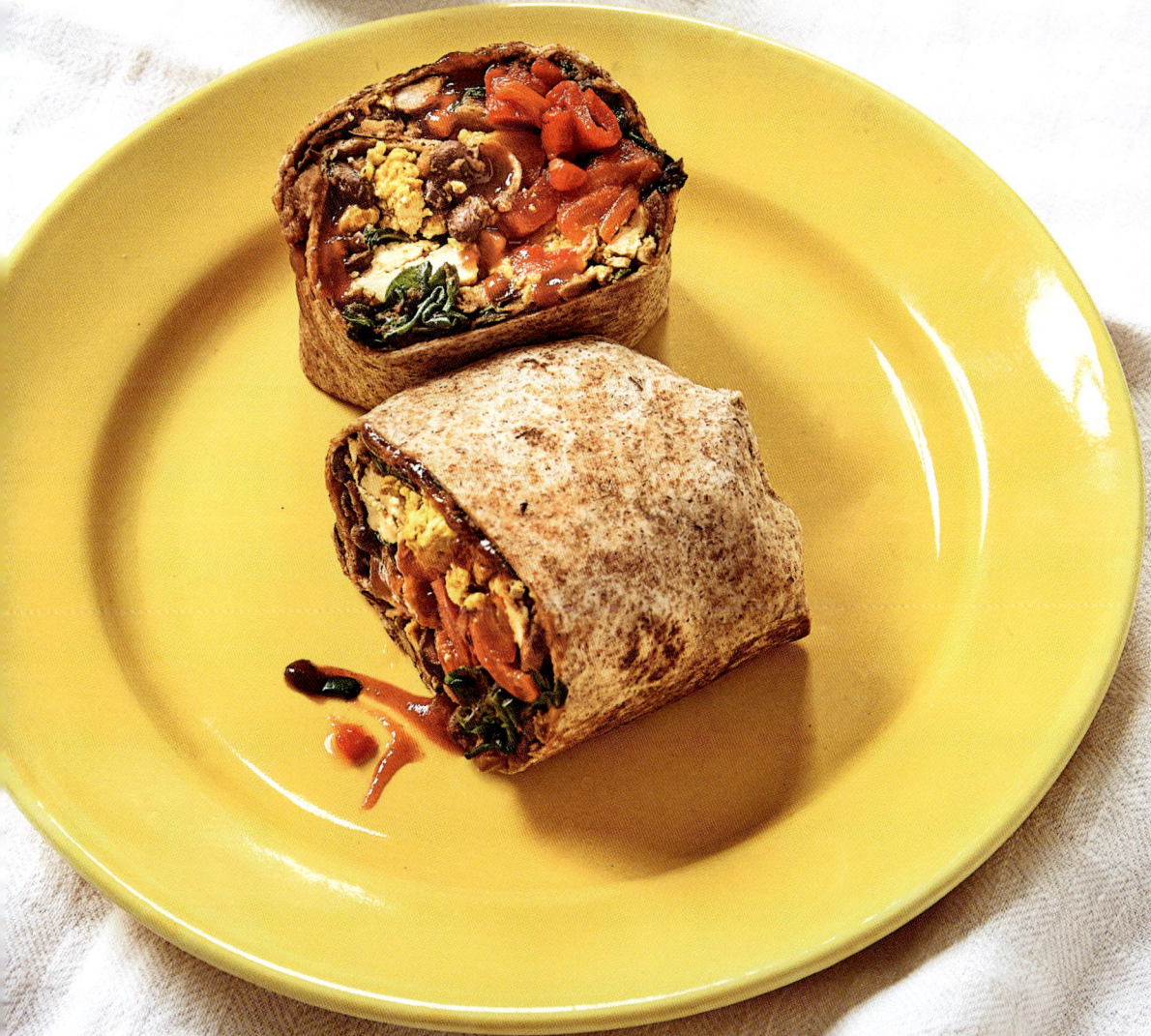

Tahini Chocolate Chip Granola

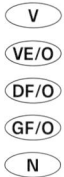

V
VE/O
DF/O
GF/O
N

I can't stop making this granola. It's crunchy, packed with flavour and just miles better than anything you'll find on any store shelves. So, if you've never made granola yourself, please go ahead and put that box down, because you're about to experience how ridiculously easy it is. The key to achieving the best, crunchy oversized clusters (because what is a good granola without these), is a secret ingredient: egg white. It sounds weird, I know, but it works like absolute magic.

large baking tray, lined (if using an oven)

air fryer basket, lined (if using an air fryer)

1 egg white

180 g/6 oz/scant 2 cup rolled/old-fashioned oats

70 g/2½ oz/½ cup almonds, roughly chopped

30 g/1 oz/¼ cup sunflower seeds

20 g/¾ oz/4 tsp chia seeds

30 g/1 oz/4 tbsp hemp seeds

¼ tsp fine sea salt

1 tsp ground cinnamon

50 ml/1½ fl oz/3½ tbsp maple syrup

1 tsp vanilla extract

50 g/1¾ oz/¼ cup tahini

40 g/1½ oz/3 tbsp coconut oil, melted and cooled

30 g/1 oz/3 tbsp dark/bittersweet chocolate chips

Greek yogurt, to serve

fruit, to serve

1 Preheat the air fryer or oven to 175°C fan/195°C/375°F/gas mark 5.

2 In a small bowl, whisk the egg white for about 1 minute until it becomes light and frothy.

3 In a separate large bowl, combine the oats, almonds, sunflower seeds, chia seeds, hemp seeds, salt, cinnamon, maple syrup, vanilla, tahini and coconut oil. Add the whisked egg white and give everything a good mix until thoroughly combined. We're not adding in the chocolate chips until after the granola has baked, so they don't melt or burn.

4 Spread the mixture evenly onto the lined baking tray or air fryer basket, pressing it down slightly to help it stick together. Bake for 25 minutes, gently turning it with a spatula halfway through (being careful not to break up the clusters more than necessary), until the granola is golden all over. If you notice some parts browning too quickly, move them to the middle of the tray, and shift the paler parts to the edges.

5 Allow the granola to cool for at least 30 minutes on the tray before touching it – this will help to create the best clusters. Once the granola has fully cooled, stir in the chocolate chips.

6 Serve the granola alongside a helping of your favourite yogurt and fresh fruit.

Substitutions:

● **Vegan?** Omit the egg white and serve with dairy-free yogurt. ● **Gluten-free?** Ensure your oats are gluten-free. ● **Nut-free?** Use pumpkin seeds instead of almonds.

Future you:

🍲 Place in an airtight container, storing at room temperature for up to 3 weeks.

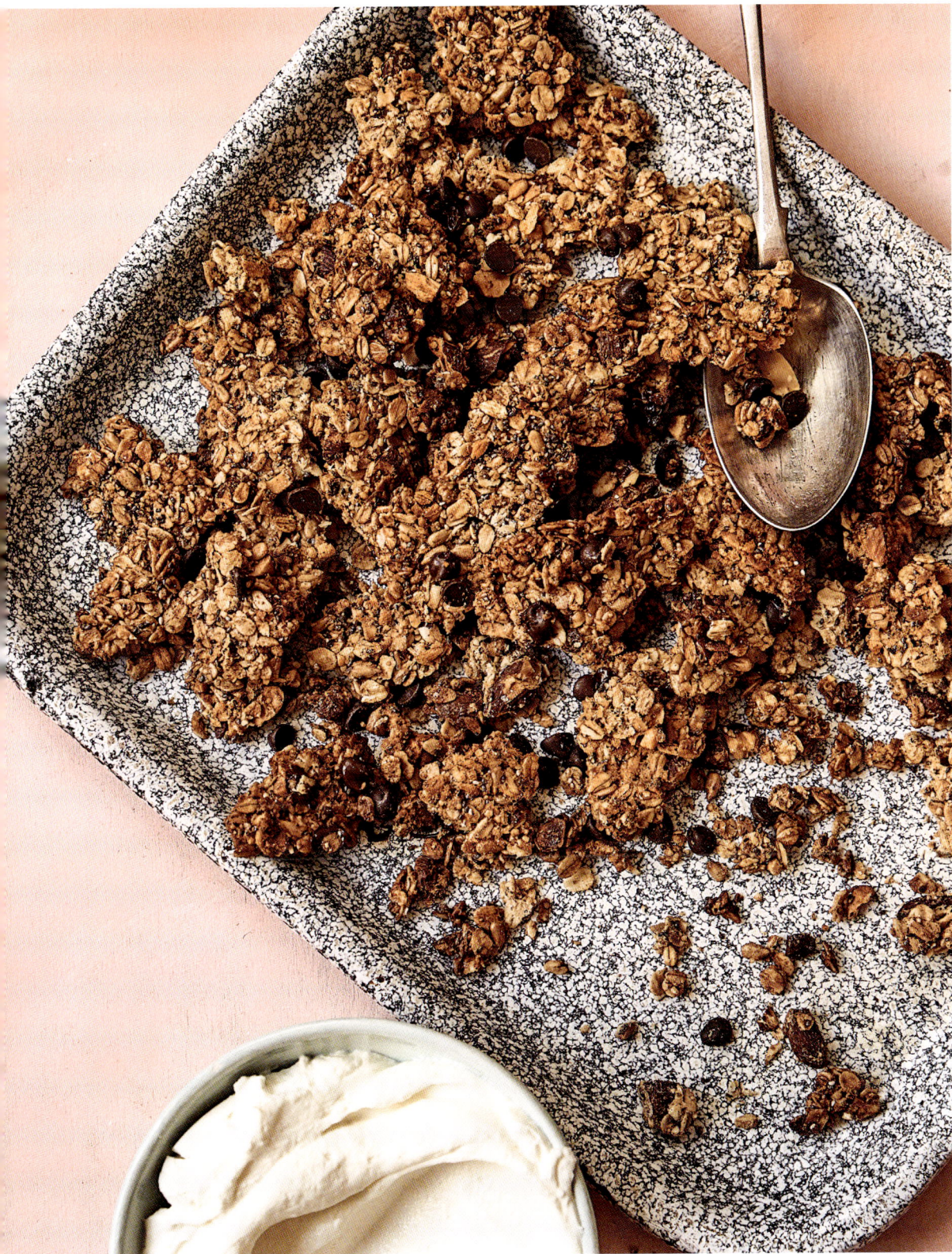

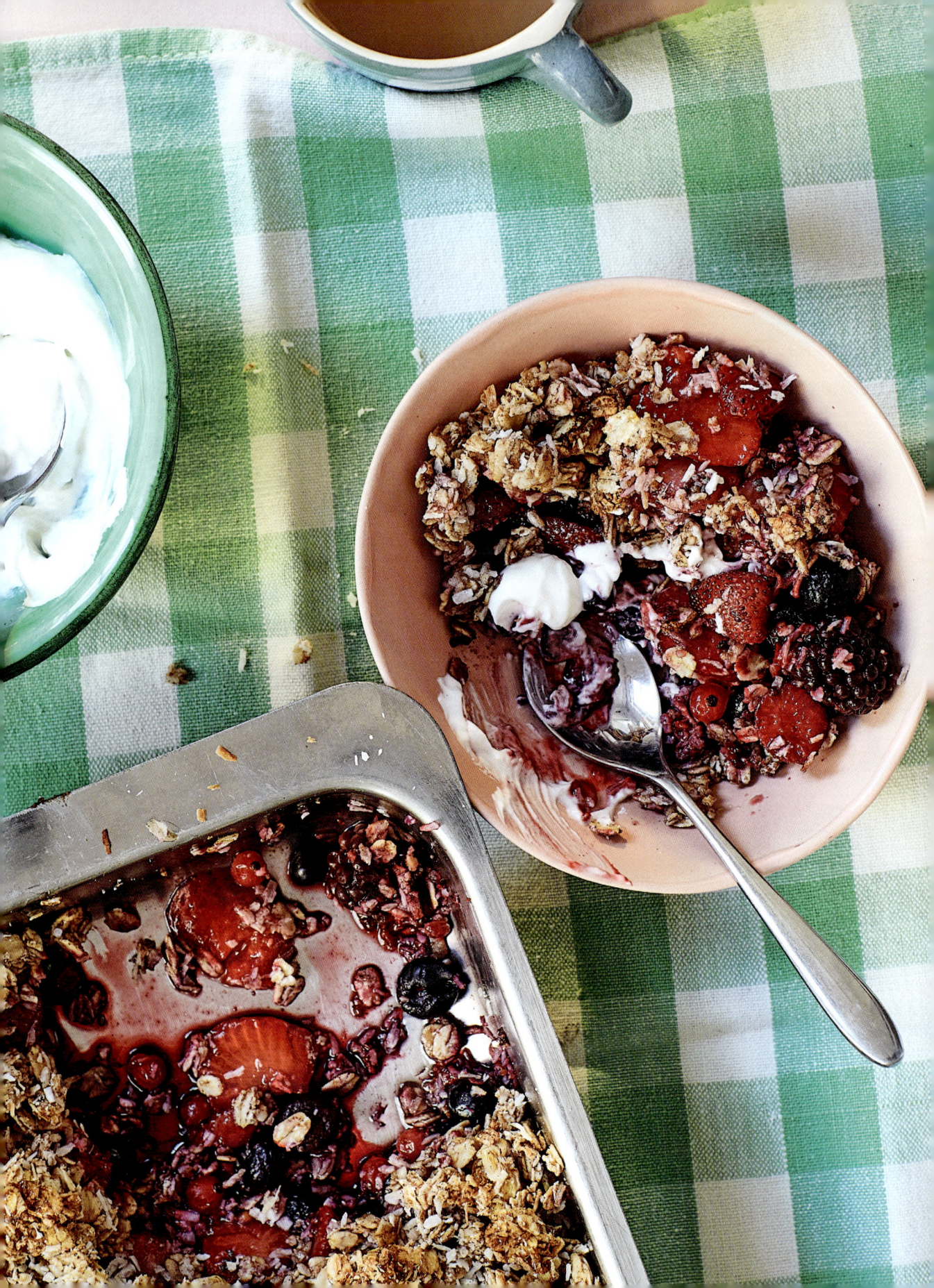

Frozen Berry + Coconut Breakfast Crumble

(V)
(VE/O)
(DF/O)
(GF/O)
(N)

Over the years I've become pretty good at turning desserts into healthy, higher protein breakfasts. From the likes of carrot cake oats and breakfast cookies to glorious stuffed muffins and now crumble. You. Are. Welcome. It's comforting, brilliantly easy to make and, despite looking and tasting like dessert, it's made with nutritious ingredients and is perfect to kick-start the day. Simply dollop some yogurt on the side, and tuck in.

23 x 15-cm/9 x 6-in baking dish

45 g/1½ oz/3 tbsp natural peanut butter

2 tbsp maple syrup

120 g/4 oz/1⅓ cups rolled/old-fashioned oats

1 tsp ground cinnamon

a pinch of salt

30 g/1 oz/scant ½ cup desiccated/dried unsweetened shredded coconut

500 g/1 lb 2 oz/3 cups any frozen berries

1 tsp chia seeds

yogurt, to serve

honey or maple syrup, to serve

1   Preheat the air fryer or oven to 180°C fan/200°C/400°F/gas mark 6.

2   In a small bowl, whisk together the peanut butter, maple syrup and 2 tablespoons of water until completely smooth. Add the oats, cinnamon, salt and most of the coconut, saving some back for the topping. Mix until combined. You're aiming for a crumble consistency that has a few big clumps and no dry patches. If the mix is still too dry, add a touch more water. If it's too wet, add a few more oats.

3   Tip the frozen berries into the baking dish and shake to spread them out in an even layer. Scatter the chia seeds evenly over the top. Sprinkle the crumble topping evenly over the berries and add the reserved coconut on top.

4   Pop the dish into the preheated air fryer or oven and cook for 20 minutes, or until the top is golden and crisp and the berries bubbling.

5   While still warm, dish up with yogurt and a drizzle of honey or maple syrup.

Substitutions:

● **No coconut?** Omit. ● **No chia seeds?** Omit. ● **Gluten-free?** Ensure your oats are gluten-free. ● **Nut-free?** Use tahini instead of peanut butter.

Future you:

🥡 Cool and place in an airtight container, storing in the fridge for up to 4 days.
❄ Cool and freeze for up to 2 months.
💧 Thaw in the fridge overnight, or on low power in the microwave.
🔥 Microwave a portion for 60–90 seconds.

Stuffed Blueberry Muffins

V

VE/O

DF/O

I see your standard, run-of-the-mill blueberry muffin and raise you these. This is my way of offering you an escape from your usual mundane grab-and-go breakfast options, because, let's face it, there is nothing satisfying or healthy about grabbing a solitary banana or cereal bar on your way out, and you deserve better than that, too.

6-hole extra-deep muffin tray, lined with muffin cases (or use a regular 12-hole muffin tray and line with 9 muffin cases)

180 g/6 oz/1⅓ cups plain/all-purpose flour

1 tsp baking powder

½ tsp bicarbonate of soda/baking soda

¼ tsp fine sea salt

120 g/4 oz/1 cup blueberries (fresh or frozen)

2 large/US extra-large eggs

1 tsp vanilla extract

60 g/2 oz/¼ cup coconut oil, melted and cooled

60 ml/¼ cup maple syrup

grated zest of 1 lemon

1 tsp freshly squeezed lemon juice

40 ml/1⅓ fl oz/2½ tbsp milk

For the cream cheese filling

60 g/2 oz/generous ¼ cup cream cheese

1 tsp maple syrup

½ tsp freshly squeezed lemon juice

For the toppings (optional)

jumbo oats

coconut sugar

1   Preheat the oven to 190°C fan/210°C/400°F/gas mark 6.

2   First up, prepare the cream cheese filling. Grab a small bowl and combine the cream cheese, maple syrup and lemon juice (be sure to zest the lemon for the muffin batter first). Set aside.

3   In a large mixing bowl, mix together the flour, baking powder, bicarbonate of soda and salt until well combined. Gently stir through the blueberries to coat them in the flour mixture (this helps prevent them sinking to the bottom of the muffins during baking).

4   In another bowl, whisk together the eggs, vanilla, oil, maple syrup, lemon zest, lemon juice and milk until well combined.

5   Pour the wet ingredients into the bowl with the dry ingredients. Using a flat rubber spatula, gently fold the mixture until just combined. Be careful not to overmix here as this will cause the muffins to be dense and dry; it's okay if the batter still has a few small lumps.

6   Divide three-quarters of the batter evenly among the muffin cases, making a small well in the centre of each with the back of a teaspoon.

7   Grab the bowl of cream cheese filling and drop a spoonful of the filling into each well. Use the remaining muffin batter to cover the tops of the muffins, ensuring the cream cheese filling is fully enclosed. Top the muffins with a few extra blueberries, a sprinkle of oats and a light dusting of coconut sugar, if using.

8   Pop the muffins into the oven for 20 minutes (if using a deep tray), or until a toothpick inserted into the centre comes out clean. If you are using a regular muffin tray, bake for 16 minutes and try the cocktail stick test. Allow the muffins to cool in the tray for a few minutes before transferring them to a wire rack to cool completely. The longer you leave them, the easier the cases will be to remove.

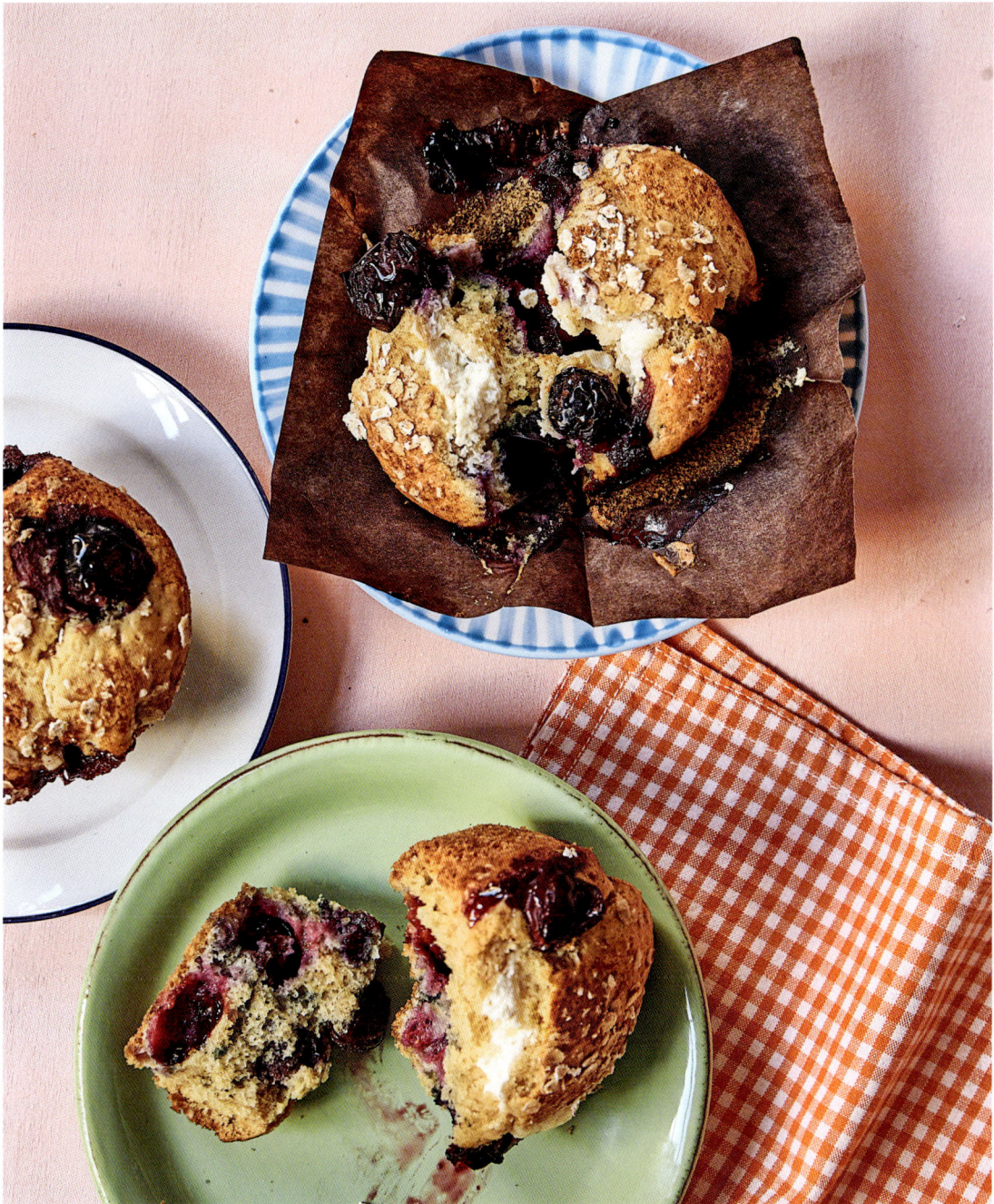

Substitutions:

● **No coconut oil?** Replace with a neutral oil, like vegetable or mild olive oil. ● **Vegan?** Make flaxseed 'eggs' by mixing 2 tbsp milled flaxseed with 5 tbsp water and use dairy-free milk and cream cheese. ● **Dairy-free?** Use dairy-free milk and cream cheese.

Future you:

🍱 Cool and place an airtight container, storing in the fridge for up to 5 days.
❄️ Cool and freeze for up to 2 months.
💧 Thaw overnight at room temperature, or on low power in the microwave.
🔥 Enjoy at room temperature, or microwave for 15 seconds.

One-Tray Protein Pancake

It's no secret that I'm a big fan of protein pancakes – so much so that this is one of two pancake recipes in this book (flip ahead to page 48 for Fluffy Protein Pancakes with Healthy-ish Chocolate Sauce). But this one is my lazy-day hero. No pan, no flipping, just a layer of batter baked with your favourite toppings. Essentially, it's one big ol' giant pancake that can then be portioned, which is not only a huge time saver but also perfect whether you're meal-prepping for the week or putting on a brunch spread for friends and family.

(V)
(VE/O)
(DF/O)
(GF/O)

23 x 33-cm/9 x 13-in baking tray, lined

400 ml/14 fl oz/1¾ cups milk

2 tsp apple cider vinegar

200 g/7 oz/1½ cups plain/all-purpose or oat flour

3 tsp baking powder

50 g/1¾ oz/generous ½ cup soy protein powder

30 g/1 oz/2 tbsp coconut oil, melted and cooled

100 g/3½ oz/⅔ cup fresh or frozen raspberries

40 g/1½ oz/4 tbsp dark/bittersweet chocolate chips

maple syrup, to serve (optional)

yogurt, to serve (optional)

fruit, to serve (optional)

1   Preheat the oven to 180°C fan/200°C/400°F/gas mark 6.

2   To start, combine the milk and vinegar in a small bowl and let it sit for 5 minutes, allowing it to curdle. This will give the milk a buttermilk-like quality, helping the pancakes turn out perfectly thick and fluffy.

3   While the buttermilk forms, grab a large mixing bowl and whisk together the flour, baking powder and protein powder. Pour in the curdled milk mixture and the melted oil, and gently fold everything together with a flat rubber spatula until just combined – be careful not to overmix to keep the batter light and airy.

4   Add in half of the raspberries and chocolate chips, folding a few more times to distribute them evenly throughout the batter.

5   Pour the pancake batter into your prepared tray, spreading it evenly to the edges with a spatula or the back of a spoon. Scatter over the remaining raspberries and chocolate chips.

6   Place the tray on the middle shelf of the oven and bake for 10–12 minutes, or until the pancake is fully cooked and springs back when touched lightly in the centre.

7   Cut the pancakes into squares while still in the tray. Place the squares on top of each other to form a stack, and serve warm with either a drizzle of syrup, your favourite yogurt or a handful of fruit.

Substitutions:

● **No coconut oil?** Use a neutral oil, i.e. vegetable or mild olive oil instead.
● **Gluten-free?** Use oat flour and ensure it is gluten-free.

Future you:

🥡 Cool and place in an airtight container, storing in the fridge for up to 4 days.
❄ Cool and insert a piece of parchment paper between each. Stack and freeze for up to 1 month.
💧 Thaw slowly in the microwave or in the fridge overnight.
🔥 Reheat each portion of pancakes in the microwave for 30 seconds.

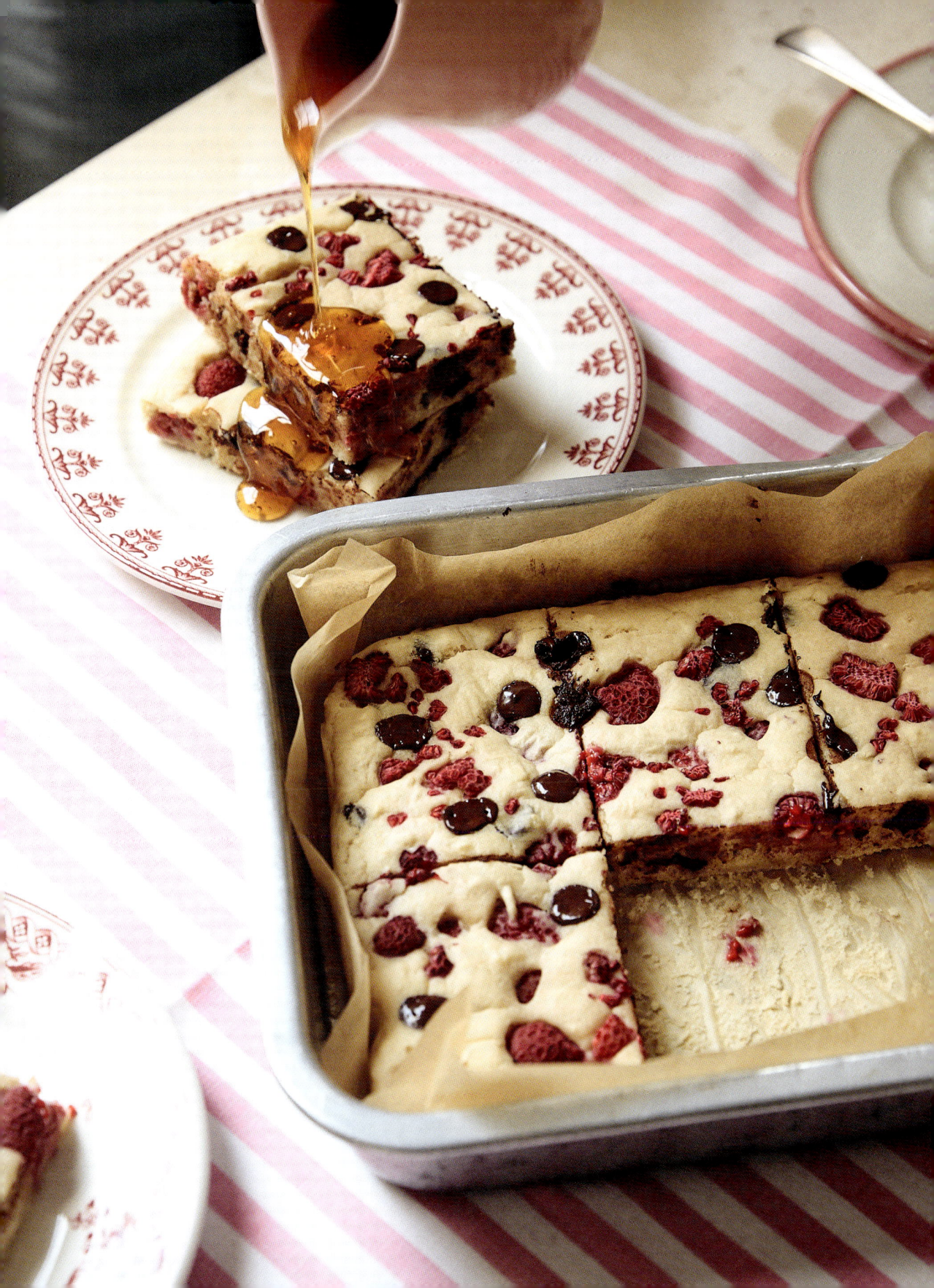

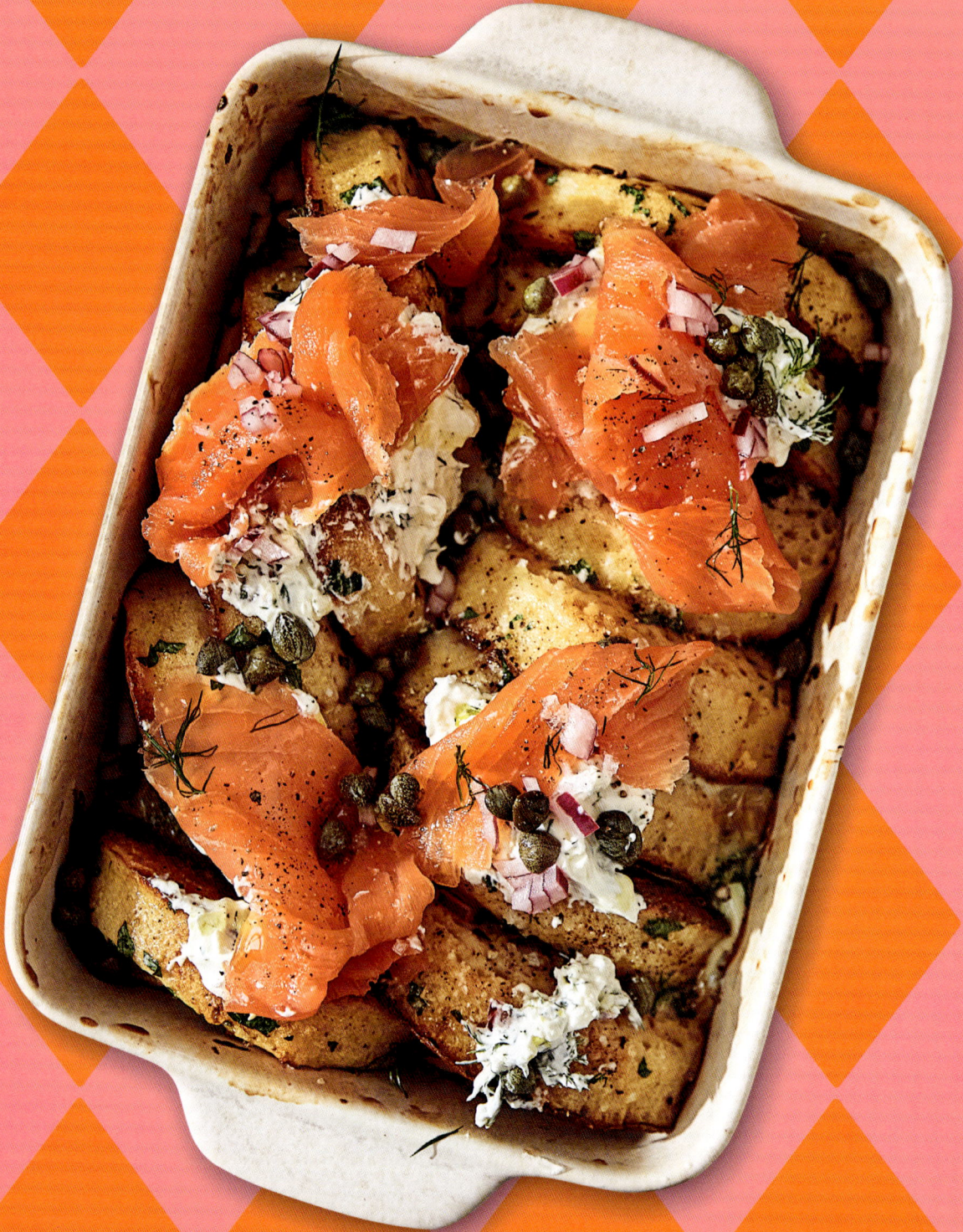

Weekend Brunch

Breakfast and Brunch Recipes to Start Your Day Right

Nothing beats starting the day with something equally as nutritious as it is yummy. Hitting that brief, these are all recipes I love to make on those long-awaited slower mornings – in my pyjamas, with a cup of coffee in hand and the TV on in the background. Each and every one packs a flavour punch and is incredibly easy to make.

Crumpet Casserole with Smoked Salmon

(V/O)
(DF/O)
(GF/O)

I don't like to play favourites, but this eggy crumpet casserole is up there. It's a perfect, easy recipe to add something a little bit different to your brunch table, all while still using our favourite brunch ingredients. Think of it as an amalgamation of humble eggy bread (which will always bring me nostalgia, as I used to request it for brekkie most weekends as a child) and a posh smoked salmon brunch. The star of the show, though, has to be the crumpets, as they take on the most divine texture when baked.

23 x 18-cm/9 x 7-in baking dish

3 large/US extra-large eggs

50 ml/1½ fl oz/3½ tbsp milk

1 tbsp roughly chopped parsley

6 sourdough crumpets

80 g/3 oz smoked salmon

¼ red onion, finely diced

1 tbsp capers

salt and pepper

lemon wedges, to serve

For the herby crème fraîche

100 g/3½ oz/½ cup crème fraîche or sour cream

grated zest and juice of ½ lemon

1 tbsp roughly chopped dill, plus extra to garnish

1   Preheat the air fryer or oven to 190°C fan/210°C/400°F/gas mark 6.

2   Crack the eggs into a large measuring jug/cup or mixing bowl, add the milk, and use a fork to beat them together until no streaks of yolk remain. Stir in the parsley and season generously with salt and pepper.

3   Cut the crumpets in half down the centre to make half-moons and stack them cut-side down in the baking dish. If you think your baked crumpets might stick to the dish, first grease the bottom with a drizzle of oil or line with parchment paper. Pour the egg mixture over the crumpets, making sure they're evenly coated. Use your hands to rearrange the crumpets if necessary to make sure each piece is well-soaked. Let the crumpets sit for about 5 minutes to absorb most of the egg.

4   Place the dish in the preheated air fryer or oven for 15–20 minutes, or until the crumpets are golden and crispy around the edges and any egg at the bottom is fully set.

5   While the crumpets are cooking, get the herby crème fraîche ready by combining the crème fraîche, lemon zest, lemon juice and dill in a small bowl. Season to taste with salt and pepper.

6   When the crumpets are ready, remove the dish from the air fryer or oven. Spoon on dollops of the herby crème fraîche and arrange the slices of smoked salmon on top. Sprinkle with the red onion, capers and extra dill. Serve with lemon wedges.

Substitutions:

● **Dairy-free?** Use dairy-free milk and sub the crème fraîche for dairy-free cream cheese. ● **Gluten-free?** Use gluten-free crumpets. ● **Vegetarian?** Omit the smoked salmon.

Future you:

🝤 Cool and place in an airtight container, storing in the fridge for up to 3 days.
🔥 First remove any smoked salmon and crème fraîche, then microwave the crumpets for 30 seconds on full power. Re-assemble and enjoy!

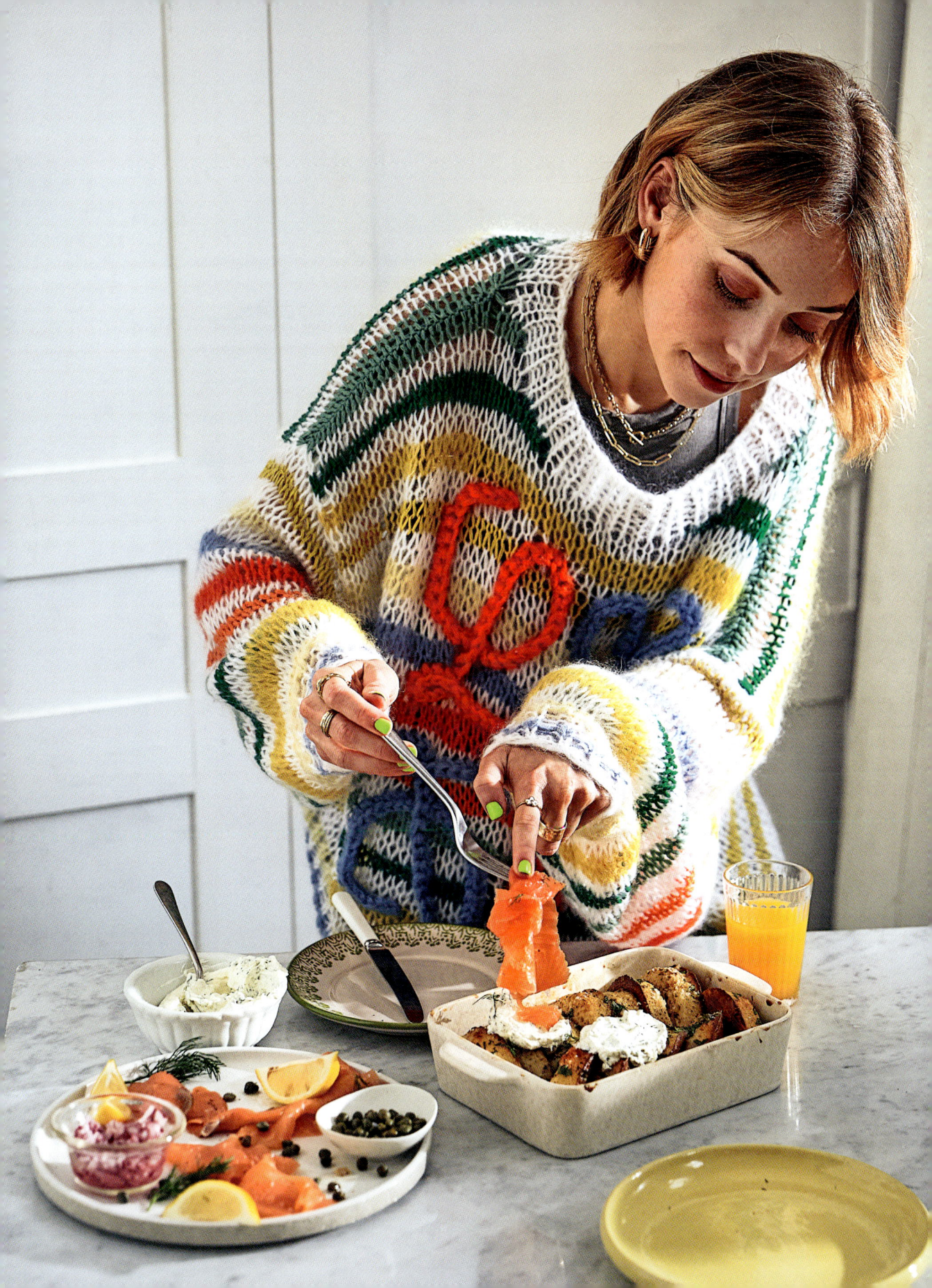

Harissa Chickpea Shakshuka + Za'atar Flatbreads

V
VE/O
DF/O
GF/O

While I love going out for a (cough, bottomless) brunch every now and again, from a food perspective, nothing will satisfy me more than making something at home for a quarter of the price, and quadruple the flavour and nutrients. There's a little bit of multitasking needed to make the flatbreads while you cook the shakshuka, so if you know that will stress you out, make the flatbreads first and reheat them when you're ready to serve up.

½ onion, finely diced

2 red (bell) peppers, finely diced

2 garlic cloves, minced

2 tsp smoked paprika

1 tsp ground cumin

1½ tbsp rose harissa paste

1 x 400-g/14-oz can chickpeas/garbanzo beans, drained

2 x 400-g/14-oz cans chopped tomatoes

4 large/US extra-large eggs

1 ripe avocado, mashed

20 g/¾ oz/scant ¼ cup feta, crumbled

a pinch of crushed chilli flakes/hot red pepper flakes

a handful of roughly chopped coriander/cilantro

salt and pepper

olive oil, for cooking

For the flatbreads

175 g/6 oz/1⅓ cups self-raising/self-rising flour, plus extra for dusting

160 g/5½ oz/¾ cup low-fat yogurt

½ tsp fine sea salt

1½ tbsp olive oil

½ tsp za'atar

½ tsp garlic granules

a pinch of flaky sea salt

1   You can make this recipe on the hob/stovetop, or in the oven. If using the oven, preheat to 180°C fan/200°C/400°F/gas mark 6 on an oven grill/broiler setting.

2   In an ovenproof frying pan/skillet, heat 1 tablespoon of olive oil over medium heat. Add the onion and cook for a minute, then stir in the peppers, garlic, paprika and cumin. Sauté for 5 minutes, until the peppers soften, then mix in the harissa.

3   While the onion mix cooks, make the flatbreads. Mix the flour, yogurt and salt in a bowl until a rough dough forms. Knead the dough on a floured surface, then divide it into four. If the dough is too sticky, sprinkle over a little extra flour. Flatten each piece into a thin circle (as thin as you can without it tearing) and set aside.

4   Going back to the pan, turn the heat down slightly, then tip in the chickpeas and canned tomatoes, and season. Simmer for a couple of minutes until thickened, then make four wells in the sauce and crack an egg into each. Reduce the heat to low.

5   For the hob-/stovetop-based option, cover and cook for 8 minutes, or until the egg whites are set. For the oven- based option, leave the pan uncovered and bake on the middle shelf of your oven for 8–10 minutes, or until the egg whites are set.

6   While the shakshuka cooks, fry the flatbreads in a separate pan over medium-high heat with a little oil for 1–2 minutes on each side until golden and nicely puffed up. Combine the oil, za'atar and garlic granules in a small bowl and brush over the warm flatbreads. Finish with a pinch of salt.

7   Top the shakshuka with the mashed avocado, crumbled feta, chilli flakes and coriander. Serve with the flatbreads to mop up the sauce.

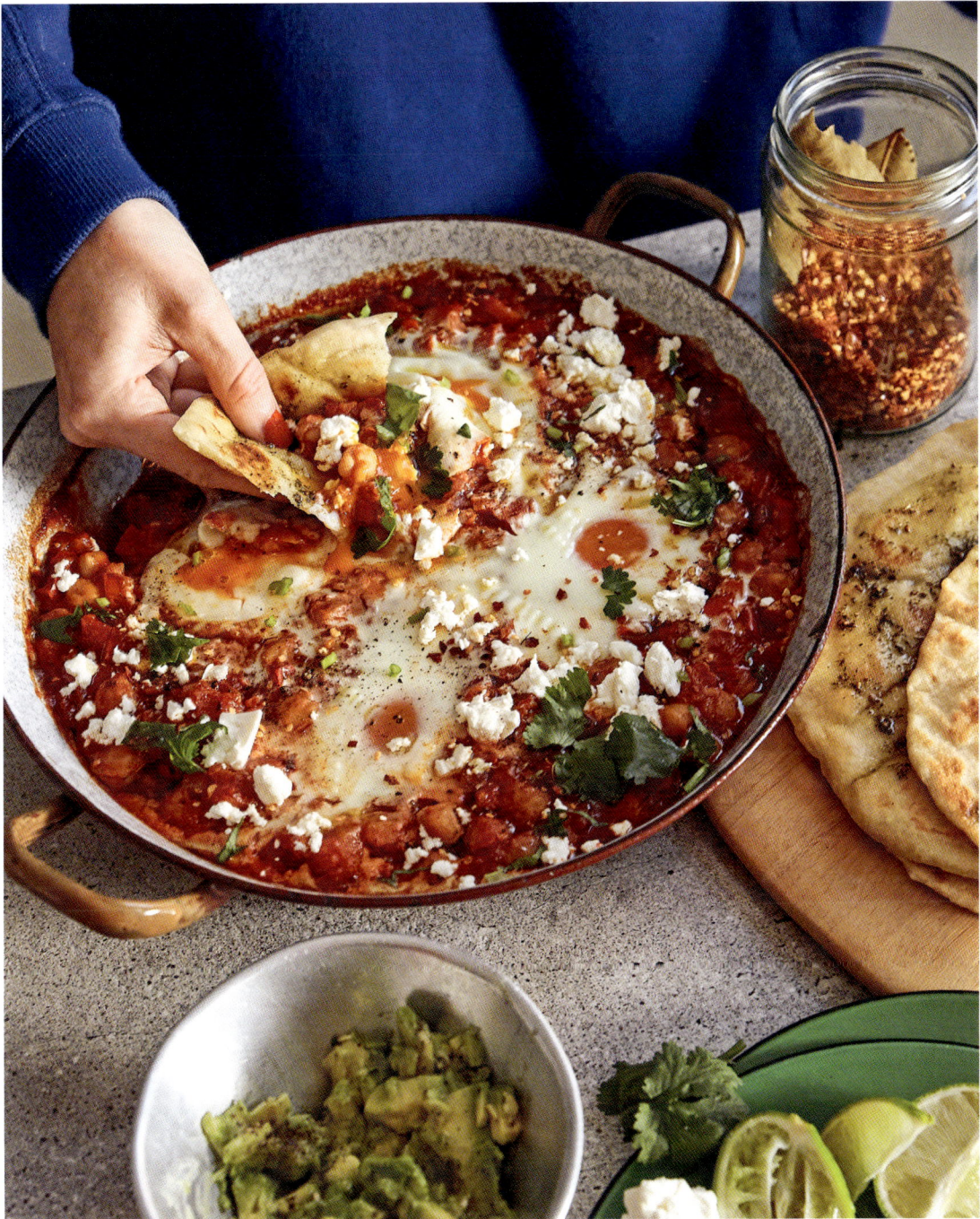

Substitutions:

● **No chickpeas?** Omit, or sub for any other bean of your choice. ● **Vegan?** Omit the eggs and feta. ● **Dairy-free?** Use a feta alternative. ● **Gluten-free?** Serve with gluten-free flatbreads.

Future you:

☕ Cool and place in an airtight container, storing in the fridge for up to 2 days.
❄ You can freeze the sauce (without the eggs) for up to 1 month.
💧 Thaw in the fridge overnight, or on low power in the microwave.
🔥 Warm to reheat, adding a splash of water if the sauce has become thick. To warm the flatbreads, heat one at a time in the microwave for 30 seconds.

Edamame Smash on Toast

(V) (VE) (DF) (GF/O)

Avocado toast is a staple, but, dare I say, it can be a little bit... boring. So, I'm defying the laws of 'if it ain't broke, don't fix it', and giving it an upgrade. Yes, it may still look like your ordinary avo smash, but, trust me, this version is higher in protein and tastes way, way better. All you need to do is blend and pile it high onto your favourite bread. When I'm feeling fancy I like to top it off with fried mushrooms, seeds and a little drizzle of hot honey. The extra touches take it to a whole new level.

200 g/7 oz mushrooms of choice, thinly sliced

a handful of pumpkin and sunflower seeds

2–3 slices bread (I like sourdough)

olive oil, for cooking

For the edamame smash

150 g/5½ oz/generous 1 cup shelled edamame beans

1 large ripe avocado

1 garlic clove

1 tbsp nutritional yeast

1 tbsp tahini

1 tbsp chopped coriander/cilantro

juice of ½ lime

salt and pepper

For the hot honey

1 tsp crispy chilli/chili oil

1 tsp honey or maple syrup

1   First up, the edamame smash. In a food processor (not a blender, as we want it to have texture), combine the edamame, avocado, garlic, nutritional yeast, tahini, coriander, lime juice and a good pinch each of salt and pepper. Pulse until the mixture is well combined, but not completely smooth. Set aside.

2   Heat a drizzle of olive oil in a frying pan/skillet over medium heat. Once hot, add the mushrooms and a good pinch each of salt and pepper. Cook for about 4 minutes, stirring often, until the mushrooms release their water and become golden. When the mushrooms are done, remove them from the pan and sprinkle in the seeds. Toast for a couple of minutes until fragrant, then remove the pan from the heat.

3   Toast the bread and prepare the hot honey simply by mixing together the chilli oil and honey or maple syrup in a small bowl.

4   To assemble, smear a generous layer of edamame smash onto your toasted bread, followed by some fried mushrooms, an extra sprinkle of toasted seeds and a drizzle of hot honey. Serve immediately.

Substitutions:

● **Gluten-free?** Use gluten-free bread.

Future you:

🍲 Place in an airtight container and store in the fridge for up to 3 days.

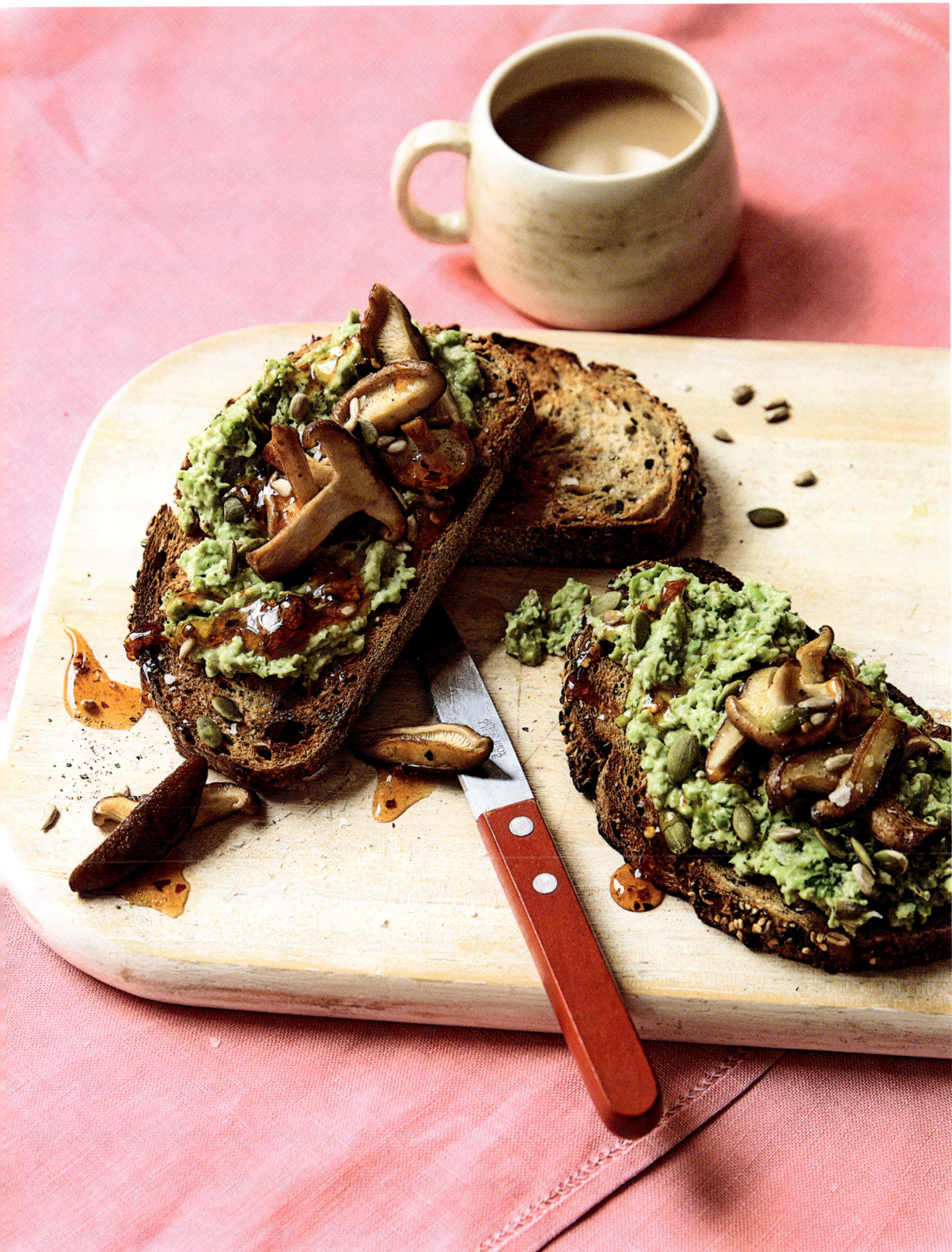

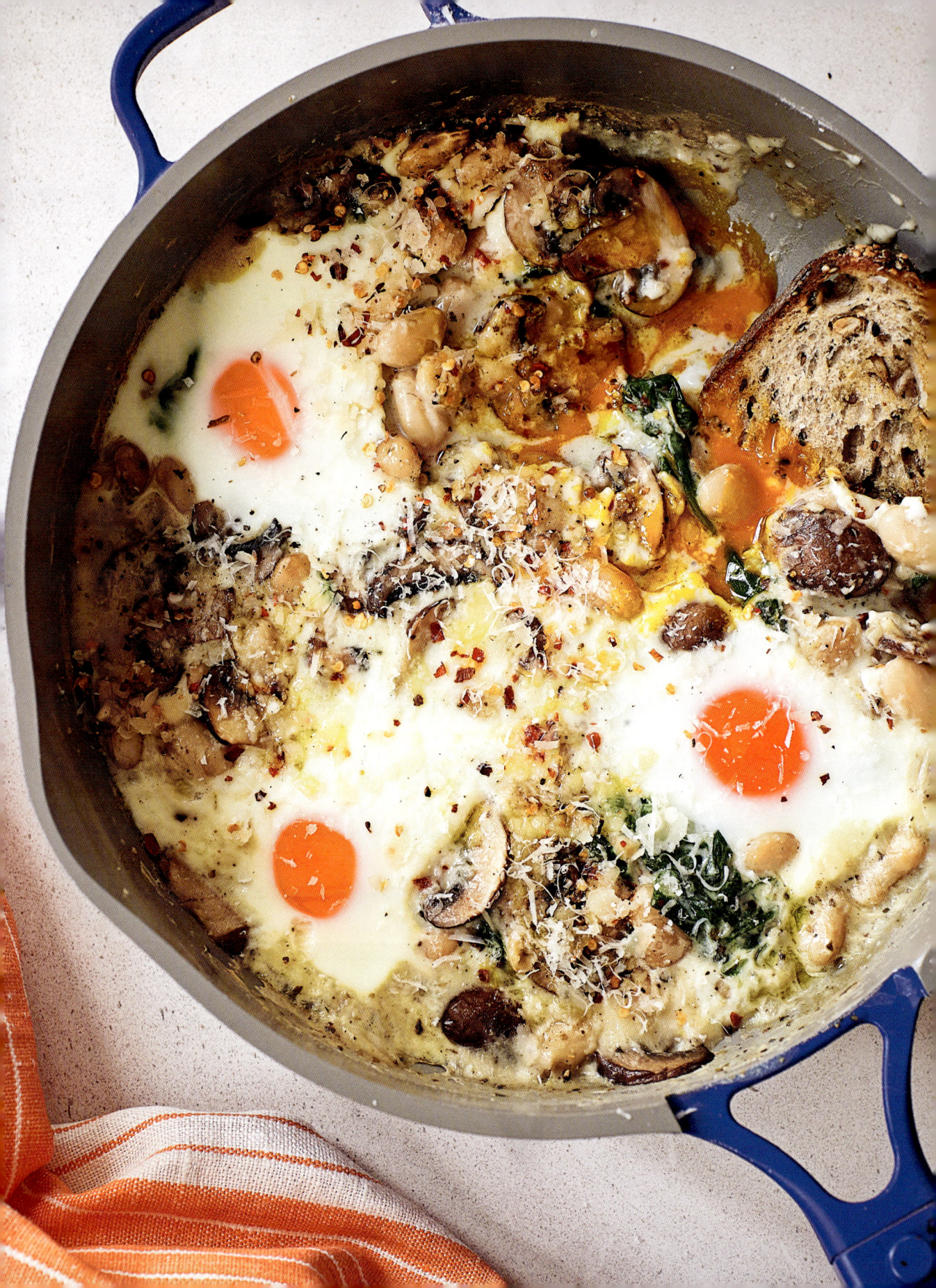

Creamy Mushroom + Butter Bean Baked Eggs

(V)
(DF/O)

A twist on the usual tomato-based shakshuka (which of course I have a recipe for too, see page 38) and it is oh so good. We've got butter beans, mushrooms, garlic, spinach and Parmesan – making it more decadent in taste, but just as quick and easy as the classic.

½ onion, finely diced

2 garlic cloves, minced

200 g/7 oz chestnut mushrooms, thinly sliced

1 tsp dried thyme

1 x 400-g/14-oz can butter beans/ lima beans, drained

2 tbsp crème fraîche or sour cream

50 g/1¾ oz/scant 1 cup spinach, roughly chopped

salt and pepper

4 medium eggs

a handful of grated Italian hard cheese

a pinch of crushed chilli flakes/hot red pepper flakes

olive oil, for cooking

crusty bread, to serve

1 You can make this recipe fully on the hob/stovetop, or in the oven. I prefer to do it in the oven because it's far easier to achieve runny yolks, but I'll let you decide. If using the oven, preheat it now to 180°C fan/200°C/400°F/gas mark 6 on an oven grill/broiler setting.

2 Heat 1 tablespoon of olive oil in an ovenproof frying pan/skillet over medium heat. Add the onion and sauté for about a minute, then stir in the garlic. Continue cooking for another couple of minutes, stirring frequently, until the onion has softened.

3 Increase the heat slightly and add the mushrooms and thyme. Cook for about 3 minutes until the mushrooms release their moisture and start to brown.

4 Lower the heat again and stir in the beans. Fill the empty bean can with 50 ml/1½ fl oz/3½ tablespoons water and pour it into the pan. Add the crème fraîche, spinach and a generous pinch each of salt and pepper, stirring until the spinach begins to wilt.

5 Make four wells around the edges of the pan with the back of your spoon or spatula. Crack the eggs into the wells.

6 For the entirely hob-based option, place the lid on the pan, reduce the heat to low, and cook, covered, for 8 minutes, or until the egg whites are set. For the oven-based option, leave the pan uncovered and slide it onto the middle shelf of your preheated oven grill for 8–10 minutes, or until the egg whites are just set.

7 Sprinkle the grated Italian hard cheese all over the top along with the crushed chilli flakes. Serve immediately with crusty bread on the side.

Substitutions:

● **Dairy-free?** Use soy cream or dairy-free cream cheese in place of the crème fraîche. Omit the Italian hard cheese.

Future you:

☕ Cool and place in an airtight container, storing in the fridge for up to 2 days.
❄ You can freeze the sauce (without the eggs) for up to 1 month.
◐ Thaw in the fridge overnight, or on low power in the microwave.
◑ Warm to reheat, adding a splash of water if the sauce has become thick.

French Toast

V

DF/O

GF/O

This breakfast feels like an indulgent treat, yet it's packed full of wholesome goodness. It delivers pillows of French toast that are perfectly crisp on the edges, topped with warm, jammy blueberries and a big dollop of yogurt for an extra protein boost. I like to opt for a thick granary or wholemeal sandwich bread because it has no trouble soaking up the custard and adds a gorgeous subtle nutty flavour, but if you've got some sourdough or brioche lying around, those will be delicious, too.

1 large/US extra-large egg

40 ml/1⅓ fl oz/2½ tbsp milk

1 tsp maple syrup, plus extra for drizzling

1 tsp ground cinnamon

2 slices thick sandwich bread

1 tsp coconut oil

50 g/1¾ oz/¼ cup frozen blueberries

3 tbsp yogurt

1   Crack the egg into a wide, shallow bowl. Whisk in the milk and maple syrup, until no yolk remains. Sprinkle in the cinnamon and give the mixture a good stir to combine.

2   Submerge each slice of bread in the batter, letting it soak for around 15 seconds on each side to absorb the mixture fully. By the time both slices have soaked, no batter should remain.

3   Heat the coconut oil in a frying pan/skillet over medium heat. Once hot, carefully place both slices of soaked bread in the pan and cook for 3–4 minutes on each side, flipping occasionally, until they're golden brown and crisp on both sides.

4   While the bread is cooking, place the blueberries in a microwave-safe bowl, cover and microwave on full power for 60–90 seconds until they soften and become jammy.

5   Serve the warm toast topped with your favourite yogurt, the jammy blueberries and a drizzle of maple syrup.

Substitutions:

● Gluten-free? Use gluten-free bread.

Future you:

🍲 If you make extra portions, store the slices of cooked toast in an airtight container in the fridge for up to 2 days.

🔥 For best results, warm the slices in a hot pan, or microwave for 20 seconds.

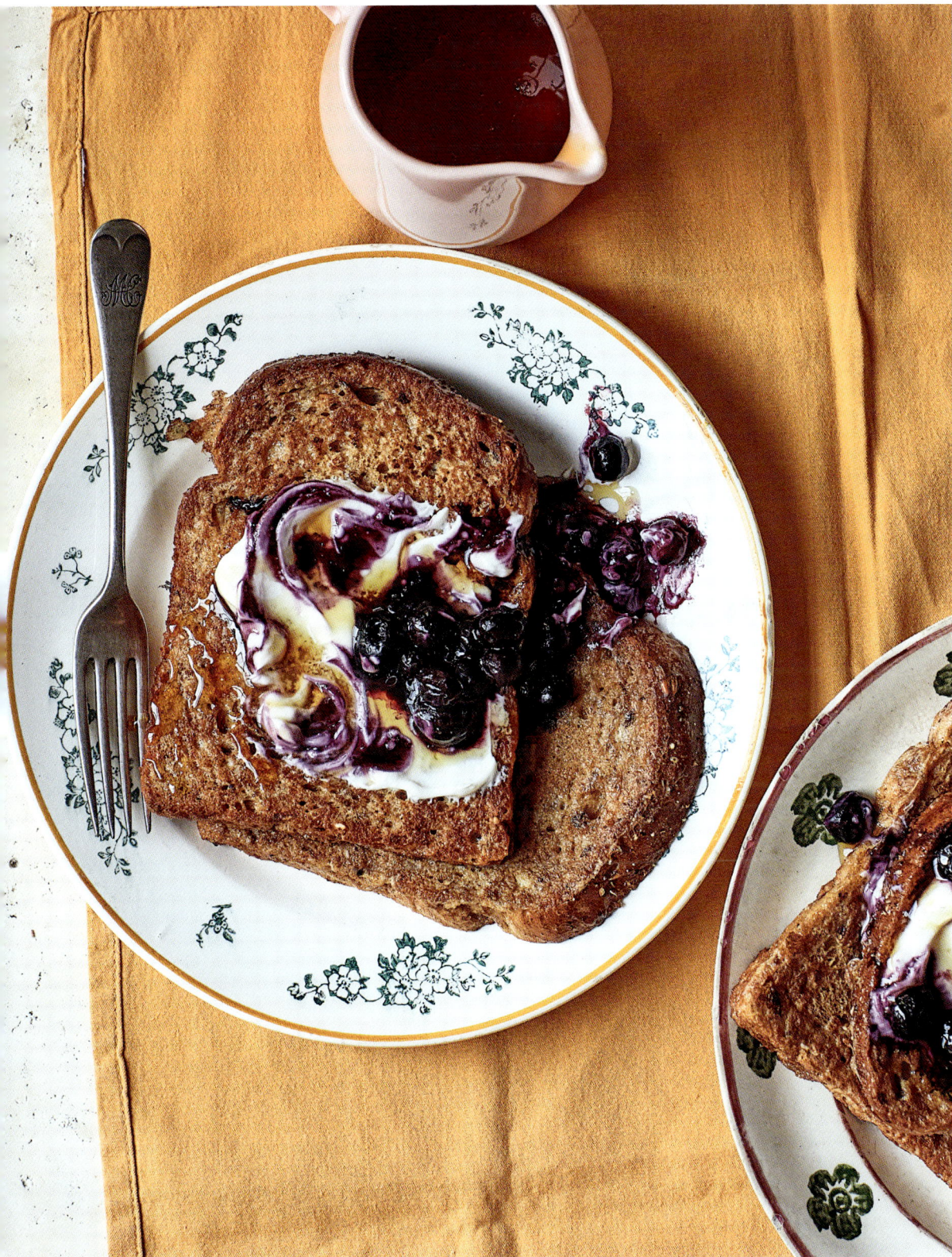

Giant Sweet Potato Rosti

V

VE/O

DF

GF/O

This rosti is essentially a giant hash brown, making it the most delicious, slightly crispy bed on which to pile high our classic brunch favourites: citrusy smashed avocado and a perfectly poached egg with a runny yolk that's waiting to spill over and mingle with all the other elements. So vibrant and packed full of nutrients, it's sure to kick off any weekend in the best way.

400 g/14 oz sweet potato, peeled and coarsely grated

½ onion, thinly sliced

1 large/US extra-large egg

2 tbsp wholemeal/whole-wheat flour

2 tsp smoked paprika

2 tsp garlic granules

2 tsp ground cumin

salt and pepper

olive oil, for cooking

To serve

2 tsp white vinegar

2 large/US extra-large eggs

1 ripe avocado

juice of ½ lime

a handful of cherry tomatoes, halved or quartered

a pinch of crushed chilli flakes/hot red pepper flakes

1   Place the grated sweet potato and sliced onion in a large mixing bowl. Add the egg, flour, paprika, garlic granules and cumin to the bowl and season everything generously with salt and pepper. Mix until well combined.

2   Heat 2 tablespoons of oil in a frying pan/skillet over medium heat. With a spatula, divide the rosti mixture into two portions in the base of the bowl (or, if you don't fancy trying your hand at flipping, make more smaller rostis instead). Carefully tip one portion into the pan and use the back of your spatula to flatten it into a 1-cm/½-in thick disk (the thinner you go, the harder it is to flip). Cook the rosti for 3–4 minutes on each side, or until it's golden and crispy around the edges. Transfer the cooked rosti to a plate lined with a paper towel to drain off any excess oil. Re-oil the pan and repeat the process with the remaining mixture.

3   While the rostis are cooking, poach the eggs to serve. Bring a saucepan of water to a simmer and add the vinegar. Crack each egg into a small bowl. Stir the simmering water to create a gentle whirlpool and carefully pour one egg into the centre. Let it cook undisturbed for 3 minutes (for a runny yolk). Use a slotted spoon to transfer the poached egg to a plate lined with a paper towel. Repeat with the second egg.

4   In a small bowl, mash the avocado with the lime juice and season to taste with salt and pepper. With all the components ready, it's time to assemble. Place a helping of smashed avocado on each rosti, followed by the cherry tomatoes, poached egg and a sprinkle of chilli flakes.

Substitutions:

● **No sweet potato?** Use white potato instead. ● **Vegan?** Replace the egg in the rosti mixture for 50 ml/1½ fl oz/3½ tbsp dairy-free milk. Swap the poached egg for Tofu Scramble (see page 24). ● **Gluten-free?** Use gluten-free flour.

Future you:

☗ Cool and place rostis in an airtight container, storing in the fridge for up to 3 days.
❄ Cool and freeze rostis for up to 2 months.
◗ Thaw in the fridge overnight, or on low power in the microwave.
◊ Place into an oven or air fryer at 180°C fan/200°C/400°F/gas mark 6 for 10–15 minutes, or until hot and crisp.

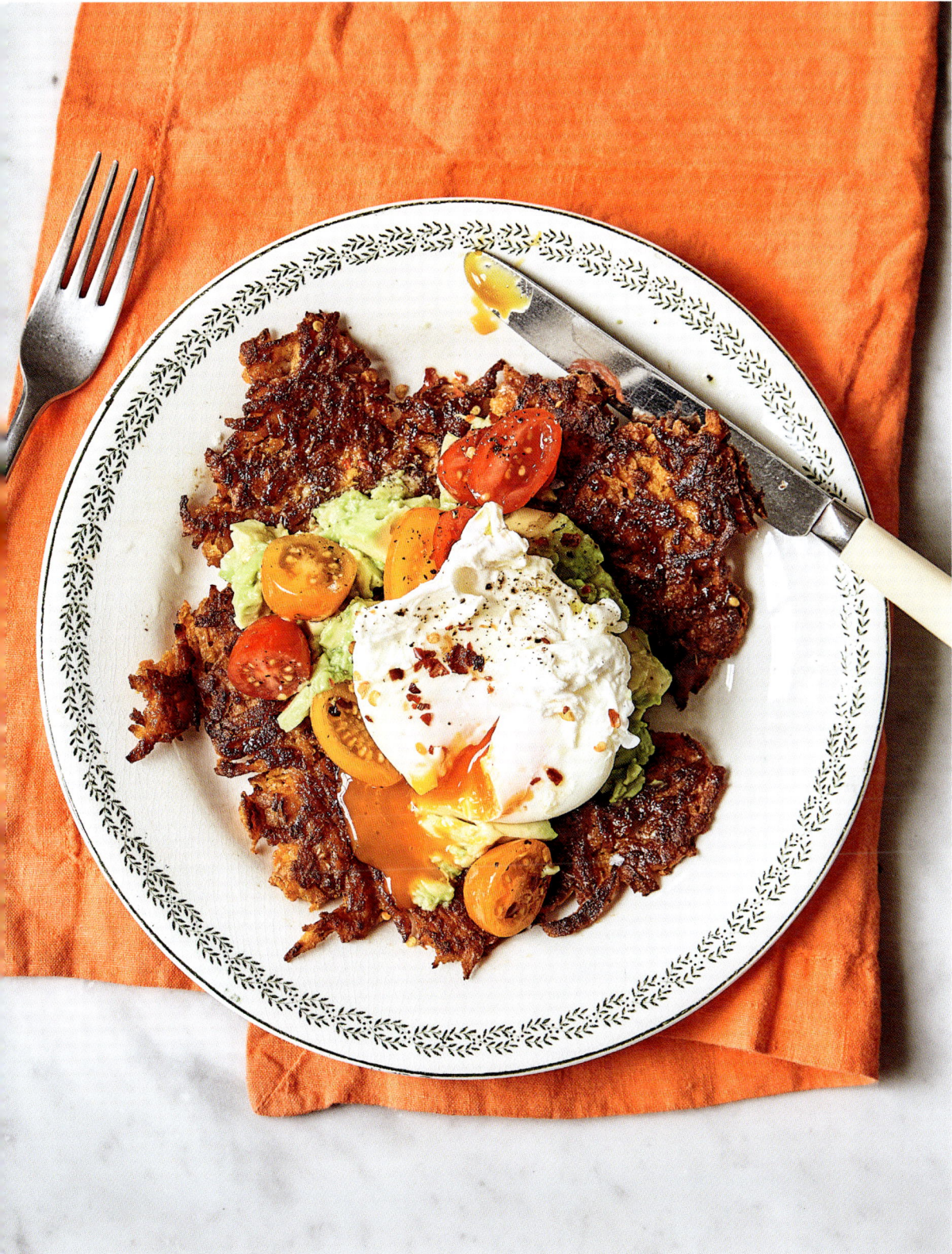

Fluffy Protein Pancakes with Healthy-ish Chocolate Sauce

(V) (VE/O) (DF/O)

Is there anything better than a towering stack of thick, fluffy pancakes smothered in chocolate sauce? I think not. Especially when they only take 20 minutes to whip up and don't require a blender (less dirties, yay!). So, stop reading and start whisking.

140 ml/4¾ fl oz/½ cup plus 1 tbsp milk

¼ tsp apple cider vinegar

60 g/2 oz/scant ½ cup wholemeal/whole-wheat flour

15 g/½ oz/generous 2 tbsp soy protein powder

1 tsp baking powder

1 tsp coconut oil, melted and cooled, plus extra for frying

1 tsp maple syrup

50 g/1¾ oz/generous ⅓ cup blueberries

yogurt, to serve

fruit, to serve

For the chocolate sauce

½ tbsp cacao powder

1 tbsp boiling water

1 tsp maple syrup

1 Combine the milk and vinegar in a small bowl and let it sit for 5 minutes to curdle. This will give the milk a buttermilk-like quality, helping the pancakes turn out gorgeously thick and fluffy.

2 In the meantime, in a large mixing bowl, measure out the flour, protein powder and baking powder. Stir together until combined.

3 Add the oil and maple syrup to the curdled milk mixture, then immediately pour the milk mixture into the bowl with the dry ingredients, whisking gently as you go. The batter will be quite thick and it's fine if a few small lumps of flour remain. After that, gently fold in the blueberries.

4 Heat 1 teaspoon of coconut oil in a large frying pan/skillet over medium heat. The batter will make 3 pancakes, so it should be possible to cook them together in one batch. Spoon the batter into the pan, forming three even-sized dollops. Use the back of the spoon to shape and smooth out each pancake. Cook for about 3 minutes on the first side, then flip and cook for an additional minute on the other side.

5 While the pancakes cook, add the cacao powder to a bowl, then slowly add in the boiling water, whisking until completely smooth. Depending on the type of cacao powder you use, you may need to adjust the amount of water to reach your desired consistency. Then, stir in the maple syrup.

6 Stack the pancakes, adding a spoonful of yogurt between each one. Pour the chocolate sauce over the top and serve immediately with fruit of your choice.

Substitutions:

● **No protein powder?** Use an extra 15 g/1/2 oz/2 tbsp flour and add an extra 1 tsp maple syrup in the batter (to compensate for the loss of sweetness from the protein powder). Reduce milk to 120 ml. ● **No wholemeal flour?** Plain/all-purpose flour will also work.

Future you:

🍲 Cool and place in an airtight container, storing in the fridge for up to 3 days.
❄ Cool and insert a piece of parchment paper between each. Stack and freeze for up to 2 months.
💧 Thaw in the fridge overnight, or on low power in the microwave.
🔥 Warm each pancake up in the microwave for 20 seconds.

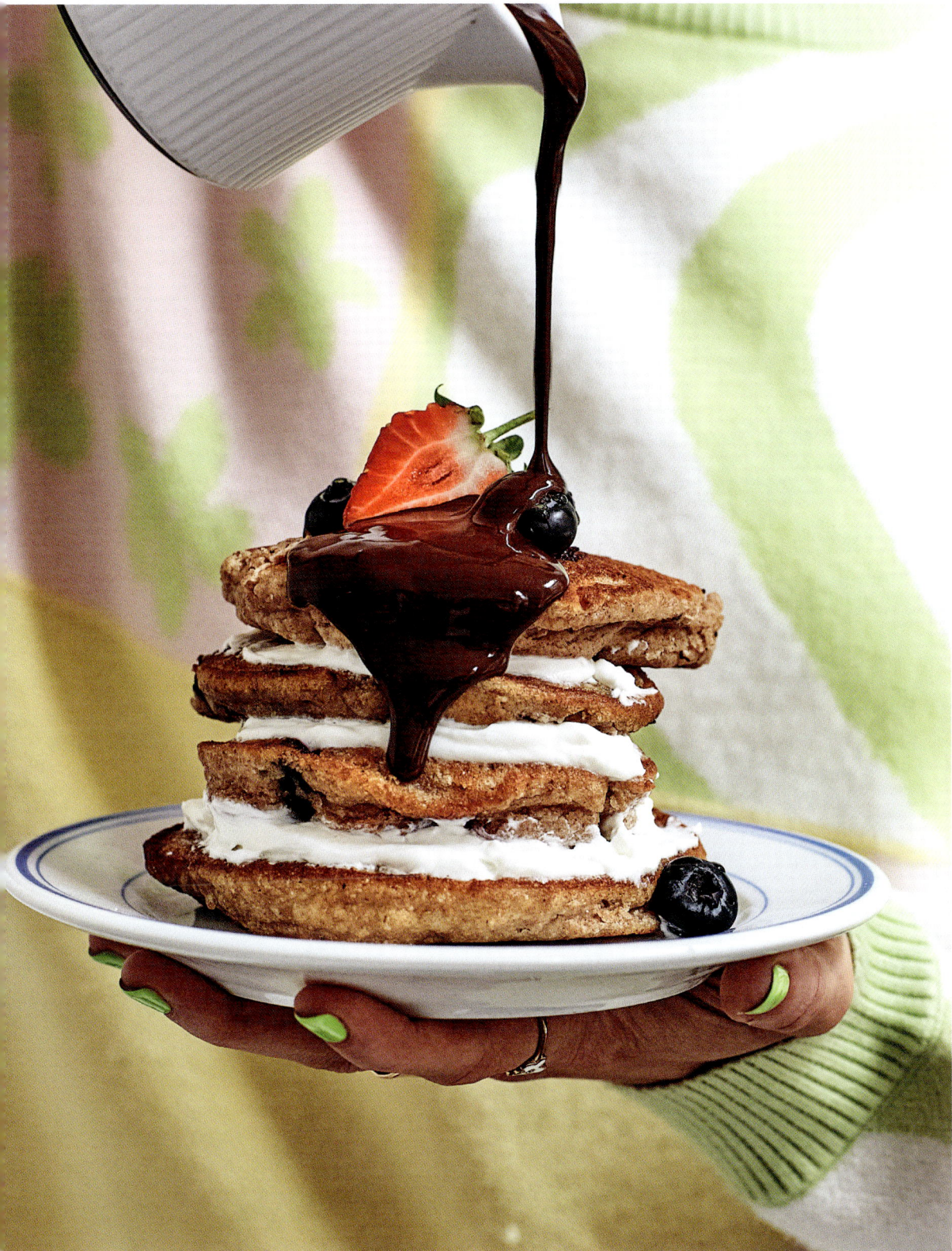

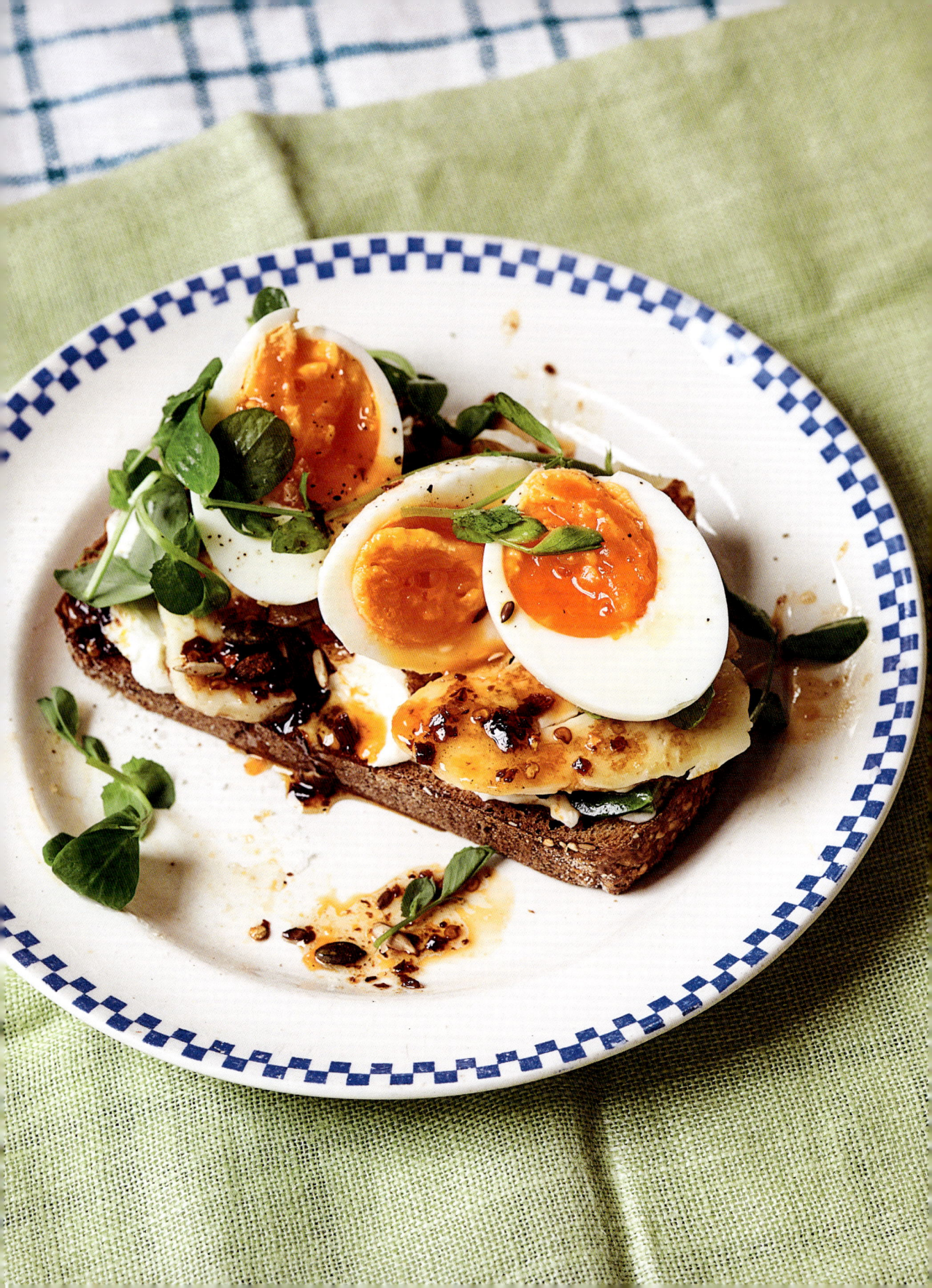

Jammy Eggs on Toast with Halloumi + Hot Honey

(V)
(VE/O)
(DF/O)
(GF/O)

This recipe takes your average eggs on toast and cranks it up several notches. The yolks are creamy, custardy and just gooey enough to moisten your toast, without too much spillage. Goldilocks eggs, if you will. Absolute magic when paired with things like salty, squeaky halloumi and a drizzle of fiery honey to marry it all together.

2 large/US extra-large eggs

45 g/1½ oz halloumi, sliced

1 thick slice sourdough bread

2 tsp cream cheese

a handful of pea shoots

½ tsp mixed seeds

salt and pepper

olive oil, for cooking

For the hot honey

½ tbsp honey

½ tsp crispy chilli/chili oil

a pinch of salt

1 Bring a small pot of water to boil over high heat. Gently lower in the eggs and boil them for exactly 6 minutes – set a timer!

2 While the eggs are boiling, heat a drizzle of olive oil in a frying pan/skillet over medium heat. Add the halloumi slices to the pan and cook for about 45 seconds on each side until nice and golden. Take the pan off the heat and set aside until later.

3 For the hot honey, combine the honey, chilli oil and pinch of salt in a small microwave-safe bowl. Microwave on full power for 15–20 seconds until the mixture is hot and bubbly. Stir well and set aside.

4 As the eggs finish boiling, take the pot over to the sink and tip as much hot water out as you can without the eggs coming out, then place the pan down in the sink. Run a steady stream of cold water from the tap into the pan for a couple of minutes – this will cool the eggs without having to faff with ice water.

5 While the eggs cool, pop the bread into the toaster and toast to your desired level of doneness.

6 Once the eggs are cool enough to handle, peel them and slice in half.

7 To assemble, spread the cream cheese on the toast in a generous layer. Lay the halloumi slices on top, then place the egg halves over the halloumi. Drizzle with the hot honey, and finish with the pea shoots, a sprinkle of seeds, a pinch of salt and a crack of black pepper.

Substitutions:

● **Dairy-free?** Use a dairy-free cream cheese and omit the halloumi. ●
Vegan? Replace the eggs with Tofu Scramble (see page 24). Omit the halloumi. Use maple syrup in place of honey. Use dairy-free cream cheese.
● **Gluten-free?** Use gluten-free bread.

Egg, Pesto + Sun-dried Tomato Buckwheat Galette

V

DF/O

GF

When I went to Paris I rightfully indulged in all the culinary delights. But amidst all the croissants, baguettes, profiteroles and frites I devoured, there's one food I haven't stopped craving: the unassumingly delicious buckwheat galette (savoury crêpe). Traditionally filled with cheese and ham, and topped with an egg, my version adds a little twist with sun-dried tomatoes, pesto and avocado. So tasty and, luckily for us, so easy to make too. Bon appétit!

60 g/2 oz/½ cup buckwheat flour

¼ tsp fine sea salt

3 medium eggs

2 tsp pesto (see Homemade Pesto, page 21, or use store-bought)

40 g/1½ oz/scant ½ cup grated cheese (I like cheddar or Gruyère)

30 g/1 oz/⅓ cup sun-dried tomatoes, finely chopped

1 ripe avocado, sliced

black pepper

olive oil, for cooking

1   In a large mixing bowl, combine the buckwheat flour and salt. Create a well in the centre, then crack in 1 egg. As you begin to whisk, slowly pour in 140 ml/4¾ fl oz/½ cup of cold water, mixing vigorously until you have a smooth batter. Transfer the bowl to the fridge to rest while you prepare the other ingredients.

2   Place a large frying pan/skillet or crêpe pan over medium–high heat and lightly coat the surface with oil. You want the pan to be hot enough that the oil just starts to smoke. Using a ladle, pour half the batter into the pan, and quickly swirl it around to spread the batter evenly over the surface of the pan – the thinner the better. Cook for 1 minute on the first side, or until the edges of the galette start to lift, then flip it over and cook for another minute.

3   Just after flipping, roughly smear the pesto across the surface of the galette and sprinkle the cheese on top. Once cooked, transfer the cooked galette to a plate (don't worry if the cheese hasn't fully melted yet; it will once the egg is added on top). Re-coat the pan with oil and repeat the process with the remaining batter.

4   While the galettes are cooking, heat 1 tablespoon of olive oil in a separate frying pan over medium–high heat. Add the sun-dried tomatoes, spreading them out evenly, then crack the remaining 2 eggs on top. Cook for a few minutes until the eggs are done to your liking.

5   To assemble, place one of your tomato-ey fried eggs in the centre of each galette, then fold the edges over to form a square. Finish by topping each galette with avocado slices and a good crack of black pepper.

Substitutions:

● **Dairy-free?** Use a dairy-free cheese and pesto.

Future you:

🗑 Untopped, the galettes can be stored in the fridge for up to 3 days.

❄ Freeze untopped galettes for up to 3 months, inserting a piece of parchment paper between each before stacking.

💧 Thaw in the fridge overnight, or at room temperature for a few hours.

🔥 Heat in a frying pan over low–medium heat, or microwave for 20–30 seconds.

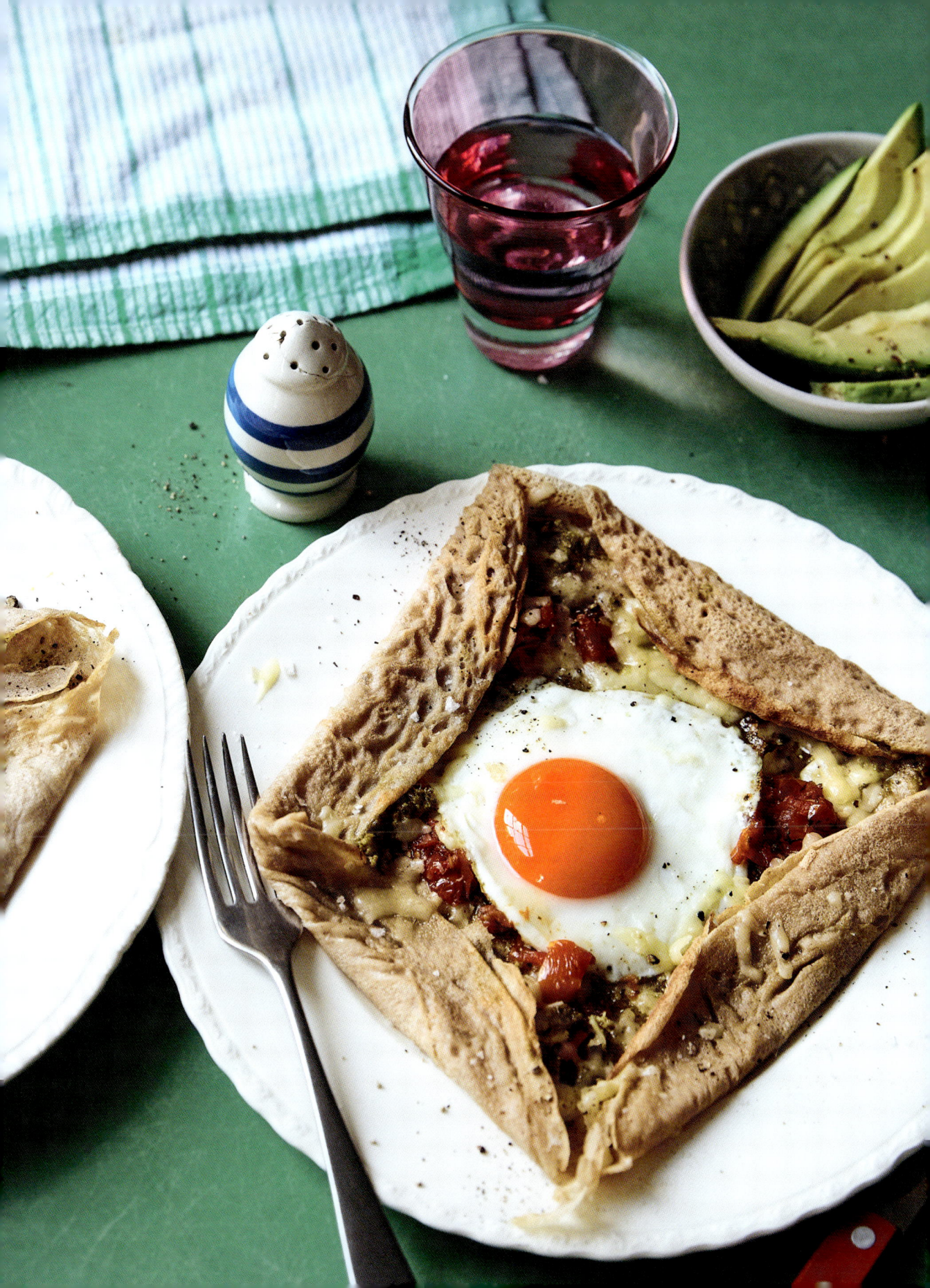

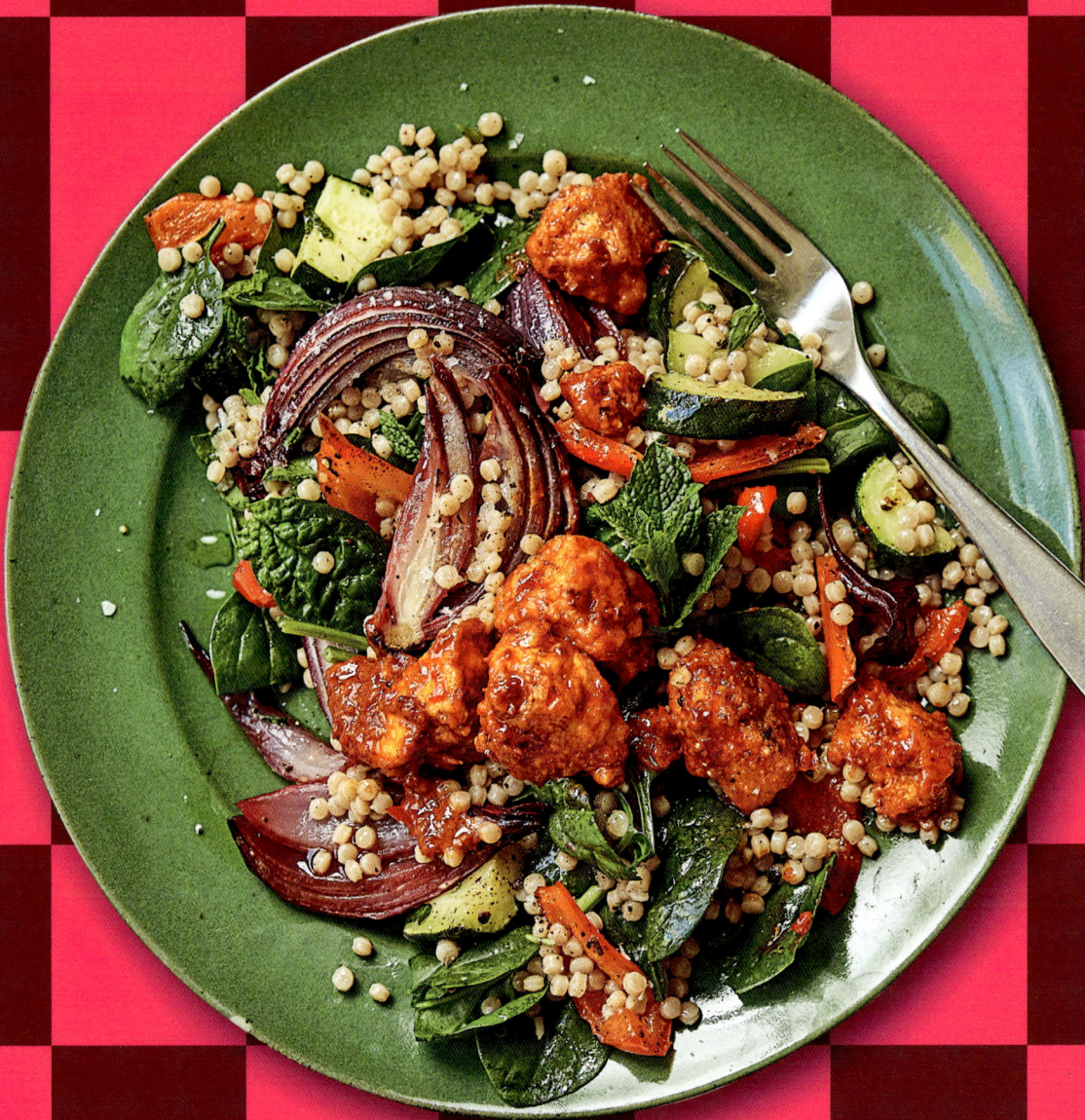

Simple Lunches

Nourishing Lunches to Fuel You, Fast

Lunch can often be a forgotten and uninspiring meal, which is why I like my lunch recipes to prioritize speed and ease. Most are optimized for meal-prepping and can be served warm or cold, making them perfect grab-and-go options for a busy work day.

PORTABLE PREP JAR:
Peanut Tofu Noodles with Edamame + Crunchy Veggies

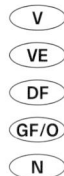

V
VE
DF
GF/O
N

This recipe kicks off a line-up of 5 Portable Prep Jars — your secret weapon for eliminating boring lunches. The beauty of this layered jar concept is in its convenience (3-4 days of lunches in 10-30 minutes) and its solution to dreaded Tupperware sogginess. You just layer them up, flip, mix, and enjoy. I have no favourite, but if you try only one, start with this. The combinations are top tier, and the peanut sauce is downright drinkable. The kind of lunch you'll look forward to tucking into all morning.

125 g/4 oz noodles of your choice

½ tsp sesame oil

1 x 300-g/10½-oz block extra-firm smoked tofu, cut into small cubes

50 g/1¾ oz/generous ⅓ cup shelled edamame beans

¼ red cabbage, shredded

1 carrot, grated

1 red (bell) pepper, thinly sliced

2 spring onions/scallions, thinly sliced

1 tbsp roughly chopped coriander/cilantro

sesame seeds, to serve (optional)

For the peanut sauce

65 g/2 oz/4½ tbsp natural peanut butter

1 thumb-sized piece ginger, grated

1½ tbsp honey or maple syrup

4 tbsp soy sauce

1½ tbsp rice vinegar

¼ tsp garlic granules

60 ml/2 fl oz/¼ cup hot water

1   Bring a small pan of water to the boil and cook the noodles according to the packet instructions. Once tender, drain and rinse them under cold water to cool. Toss the noodles with the sesame oil to prevent them from sticking together, and set aside.

2   While the noodles are cooking, grab a small jar to make the peanut sauce. Add the peanut butter, ginger, honey, soy sauce, rice vinegar, garlic granules and hot water. Seal the jar tightly and shake vigorously until the sauce is smooth and well combined.

3   To assemble your three jars (or containers), start by spooning a generous layer of peanut sauce into the bottom, then layer in the noodles. Follow with the tofu, edamame beans, cabbage, carrot, red pepper, spring onion and a sprinkle of fresh coriander.

4   When you're ready to eat, simply flip the jar or container upside down into a bowl and toss everything together, so the peanut sauce coats all the ingredients. Top with sesame seeds, if you like.

Substitutions:

● **Gluten-free?** Swap soy sauce for tamari. Use gluten-free noodles.
● **Nut free?** Swap the peanut butter for tahini.

Future you:

🍱 Store the airtight jars or containers in the fridge for up to 3 days.
❄ Freeze the peanut sauce for up to 1 month.
💧 Defrost by thawing in the fridge overnight, at room temperature for a few hours, or on low power in the microwave.

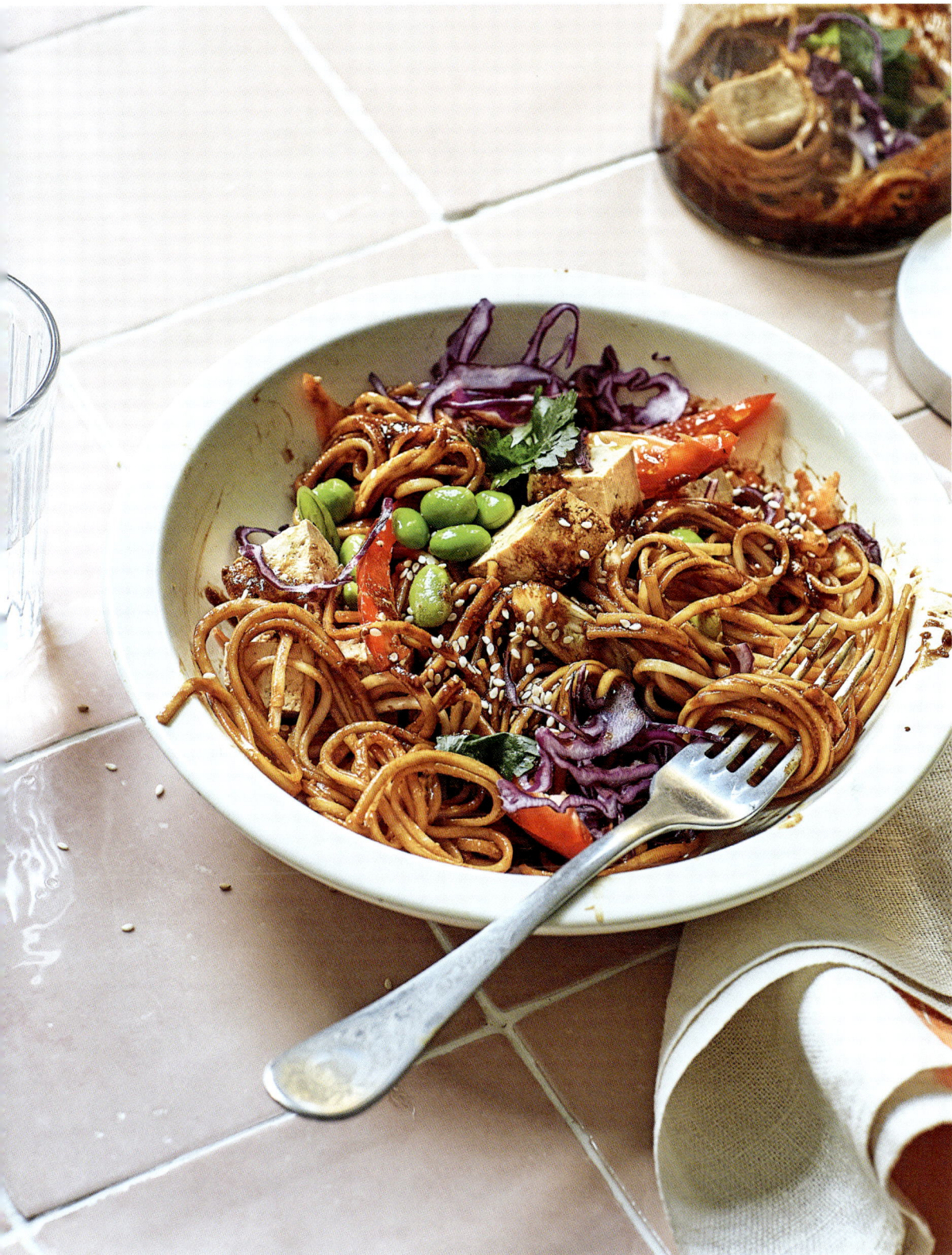

PORTABLE PREP JAR:
Lemon Herb Chicken with Quinoa Salad + Hummus

V/O
VE/O
DF
GF

One word: yum. This jar packs in so many delicious things, all stacked in one portable, protein- and flavour-packed vessel. Depending on my mood, I'll either mix it all together for a perfectly blended bite, or tip it upside down and leave it as is with the generous splodge of hummus on top, making each mouthful a little different from the last.

grated zest and juice of 1 lemon

1 tsp extra virgin olive oil

1 tsp dried oregano

1 tsp dried thyme

½ tsp garlic granules

2 skinless chicken breasts

100 g/3½ oz red pepper hummus (see 5-minute Hummus, page 78, or use store-bought)

80 g/3 oz salad leaves

salt and pepper

olive oil, for cooking

For the quinoa

1 x 250-g/9-oz pouch cooked quinoa, or 150 g/5½ oz/1 cup minus 2 tbsp quinoa cooked according to packet instructions

100 g/3½ oz cucumber, finely diced

60 g/2 oz/generous ½ cup pitted Kalamata olives, roughly chopped

¼ red onion, finely diced

1 tbsp extra virgin olive oil

juice of ½ lemon

1 garlic clove, minced

1½ tbsp finely chopped parsley

1 tbsp finely chopped mint

1   In a large, shallow bowl, combine the lemon zest and juice, extra virgin olive oil, oregano, thyme and garlic granules, along with a generous pinch each of salt and pepper.

2   Using a sharp knife, butterfly the chicken breasts by slicing them in half horizontally, taking care not to cut all the way through, so you can open them up like a book. Add the butterflied chicken breasts to the bowl and gently toss to coat them evenly in the marinade.

3   Heat 1 tablespoon of olive oil in a frying pan/skillet over medium heat. Once hot, cook the chicken breasts for 5 minutes on each side, until browned and fully cooked. Transfer the chicken to a clean plate or wooden board and let rest for a few minutes before chopping into bite-sized pieces.

4   While the chicken is cooking, heat the quinoa in the microwave according to the packet instructions, usually about 2 minutes.

5   In a large mixing bowl, combine the cooked quinoa, cucumber, olives and red onion. In a small jar, combine the extra virgin olive oil, lemon juice, garlic, parsley, mint and a good pinch each of salt and pepper. Secure the lid and shake briefly until the dressing is emulsified. Pour the dressing over the quinoa mixture and toss to combine.

6   To assemble your three jars (or containers), start with a generous layer of red pepper hummus, then follow with a layer of the quinoa salad, lemony chicken and finally a handful of salad leaves.

7   When you're ready to eat, simply flip the jar or container upside down into a bowl, allowing the layers to mix, and toss everything together.

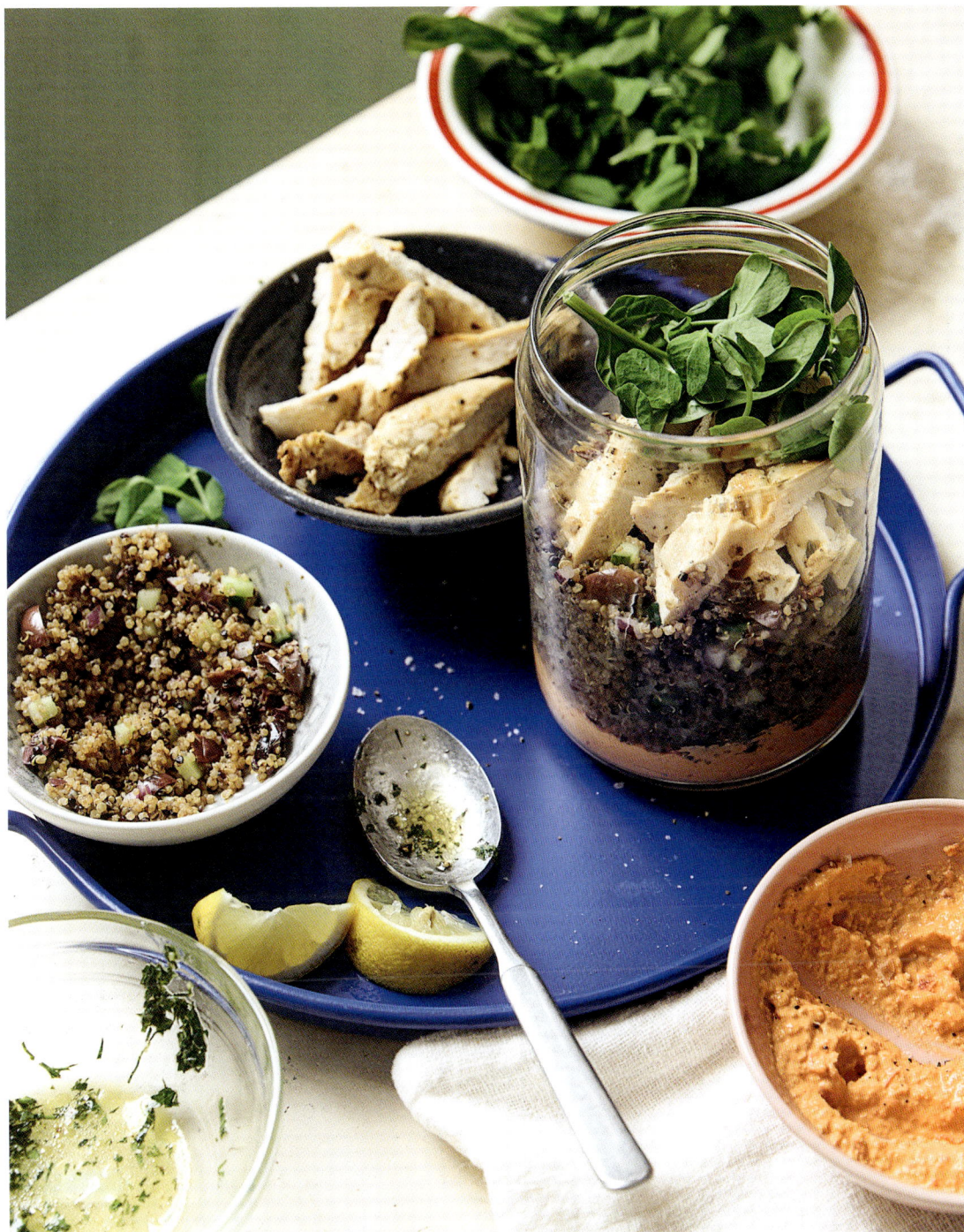

Substitutions:

● **Vegetarian or vegan?** Swap the chicken for tofu, or your favourite meat-free protein alternative. ● **No quinoa?** Use a pouch of cooked rice, or your favourite cooked grains instead.

Future you:

🍱 Store the airtight jars or containers in the fridge for up to 3 days.

PORTABLE PREP JAR:
Pesto Prawns with Herby Lentils + Sun-dried Tomato Dip

V/O
VE/O
DF/O
GF

Yes – this jar really does deliver 4 days' worth of lunches in just 10 minutes! With zero actual cooking involved, it's the jar to turn to when even thinking about the kitchen feels like too much. The flavours here are as vibrant as they are simple, but the star of the show has to be the saucy base of the sun-dried tomato and cannellini bean dip (see page 80). It pairs beautifully with the pesto prawns and herby lentils, creating a fresh, flavoursome lunch that tastes far greater than the sum of its parts.

2 x 400-g/14-oz cans green lentils in water

2 tbsp finely chopped parsley

300 g/10½ oz cooked king prawns/jumbo shrimp

3 tbsp pesto (see Homemade Pesto, page 21, or use store-bought)

120 g/4 oz/1¼ cup Spicy Sun-dried Tomato Cannellini Bean Dip (see page 80)

250 g/9 oz vine cherry tomatoes, halved or quartered

80 g/3 oz rocket/arugula

salt and pepper

1 Empty the cans of lentils into a microwave-safe bowl, cover and microwave on full power for 2 minutes, stirring halfway through. Once warmed, drain away any excess liquid and stir in the parsley, along with a good pinch each of salt and pepper.

2 While the lentils are heating, toss the cooked prawns in the pesto until they are well coated. That really is all of the work done!

3 So, now it's time to assemble your four jars (or containers). Start with a generous layer of sun-dried tomato dip at the bottom, then follow with a layer of the herby lentils, pesto-coated prawns, vine tomatoes and a handful of rocket.

4 When you're ready to eat, simply flip the jar or container upside down into a bowl and toss everything together, letting the flavours meld.

Substitutions:

● **No lentils?** Sub for cannellini beans, chickpeas/garbanzo beans, butter beans/lima beans or a cooked grain like quinoa or rice. ● **Vegetarian?** Swap the prawns for tofu, or your favourite meat-free protein alternative. ● **Vegan?** Swap the prawns for tofu. Use dairy-free pesto. ● **Dairy-free?** Use dairy-free pesto.

Future you:

🥡 Store the airtight jars or containers in the fridge for up to 4 days. However, please ahere to best before end (BBE) date on the packaging of your prawns.

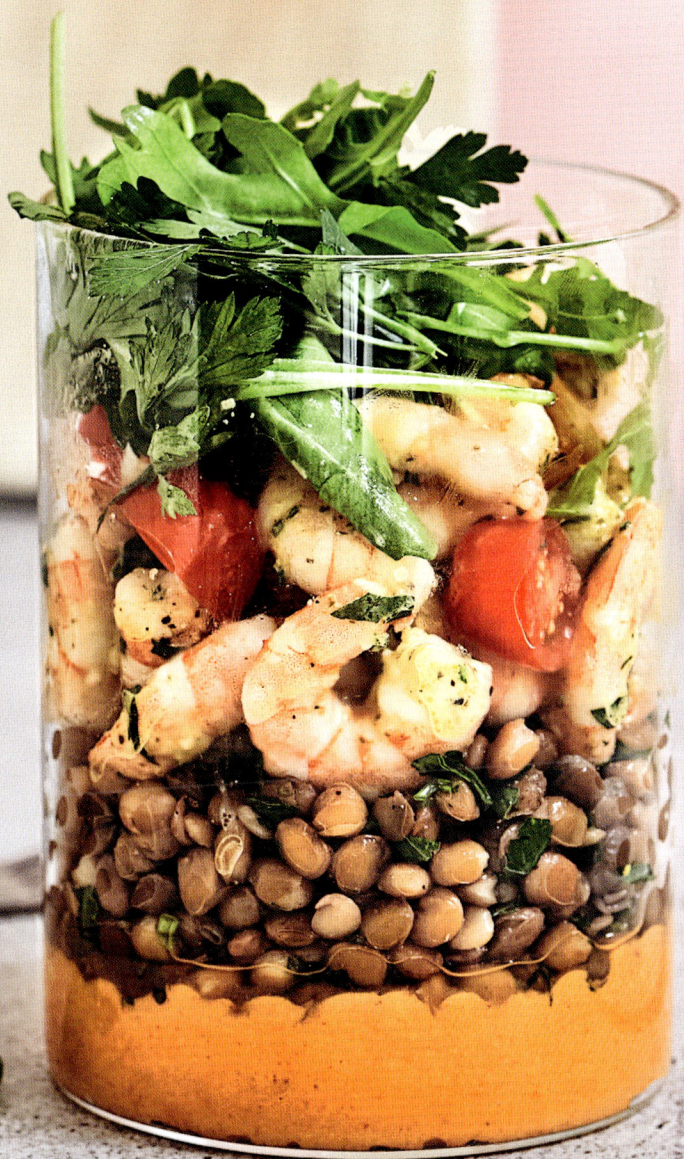

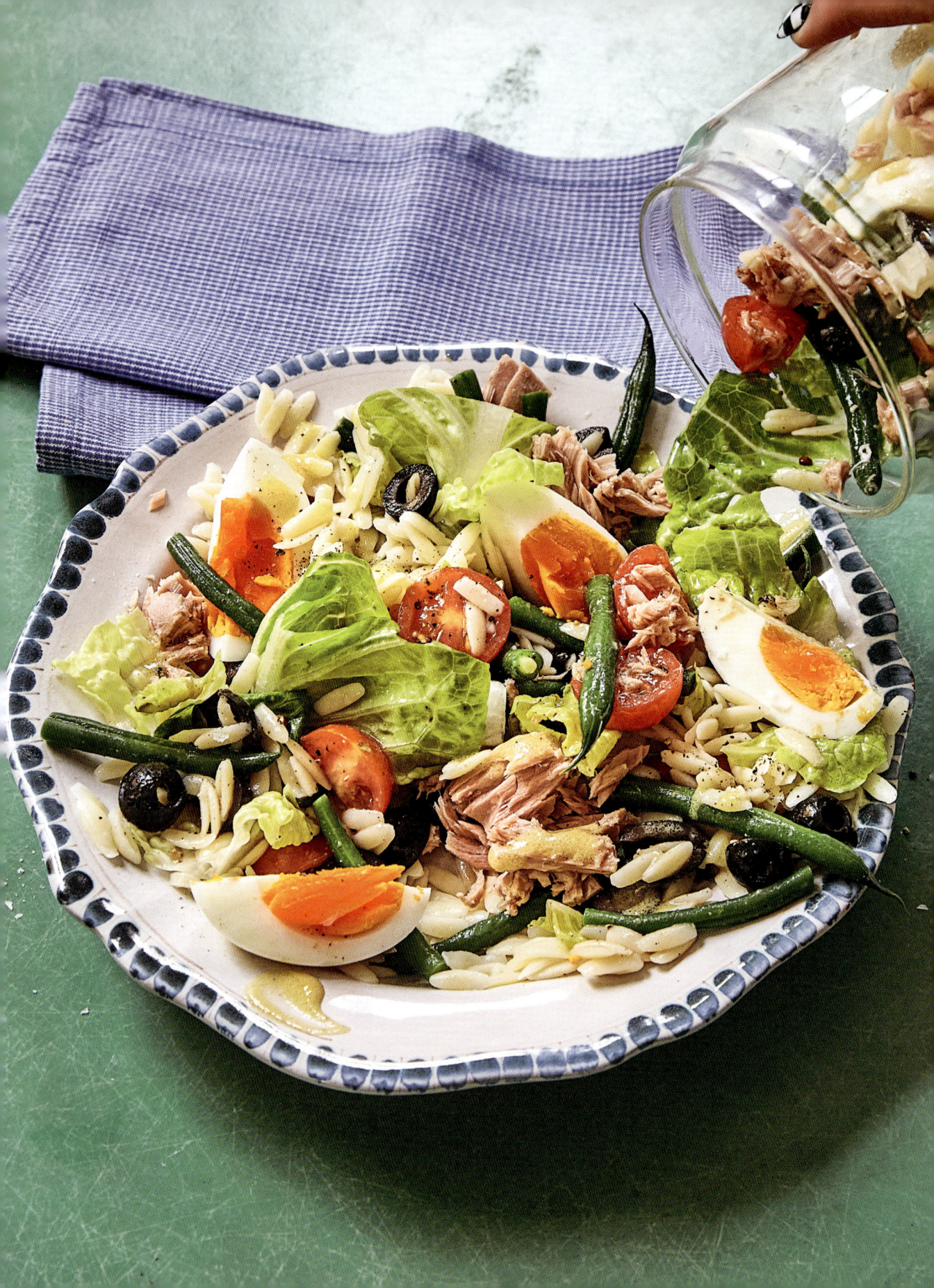

PORTABLE PREP JAR:
Tuna Niçoise

V/O
VE/O
DF
GF/O

This is my version of a tuna niçoise. The orzo adds a lovely chewy base, carrying all the flavours without feeling the least bit heavy. Then, there are the usual suspects: tuna, briny olives, crisp green beans, and juicy tomatoes, all nestled alongside perfectly cooked hard-boiled eggs, while a gorgeously zingy mustard vinaigrette waits to bring it all together. Again, layered jar-style, so it stays fresh and vibrant no matter where you take it.

80 g/3 oz orzo
50 g/1¾ oz fine green beans, cut in half
3 large/US extra-large eggs
125 g/4 oz cherry tomatoes, halved
1 shallot, thinly sliced
90 g/3 oz/scant 1 cup pitted black olives, halved
2 x 200-g/7-oz cans tuna steak in olive oil
80 g/3 oz salad leaves
salt and pepper

For the dressing

2 tbsp extra virgin olive oil
1 tbsp white wine vinegar
1 garlic clove, minced
1 tsp Dijon mustard
salt and pepper

1   Bring two small pots of water to the boil. In the first pot, add a pinch of salt, then tip in the orzo. Cook per the packet instructions, stirring occasionally, until al dente. A few minutes before the orzo is done, add the green beans to the same pot so they can cook simultaneously.

2   In the second pot, carefully lower in the eggs using a spoon to avoid cracks. Let them boil for exactly 9 minutes (set a timer!) for a perfectly set yolk.

3   While the eggs and orzo bubble away, combine the dressing ingredients in a small jar, secure the lid and shake until the dressing is emulsified.

4   Once the 9 minutes on the eggs are up, drain and rinse the eggs under a steady stream of cold water for a couple of minutes – this will cool them. By this time, the orzo and green beans should be ready. Drain them in a colander and run under cold water to cool.

5   In a large mixing bowl, combine the orzo and green beans with the cherry tomatoes, shallot and olives. Pour in the dressing and toss everything together until well coated.

6   Peel the cooked eggs and slice them into quarters.

7   Now it's time to layer up your three jars (or containers). Begin with a helping of the orzo salad, then layer on the tuna and egg, finishing with a handful of salad leaves.

8   When you're ready to eat, simply flip the jar or container upside down into a bowl and toss everything together to combine.

Future you:

🥡 Store the airtight jars or containers in the fridge for up to 3 days.

Substitutions:

● **Vegetarian?** Swap the tuna for chickpeas/garbanzo beans, or your favourite meat-free protein alternative. ● **Vegan?** See vegetarian advice above. Omit the eggs. ● **Gluten-free?** Use a gluten-free pasta alternative. ● **No orzo?** Use your favourite pasta as an alternative.

PORTABLE PREP JAR:
Chickpea Caesar

V

VE

DF

GF/O

I love the indulgence of a classic Caesar salad, but enjoying one every day might not leave me feeling my best. That's why I created this lighter version that still delivers all the rich, tangy Caesar flavours with a nutritional boost. Don't be alarmed when you see silken tofu in the ingredients – it's a game changer. Silky and neutral in taste, it blends beautifully into creamy dressings. I sneak it into sweet and savoury recipes throughout this book to elevate the protein, and here, it makes the perfect base for our Caesar dressing.

2 x 400-g/14-oz cans chickpeas/garbanzo beans, drained

2 slices crusty bread (fine if it's stale!), torn into chunks

1 tsp dried marjoram

250 g/9 oz whole-wheat fusilli

½ red onion, finely diced

1 romaine lettuce, roughly chopped

salt and pepper

olive oil, for cooking

For the Caesar dressing

1 x 300-g/10½-oz block silken tofu

1 tsp capers

40 g/1½ oz sweet pickles or gherkins

2 tsp Dijon mustard

1 garlic clove

juice of 1 lemon

1 tbsp tahini

1 tsp extra virgin olive oil

1 tsp fine sea salt

¼ tsp pepper

1 heaped tbsp nutritional yeast (optional)

1 Preheat the air fryer or oven to 180°C fan/200°C/400°F/gas mark 6.

2 If using an air fryer, tip the chickpeas and chunks of bread into the basket. Drizzle everything with a bit of oil, then season with marjoram, salt and pepper. Cook for about 8 minutes, or until the bread is crisp. If using an oven, spread the chickpeas and bread chunks on a baking tray. Drizzle with oil and season with marjoram, salt and pepper. Cook for 10 minutes, or until the bread is crisp.

3 Meanwhile, fill a pan with boiling water and cook the pasta according to the packet instructions. Once al dente, drain the pasta in a colander and run it under cold water to cool completely.

4 Next up, prepare the Caesar dressing. In a blender combine all the dressing ingredients and blend for 1–2 minutes until the dressing is silky smooth. Have a taste for seasoning and tweak if needed.

5 Now, for the fun part: assembling the four jars (or containers). Start with a generous layer of Caesar dressing at the bottom, then follow with layers of pasta, chickpeas, onion and lettuce. I'd recommend storing the bread croutons separately and adding them on top just before serving to make sure they stay perfectly crisp.

6 When you're ready to eat, simply flip the jar or container upside down into a bowl and toss everything together to evenly coat in the dressing. Finally, add the croutons on top.

Substitutions:

● **No silken tofu?** If you have a powerful blender, use firm tofu instead and add a splash of water to loosen.
● **Gluten-free?** Use a gluten-free pasta alternative.

Future you:

🥡 Store the airtight jars or containers in the fridge for up to 4 days.
❄ Freeze the Caesar dressing for up to 1 month.
💧 Thaw in the fridge overnight, at room temperature for a few hours, or on low power in the microwave.

64

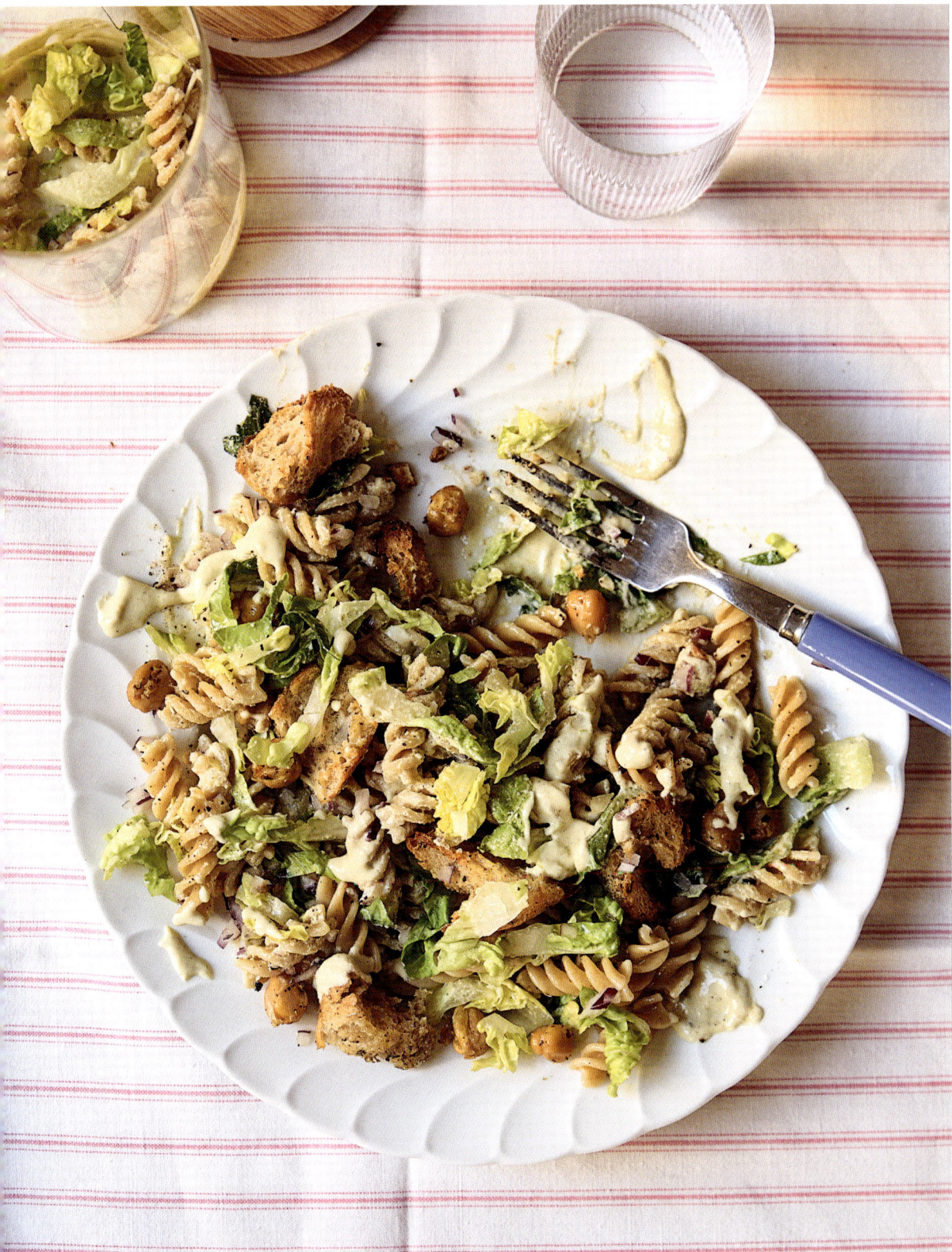

Jalapeño + Cheddar Eggs in the Hole

V

DF/O

GF/O

Get ready to have this lunch on repeat, because not only is it easy and fun to make, it's also incredibly satisfying to eat. Honestly, it might just be the easiest recipe in this whole book, so there's absolutely no excuse not to give it a go at least once. All it takes is cracking an egg into the centre of a bagel half, showering it with cheese and jalapeños, and letting the air fryer or oven do the rest of the work as it cooks to golden perfection. That's it. It's best made to order. So, if you're cooking for one, halve the ingredients and, equally, if you're feeding a crowd, fill up the whole tray with bagels and everyone will be very happy indeed.

baking sheet, lined (if using an oven)

air fryer basket, lined (if using an air fryer)

1 bagel

2 eggs

15 g/½ oz/3 tbsp grated cheddar

6 pickled jalapeño slices

salt and pepper

1 spring onion/scallion, to garnish

salad leaves, to serve

1   Preheat the air fryer or oven to 200°C fan/220°C/425°F/gas mark 7.

2   Slice the bagel in half and place it cut-side down on the lined baking sheet or in the lined air fryer basket. If the holes in the middle are too small, use a knife to hollow them out to make room for the eggs.

3   Crack an egg into the centre of each bagel half. To prevent the egg whites from overflowing too much, lift the bagel slightly to help the whites settle underneath, leaving the yolk sitting proudly on top. Sprinkle the cheese over each bagel and top with the jalapeños. Season with a pinch each of salt and pepper.

4   Cook for 8 minutes (air fryer) or 10 minutes (oven), or until the egg whites are fully set but the yolks remain runny.

5   Serve the bagel halves garnished with a sprinkle of chopped spring onion, alongside your favourite salad.

Substitutions:

● **Dairy-free?** Use dairy-free cheese.
● **No bagels?** Use a slice of thick bread (i.e. sourdough) instead and carve out a hole in the middle for the egg. ● **Gluten-free?** Use a gluten-free bagel or bread.

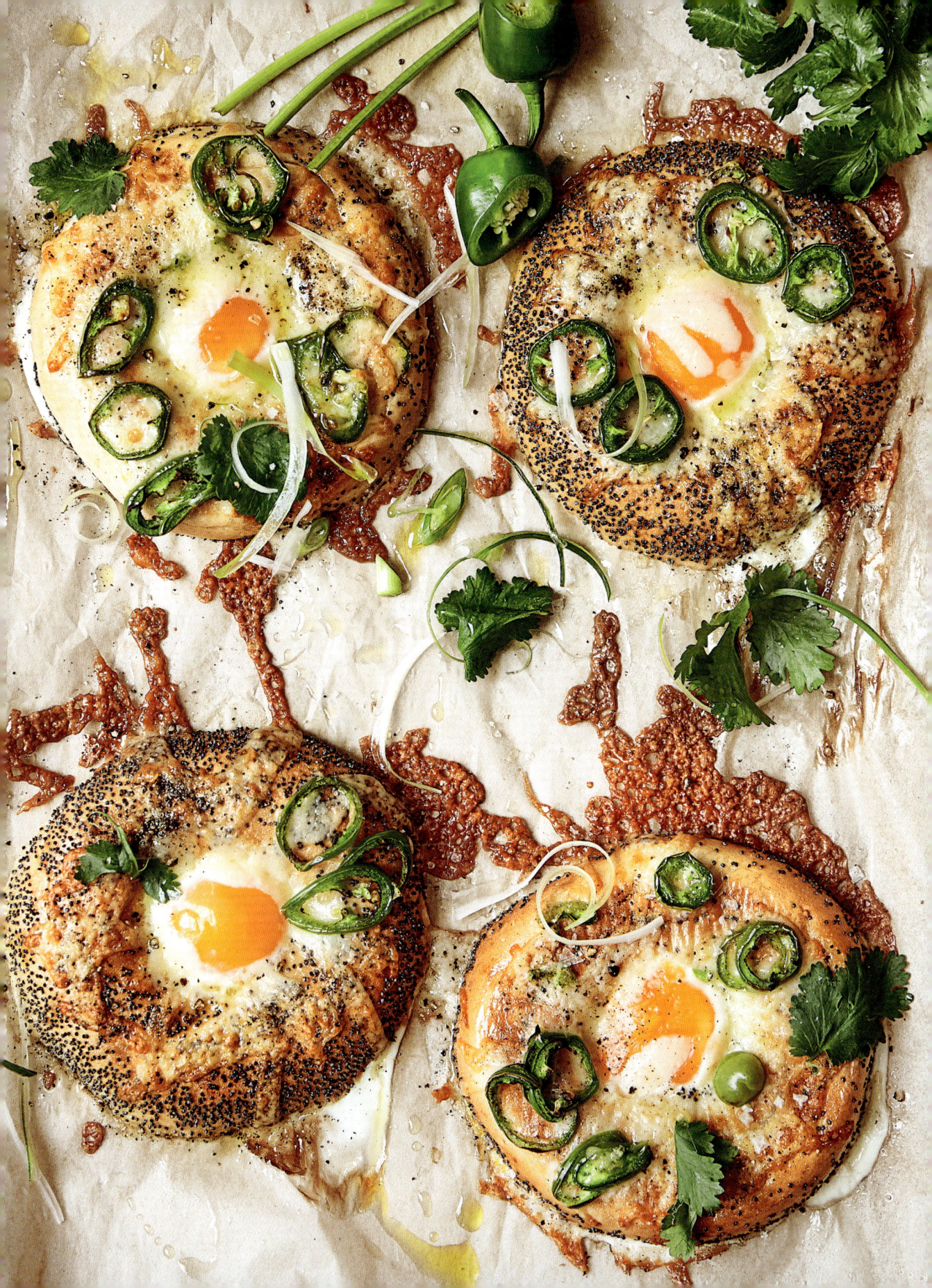

Protein-Loaded Sweet Potato

V
VE
DF
GF/O

This dish might not win any beauty contests, but oh boy does it taste good. Think of tempeh as tofu's more rugged cousin – packed with natural protein and perfect as a meat-free alternative. I'm hoping this recipe will convert you into a full-blown tempeh fan. But, if not, I understand – tofu is always waiting in the wings to be subbed back in!

baking sheet, lined (if using an oven)

air fryer basket, lined (if using an air fryer)

1 x 200-g/7-oz block tempeh

2 tbsp soy sauce

1 tbsp tomato purée/paste

½ tsp smoked paprika

½ tsp dried oregano

½ tsp dried thyme

½ tsp garlic granules

½ tsp onion granules

2 sweet potatoes (about 200 g/ 7 oz each)

4 tbsp hummus (see 5-minute Hummus, page 78, or use store-bought)

a handful of rocket/arugula leaves

salt and pepper

olive oil, for cooking

1 Begin by filling a pan with water about 2.5 cm/1-in deep and bringing it to a simmer. Add the block of tempeh, cover and allow to steam for 10 minutes – this will remove any bitterness and make it much easier to crumble. Drain and run the tempeh under cold water until it's cool enough to handle. Then, crumble it into pieces.

2 Meanwhile, in a small bowl, make the tempeh glaze by mixing together the soy sauce, tomato purée, paprika, oregano, thyme, garlic granules, onion granules and 2 tablespoons of water until combined and glossy.

3 Pierce the sweet potatoes with a fork, then wrap separately in damp paper towels. Place both potatoes into the microwave and cook for 2 minutes on full power. Turn and microwave for a further 2 minutes. They should be knife-tender; but if they're not quite there, continue to microwave in minute-long intervals. Carefully remove, unwrap and set aside to cool slightly.

4 While the potatoes are cooling, heat 1 tablespoon of olive oil in a frying pan/skillet over medium–high heat. Add the crumbled tempeh and cook for about 4 minutes, stirring often, until lightly browned. Season to taste with salt and pepper. Pour in the glaze and continue to cook for a further 3 minutes, then remove from the heat.

5 To serve, slice each cooked potato down the middle and pinch at each end to open up. Stuff with a dollop of hummus, a portion of the glazed tempeh and a handful of rocket on top.

Substitutions:

● **No tempeh?** Sub for tofu instead and skip step 1. ● **No sweet potato?** Use white potatoes instead. ● **Gluten-free?** Use tamari instead of soy sauce. Ensure your tempeh is gluten-free.

Future you:

☷ Cool and place elements in separate airtight containers, storing in the fridge for up to 4 days.

❄ Cool and freeze for up to 2 months.

💧 Thaw in the fridge overnight, or on low power in the microwave.

🔥 Reheat the potato and tempeh in the microwave for 2–3 minutes before reconstructing with hummus.

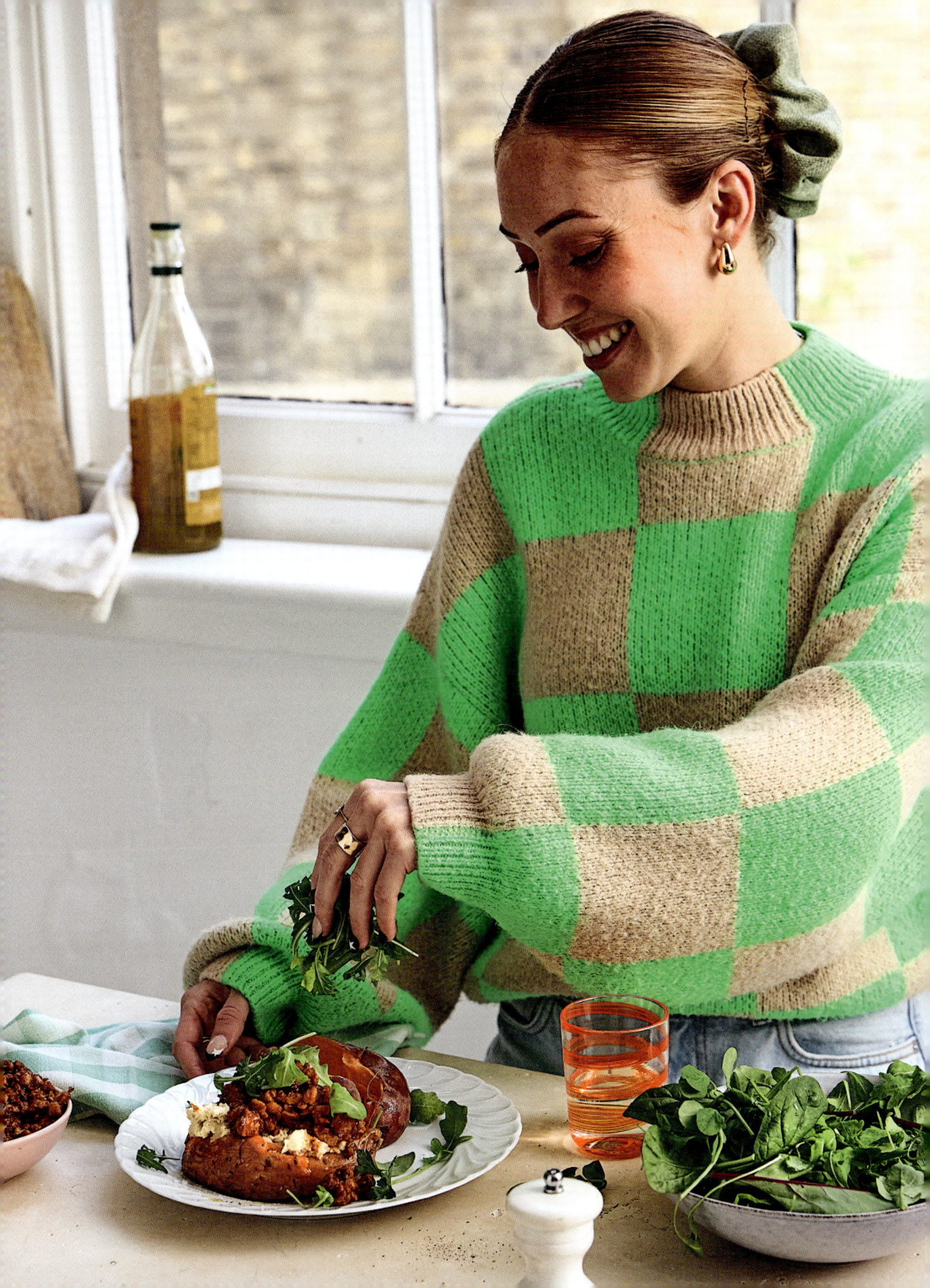

Shredded BBQ Tofu Sandwich + Pickled Slaw

(V)
(VE)
(DF)
(GF/O)

The crispy shredded tofu is bathed in a sweet, smoky homemade BBQ sauce, giving it a rich, caramelized flavour that's perfectly complemented by the acidic crunch of the quick-pickled cabbage slaw. Both the BBQ tofu and the pickle stay fresh in the fridge for up to 4 days, making those components ideal for doubling up to make delicious lunches all week.

baking sheet, lined (if using an oven)

air fryer basket, lined (if using an air fryer)

1 x 225-g/8-oz block extra-firm smoked tofu

1 tsp cornflour/cornstarch

1 large ripe avocado

squeeze of lime juice

4 slices sourdough bread, lightly toasted

salt and pepper

olive oil, for cooking

For the pickled cabbage

¼ red onion, shredded

¼ red cabbage, shredded

juice of 1 lime

1 tbsp roughly chopped coriander/cilantro

For the BBQ sauce

3 tbsp tomato purée/paste

1 tbsp maple syrup

1 tsp smoked paprika

½ tsp ground cumin

½ tsp crushed chilli flakes/hot red pepper flakes

¼ tsp garlic granules

2 tsp balsamic vinegar

Substitutions:

● **Gluten-free?** Serve in gluten-free bread. ● **No bread?** This combo is utterly delicious in tacos too!

1 Preheat the oven or air fryer to 200°C fan/220°C/425°F/gas mark 7.

2 Press out any water from the block of tofu (this will vary depending on the brand you use). Then, grate the tofu using the coarse side of a grater. In a mixing bowl, and toss the tofu with the cornflour and a generous pinch of salt and pepper until well coated.

3 If using an oven, spread out the tofu evenly on the prepared baking sheet. Drizzle with a little oil and bake for 10 minutes. If using an air fryer, add the tofu into the basket, drizzle with oil and cook for 8–10 minutes until golden and crisp.

4 While the tofu cooks, prepare the pickled cabbage. In a bowl, combine the onion, cabbage, lime juice and coriander. Season with a generous pinch of salt, then mix, massaging the mixture as you do until the cabbage and onion turn a brighter pink. Set aside to continue pickling.

5 Next, whip up the BBQ sauce. In a small jar, combine all the ingredients along with 1–2 tablespoons of water. Shake vigorously until the sauce is well mixed, then taste and adjust the seasoning if needed.

6 Finally, smash the avocado in a bowl using the back of a fork and season with salt, pepper and a squeeze of lime juice.

7 By now, your tofu should be ready. Drizzle the BBQ sauce over the tofu and use tongs to coat it evenly.

8 To assemble the sandwich, start with a layer of smashed avocado on the toasted bread, followed by the BBQ tofu. Top with the pickled cabbage.

Future you:

🥡 Store the pickle and tofu separately in an airtight container in the fridge for up to 4 days.
❄ Cool and freeze the tofu for up to 2 months.
💧 Thaw in the fridge overnight, or on low power in the microwave.
🔥 Enjoy the defrosted tofu chilled or warm in the microwave for 1–2 minutes.

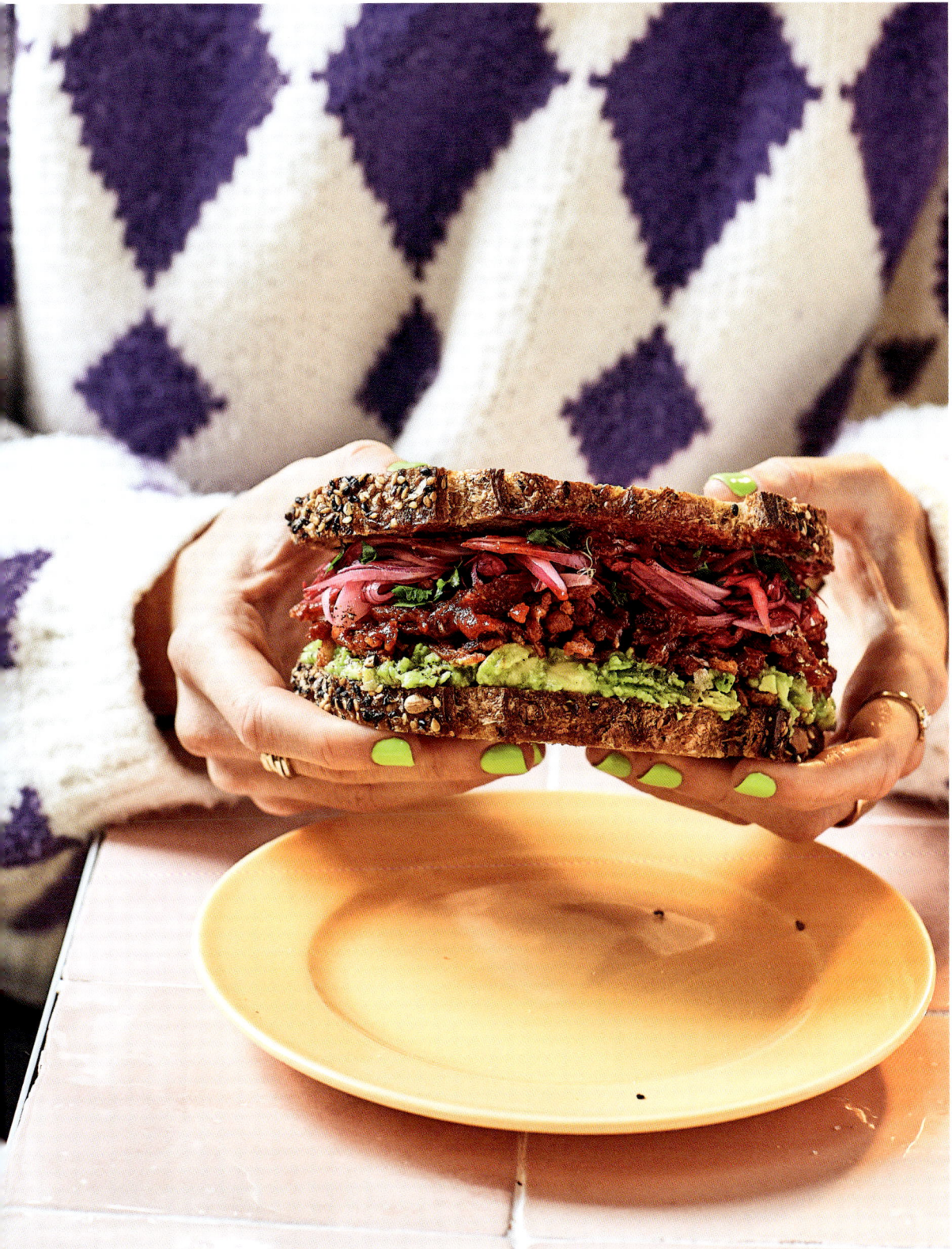

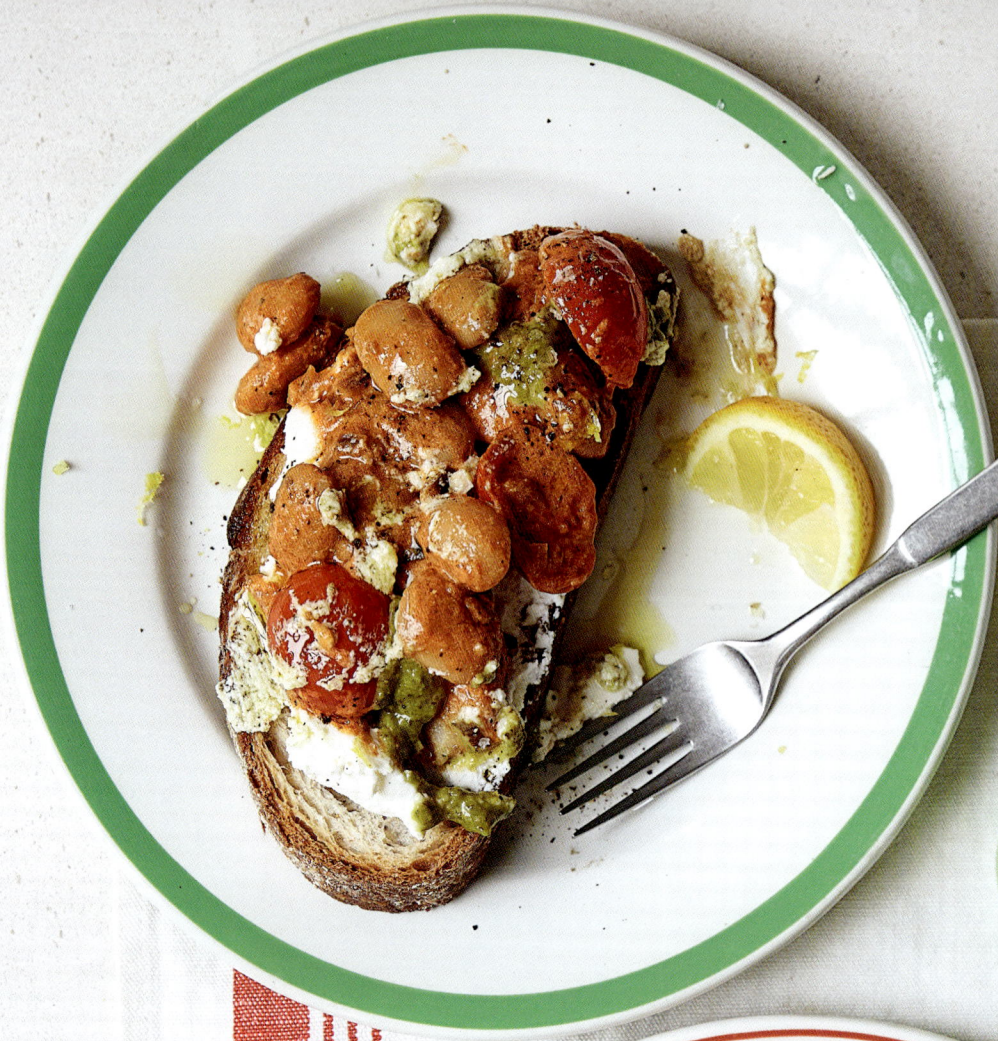

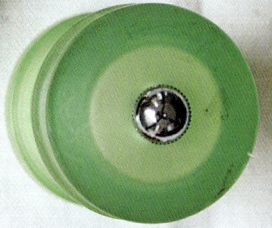

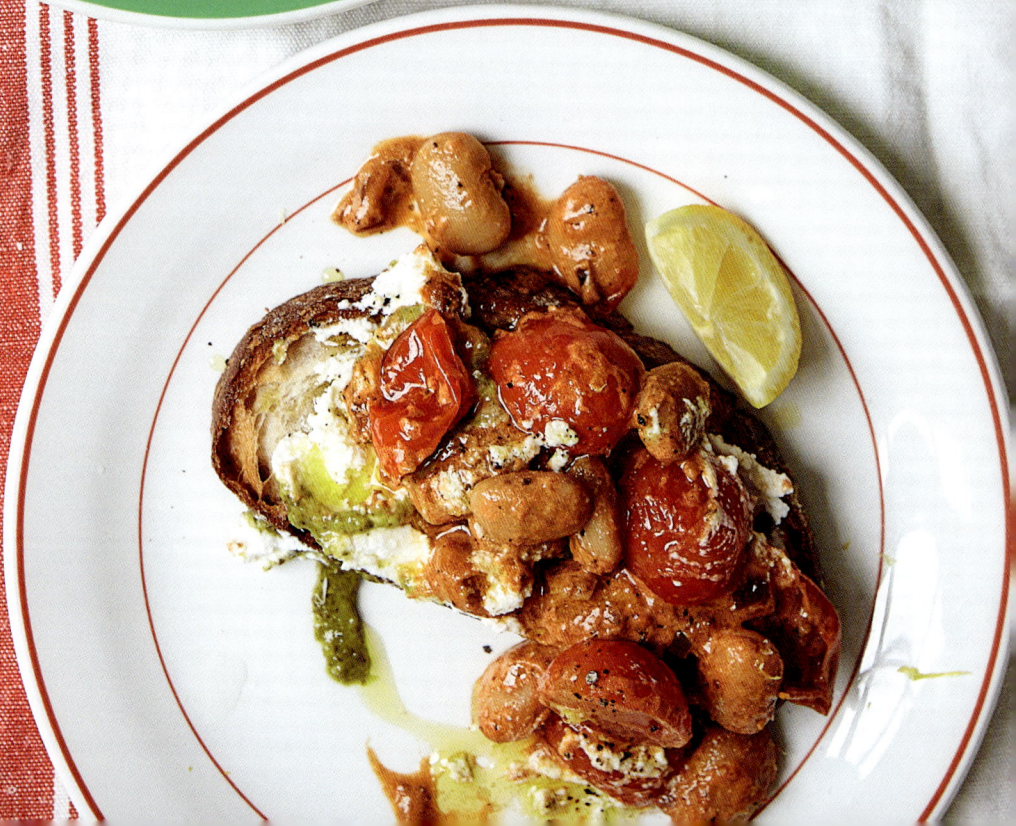

Posh Beans on Toast with Ricotta + Pesto

V

VE/O

DF/O

GF/O

N

Some days, good old classic beans from a can are more than enough to hit the spot. But sometimes we feel like treating ourselves to something a bit more special. So I'm leaving this glorious recipe here for you to pick up on one of those days, and I promise you won't regret getting the chopping board out for it. When I initially tested this recipe, the first thing I thought was: if I ever open a café, this is going straight on the menu. It's that good. It's as impressive in flavour as it is quick (just 15 minutes!) but, it comes with a warning: it will probably make you a beans on toast snob for life.

½ red onion, finely diced
1 garlic clove, minced
150 g/5½ oz cherry tomatoes, halved
1 tsp dried oregano
1 x 400-g/14-oz can butter beans/ lima beans, drained
1½ tbsp tomato purée/paste
1½ tbsp crème fraîche or sour cream
1–2 slices bread (I like sourdough or ciabatta)
2 tbsp ricotta
1 tbsp pesto (see Homemade Pesto, page 21, or use store-bought)
squeeze of lemon juice
salt and pepper
olive oil, for cooking

1 Heat 1 tablespoon of olive oil in a frying pan/skillet over medium heat. Add the onion and garlic, allowing them to cook for a couple of minutes until softened and fragrant. Toss in the cherry tomatoes and oregano and cook for another 2–3 minutes until the tomato skins begin to soften and break down. Use the back of a spatula to crush the tomatoes gently, releasing their juices.

2 Add the drained beans to the pan, along with the tomato purée, crème fraîche and a generous pinch each of salt and pepper. If the sauce seems too thick, fill the empty bean can with a splash of water and stir it into the pan to loosen the mixture and help create a creamy, saucy consistency. Turn the heat to low while you toast the bread.

3 Spread the ricotta on the toast, then add a generous helping of the beans. Finish with a drizzle of pesto and a squeeze of lemon over the top.

Substitutions:

● **No butter beans?** Use cannellini or borlotti/cranberry beans instead.
● **Dairy-free?** Use soy cream, dairy-free cream cheese or dairy-free yogurt in place of the crème fraîche. Use dairy-free pesto. ● **Gluten-free?** Use gluten-free bread. ● **Nut-free?** Use a nut-free pesto.

Future you:

☕ Cool and place in an airtight container, storing in the fridge for up to 4 days.
❄ Cool and freeze the beans for up to 2 months.
💧 Thaw in the fridge overnight, or on low power in the microwave.
🔥 Warm to reheat, adding a splash of water if the sauce has become thick.

Couscous Salad with Harissa Tofu

V
VE/O
DF/O
GF/O

Whilst tofu often gets a bad rap for being bland and boring, when it's coated in cornflour and cooked like this, it truly takes on the most amazing texture that clings to any sauce you send its way. Here, that's a sticky harissa glaze, as sweet as it is spicy, and the perfect pairing with this tangy couscous salad.

large baking sheet, lined (if using an oven)

air fryer basket, lined (if using an air fryer)

1 x 300-g/10½-oz block extra-firm tofu

1 tbsp cornflour/cornstarch

1 red (bell) pepper, cut into chunks

1 courgette/zucchini, sliced and quartered

½ red onion, cut into chunks

100 g/3½ oz/generous ½ cup giant couscous

50 g/1¾ oz/scant 1 cup spinach, roughly chopped

1 tbsp zhoug

salt and pepper

olive oil, for cooking

For the tofu glaze

1 tbsp rose harissa paste

1 tbsp maple syrup

juice of ½ lemon

½ tbsp cornflour/cornstarch

For the minted yogurt

4 tbsp runny yogurt

1½ tbsp roughly chopped mint

1   Preheat the air fryer or oven to 200°C fan/220°C/425°F/gas mark 7.

2   Press out any water from the tofu (this will vary depending on the brand you use), tear it into bite-sized chunks, and toss in a mixing bowl with the cornflour and a good pinch of salt and pepper until coated.

3   If using an oven, spread the tofu chunks, pepper, courgette and onion onto the prepared tray. Drizzle with oil, season with salt and pepper, and bake for 20 minutes. If air frying, combine the tofu and vegetables in the basket, drizzle with oil, season, and cook for 15 minutes.

4   While the tofu and veggies are cooking, grab a small jar. Into it, add the tofu glaze ingredients with 3 tbsp water. Shake until well combined.

5   In a separate bowl, stir together the yogurt and mint. Set aside for later.

6   When the tofu and vegetables have 10 minutes of cooking time remaining, cook the couscous according to the packet instructions.

7   Heat a frying pan/skillet over low–medium heat and pour in the glaze. Once it starts to bubble and thicken, stir in the tofu to coat in the glaze. Once everything is beautifully combined, take the pan off the heat.

8   With all the components ready, it's time to assemble the salad. Grab a large bowl and add in the cooked couscous, roasted vegetables, spinach and zhoug. Mix well and season with salt and pepper.

9   Plate up the couscous salad and spoon the sticky tofu on top. Finish with a generous drizzle of the minted yogurt and, if you love citrus as much as I do, a squeeze of lemon juice.

Substitutions:

● **Gluten-free?** Sub the couscous for quinoa. ● **No zhoug?** Make a dressing for the couscous with 2 tbsp olive oil, 1 minced garlic clove, 1 tbsp lemon juice, 1 tsp maple syrup, salt and pepper.

Future you:

🥡 Cool and place in an airtight container, storing in the fridge for up to 3 days.
❄ Cool and freeze (minus the dressing) for up to 2 months.
◐ Thaw in the fridge overnight, or at room temperature for a few hours.
♨ Enjoy cold or reheat in the microwave for 2 minutes, stirring halfway.

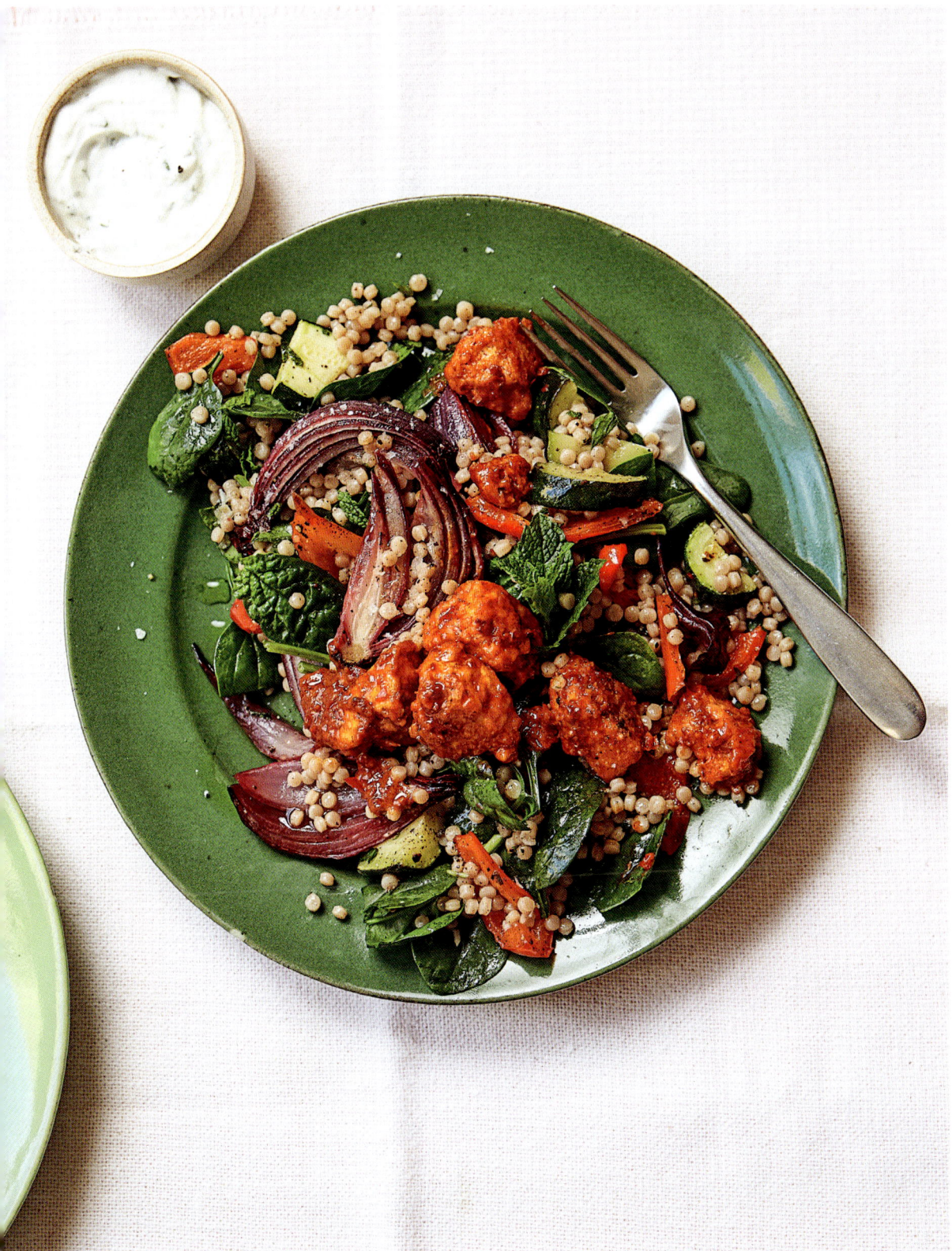

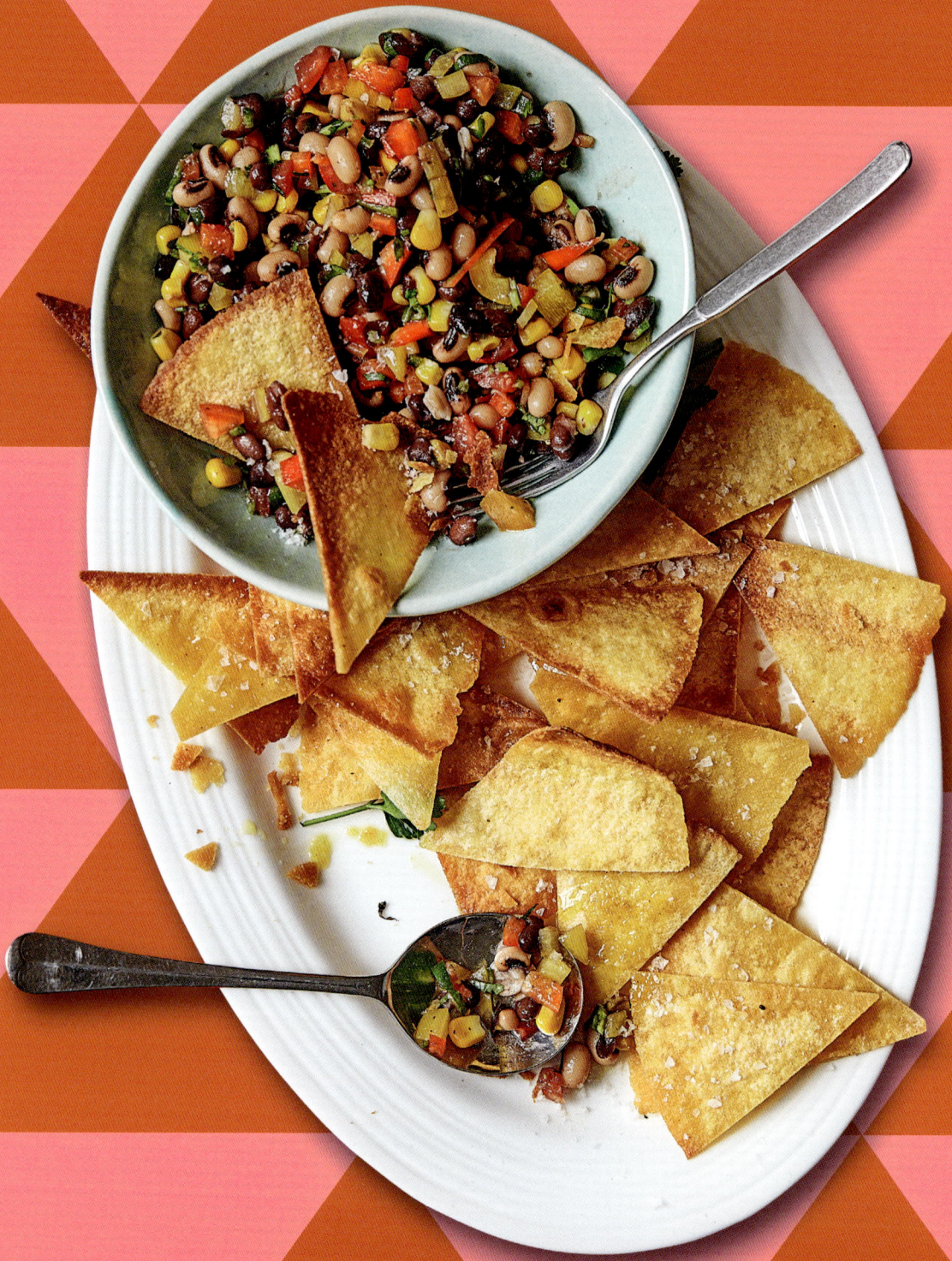

Snacks

Hanger-Saving Snacks for Between Meals

Snacks are an essential part of my diet – not only do I find they improve my concentration, productivity and mood throughout the day, but without them I face the even more ominous danger of getting hangry. Hence why I make sure I have nourishing and satisfying snacks on hand in the fridge and freezer at all times, for everyone's benefit!

5-Minute Hummus, 3 Ways

V

VE

DF

GF

There's nothing quite like homemade hummus, and this version is not only quick and easy, but also far more affordable than store-bought options. But what I love most is its versatility, which is why I had to bring you not just one, but three delicious variations. Try the jalapeño and coriander version when you're craving a kick of spice and fresh herbs; the roasted red pepper version for a smoky depth and subtle sweetness; or, stick with the timeless classic – it never disappoints. Each one is perfect for dipping with fresh veggies, pita or crackers, spreading on sandwiches, or even loading onto potatoes.

1 x 400-g/14-oz can chickpeas/ garbanzo beans, drained

50 g/1¾ oz/¼ cup tahini

juice of 1 large lemon

50 ml/1½ fl oz/3½ tbsp extra virgin olive oil, plus extra for topping

1 tsp ground cumin

1 garlic clove

1 tsp sea salt, or to taste

1–2 ice cubes

za'atar, to serve (optional)

For jalapeño + coriander

2 tbsp roughly chopped coriander/ cilantro

3 spring onions/scallions, roughly chopped

50 g/1¾ oz sliced jalapeños

chilli/chili oil, to serve (optional)

For roasted red pepper

140 g/5 oz/¾ cup jarred roasted red peppers

1 tsp smoked paprika, plus extra to serve

½ tsp onion granules

1 In a high-powered blender (for a smoother dip) or food processor (for a bit of texture), add the chickpeas, tahini, lemon juice, olive oil, cumin, garlic and salt. If making a flavoured variation, add the additional ingredients listed for those now too.

2 Blend on full power for 30–60 seconds, then pause to scrape down the sides with a flat spatula, bringing any lumpy bits back into the mix.

3 Place the lid back on, but this time without the lid cap, and start blending again. While the machine is running, feed the ice cubes through the opening. The addition of ice cubes helps to create a light, creamy texture and also thins the mixture. Blend for an additional 30 seconds to fully incorporate the ice. If at this point the hummus is still too thick for your liking, gradually add cold water, a tablespoon at a time, until you achieve your desired consistency.

4 Have a final taste and adjust the seasoning if necessary. More often than not, I give it an extra pinch of salt and squeeze of lemon juice.

5 If you've made plain hummus, serve it with an extra drizzle of olive oil and a sprinkle of za'atar. If you've made the jalapeño and coriander hummus, you can serve it with a drizzle of chilli oil on top. If you've made the roasted red pepper hummus, you can serve it with a little extra olive oil and a pinch of smoked paprika.

Substitutions:

● **No chickpeas?** Try using cannellini or butter beans/lima beans instead.

Future you:

🥡 Place in an airtight container, storing in the fridge for up to 7 days.

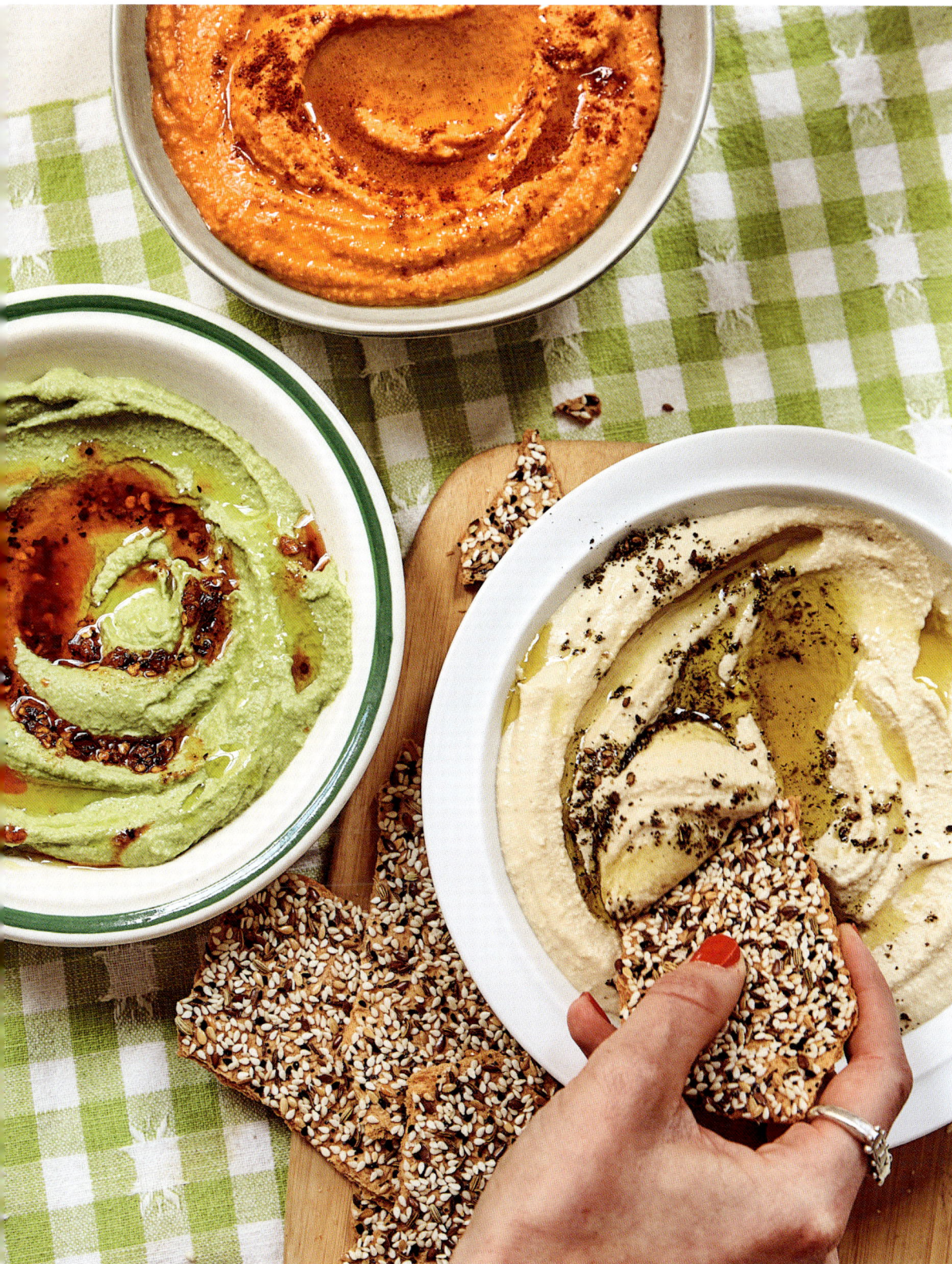

Spicy Sun-dried Tomato Cannellini Bean Dip

This cannellini bean dip was born from a near-kitchen disaster when I ran out of chickpeas just before a dinner party, but it quickly became the unexpected star of the night. So, while chickpeas and hummus may continue to steal the spotlight in the dip world (and they rightfully have their air time on page 78), this recipe is proof not to underestimate how amazing a cannellini bean dip can be. It's bold, smoky, spicy and packed with flavour – perfect for dipping and spreading to your heart's content.

1 x 400-g/14-oz can cannellini beans, drained

80 g/3 oz/generous ¾ cup sun-dried tomatoes

1 garlic clove

juice of ½ lemon

½ tsp hot chilli/chili powder

1 tsp smoked paprika

50 ml/1½ fl oz/3½ tbsp oil from the sun-dried tomatoes

a handful of basil

1 tsp sea salt, or to taste

2–3 ice cubes

extra virgin olive oil, to serve

a pinch of crushed chilli flakes/hot red pepper flakes, to serve

1   In a high-powered blender or food processor, add the cannellini beans, sun-dried tomatoes, garlic, lemon juice, chilli powder, paprika, oil, basil and salt.

2   Blend on full power for 30–60 seconds, then pause to scrape down the sides with a flat spatula, bringing any lumpy bits back into the mix.

3   Place the lid back on, but this time without the lid cap, and start blending again. While the machine is running, feed the ice cubes through the opening. The addition of ice cubes helps to create a light, creamy texture and also thins the mixture. Blend for an additional 30 seconds to fully incorporate the ice. If at this point the dip is still too thick for your liking, gradually add cold water, a tablespoon at a time, until you achieve your desired consistency.

4   Have a final taste and adjust the seasoning if necessary. More often than not, I give it an extra pinch of salt and squeeze of lemon juice.

5   Serve with a drizzle of extra virgin olive oil and a pinch of chilli flakes on top.

Substitutions:

● **No cannellini beans?** Use butter beans/lima beans or chickpeas instead.

Future you:

☕ Place in an airtight container, storing in the fridge for up to 7 days.

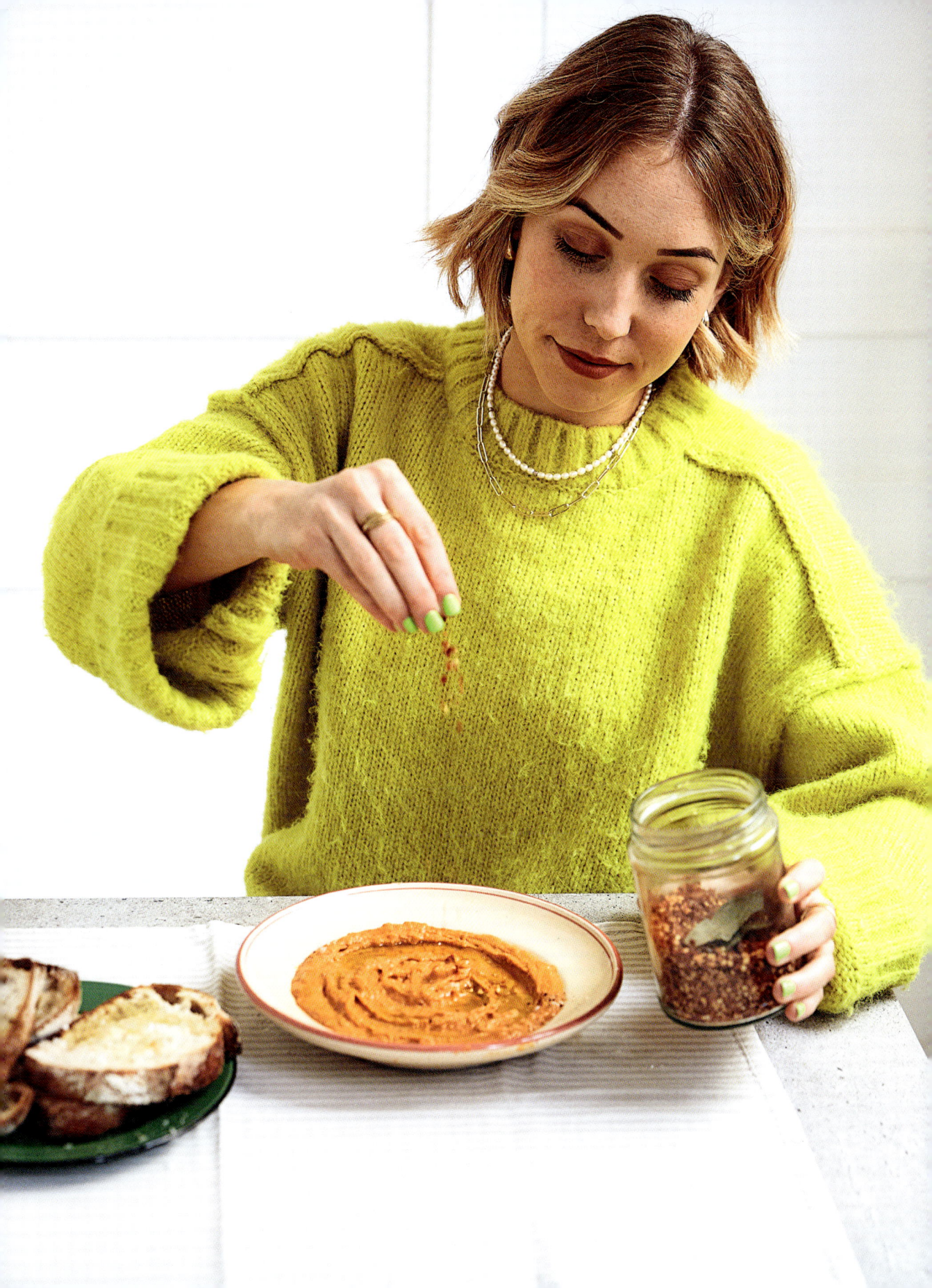

Lime + Coconut Energy Balls

V
VE
DF
GF
N

I remember energy balls being one of the first snacks I made when I decided to embrace a healthier lifestyle – they just screamed 'health', didn't they? But, and I don't know if it was just my bad luck, I found those early versions a bit uninspiring. Which is why I'm excited to reintroduce them with this zesty lime and coconut twist, complete with an optional (cough, essential) addition of dark chocolate chips. So, so good.

10 medjool dates (about 200 g/ 7 oz), pitted

50 g/1¾ oz/⅔ cup desiccated/dried unsweetened coconut

120 g/4 oz/1 cup cashews

30 g/1 oz/4 tbsp hemp seeds

1 tbsp cacao powder

grated zest and juice of 2 limes

a pinch of salt

20 g/¾ oz/2 tbsp dark/bittersweet chocolate chips (optional)

For coating

a handful of desiccated/dried unsweetened coconut

1 In a food processor, combine the dates, coconut, cashews, hemp seeds, cacao powder, lime zest, lime juice and salt. Blitz for 1–2 minutes, or until the mixture is well combined and starts to come away from the sides, but still has some texture remaining. Be careful not to over-blend, as this will make the mixture too sticky.

2 Tip in the chocolate chips, if using, and fold them in by hand. This can be done directly in the processor bowl (blade removed!) or in a separate mixing bowl, whichever you find easier.

3 Using an ice-cream scoop or spoon, portion out the mixture into 12 equal-sized portions. Roll each portion between your hands to form smooth balls.

4 Tip the desiccated coconut for coating onto a plate. One by one, roll each ball in the coconut, pressing gently to ensure an even coating. Place the coated balls on a clean plate or tray and pop them in the fridge for at least 30 minutes to firm up.

5 Once the balls are set, transfer them to an airtight container to enjoy straight from the fridge or freezer whenever you fancy one.

Substitutions:

● **Nut free?** Sub cashews for sunflower seeds.

Future you:

☕ Place in an airtight container, storing in the fridge for up to 10 days.
❄ Freeze for up to 3 months.
🌢 Thaw at room temperature for 10 minutes before eating.

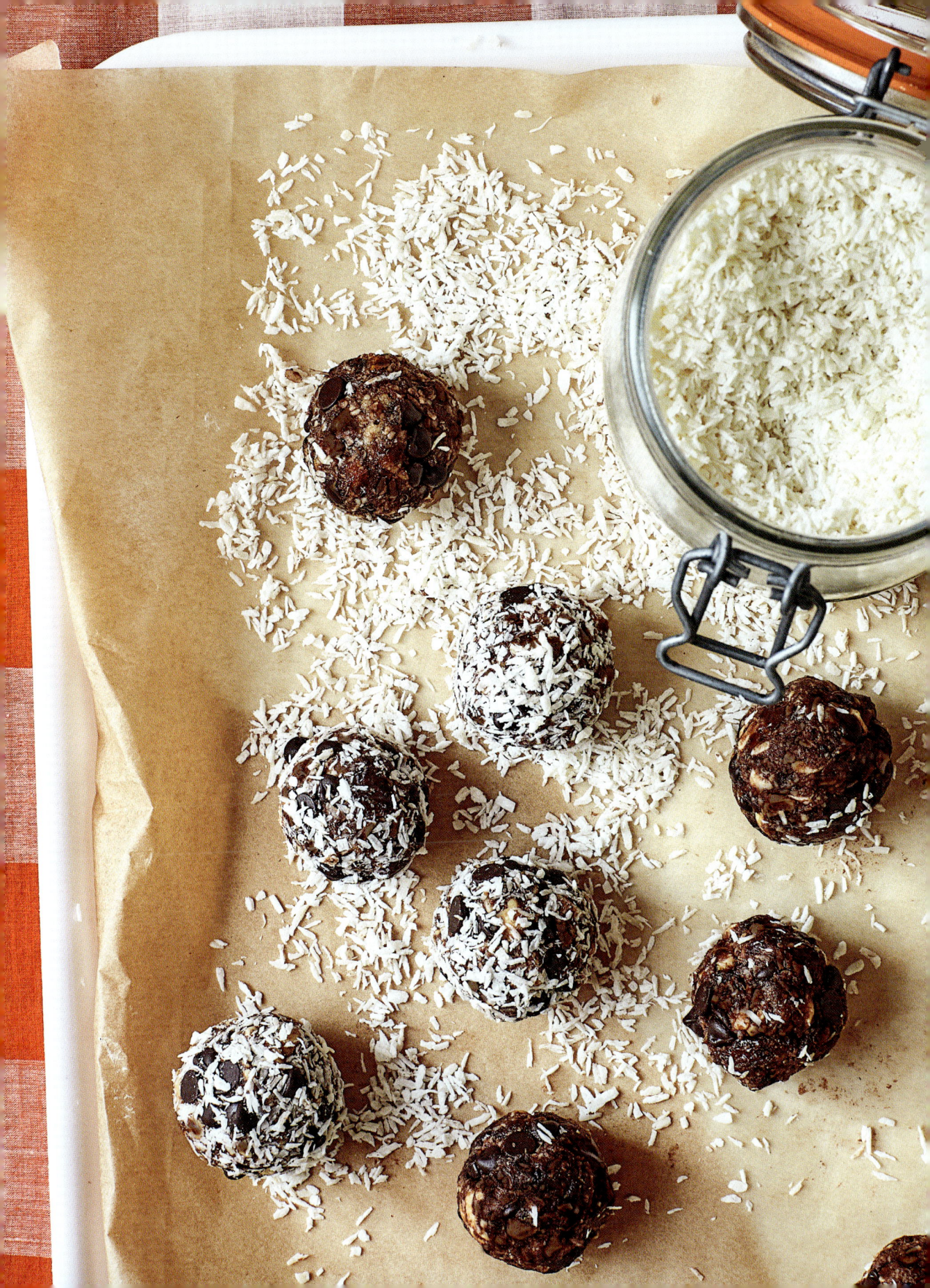

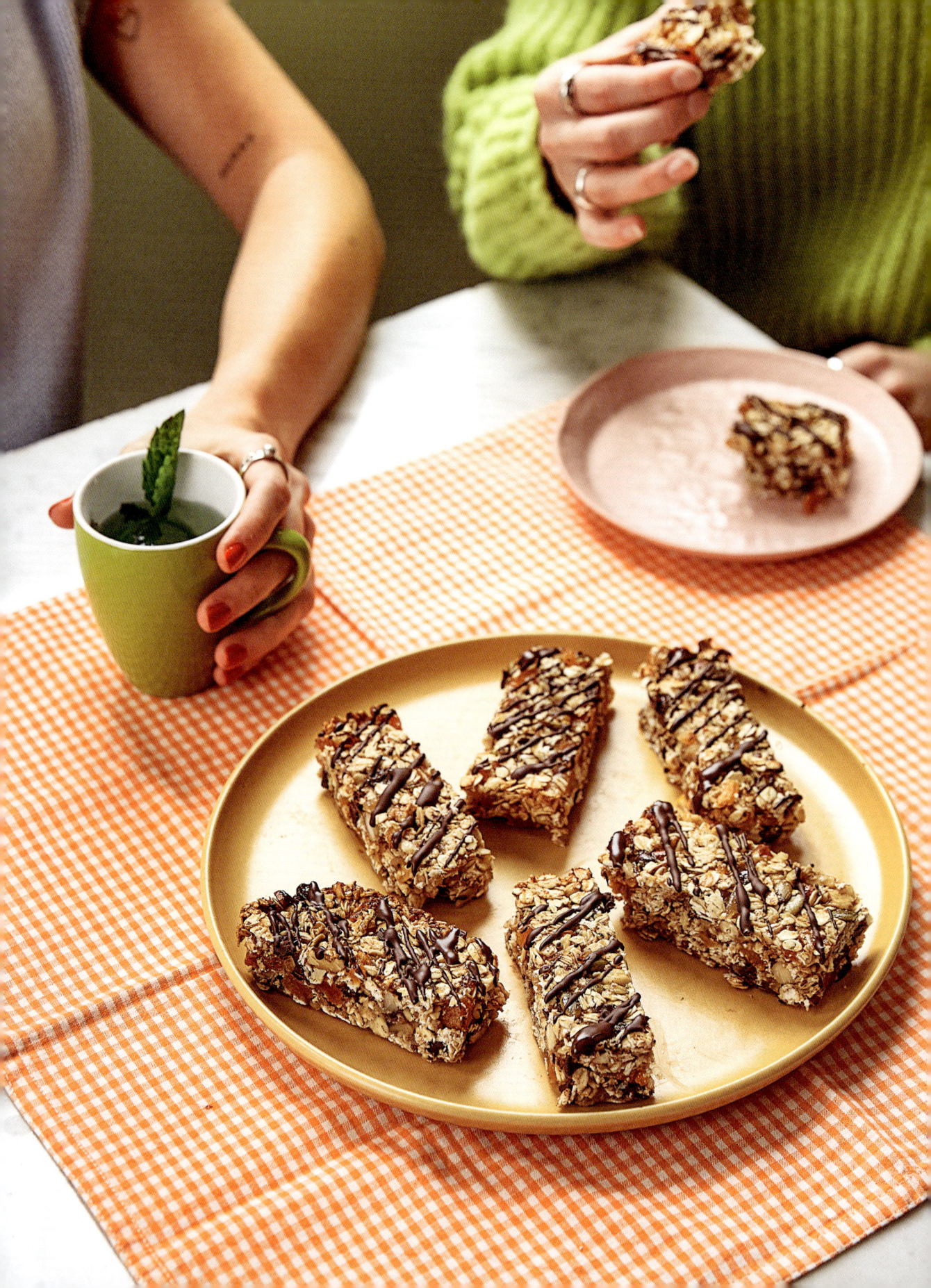

Peanut, Apricot + Chocolate Granola Bars

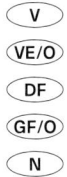

(V)
(VE/O)
(DF)
(GF/O)
(N)

These granola bars are the perfect combination of chewy, crunchy, salty and sweet, and are way tastier than anything you'd get in a packet. You can experiment with almost any variety of nuts, seeds and dried fruits based on your preferences and what you have to hand. Each bite is packed with healthy fats, complex carbs and omega-3s, making them the ultimate healthy (but totally delicious) snack to keep you going through the afternoon.

20-cm/8-in square baking tin, lined (allow the paper to overhang the edges)

280 g/10 oz/generous 1 cup apple purée/apple sauce

60 ml/2 fl oz/¼ cup honey

60 g/2 oz/4 tbsp natural peanut butter

250 g/9 oz/2⅔ cups rolled/old-fashioned oats

20 g/¾ oz/2 tbsp pumpkin seeds

15 g/½ oz/2 tbsp hemp seeds

130 g/4½ oz/1 cup roughly chopped nuts of choice (I use cashews and peanuts)

200 g/7 oz/1⅓ cups dried apricots, roughly chopped

50 g/1¾ oz/⅓ cup dark/bittersweet chocolate chips

½ tsp ground cinnamon

¼ tsp fine sea salt

40 g/1½ oz dark/bittersweet chocolate, melted

1 Preheat the oven to 170°C fan/190°C/375°F/gas mark 5.

2 In a mixing bowl, combine the apple purée, honey and peanut butter, and mix until well combined.

3 In a separate bowl, mix together the oats, pumpkin seeds, hemp seeds, nuts, chopped apricots, chocolate chips, cinnamon and salt.

4 Pour the wet ingredients into the dry ingredients and stir until everything is well combined and forms a sticky mixture.

5 Tip the mixture into your prepared tin. Use the back of a spoon or a flat rubber spatula to spread out the mixture and pack it down really tightly – this will ensure it doesn't crumble apart when sliced. Slide the tin onto the middle shelf of the oven and bake for 30 minutes, or until the top is lovely and golden.

6 Remove from the oven and, while still warm, carefully run a knife along the edges to free them. Now, unfortunately, patience is key here – you'll want to allow the bars to cool completely in the tin for at least 1 hour. And for best results, refrigerate overnight once cooled – this will improve their texture and make slicing much easier.

7 Once cool, slice into 12 equal bars and drizzle the melted dark chocolate over the top.

Substitutions:

● **Vegan?** Sub the honey for maple or agave syrup. ● **No apple purée?** Sub for an equal amount of mashed ripe banana. ● **Gluten-free?** Use gluten-free oats. ● **Nut-free?** Use only seeds instead of nuts, and tahini instead of peanut butter. ● **No apricots?** Use dates, raisins, prunes or cranberries instead.

Future you:

🥡 Cool and place in an airtight container, storing in the fridge for up to 5 days.
❄ Cool and freeze for up to 2 months.
💧 Thaw in the fridge overnight, or at room temperature for a few hours.

Broccoli Cheese Egg Bites

(V)
(DF/O)
(GF)

These egg and broccoli bites are the ultimate on-the-go snack – easy to throw together, loaded with protein and perfect for meal-prepping. All you have to do is mix beaten eggs with broccoli (or whichever other veggies you have on hand, as these are perfect for clearing out the fridge) and your favourite cheeses, then pop them in the oven or air fryer until they're golden and cooked through. Such a sneaky way to get veggies and protein in, all while delivering the best cheesy, comforting hit.

12-hole muffin tray, lightly oiled (if using an air fryer, ensure the muffin tray can fit inside)

300 g/10½ oz broccoli florets

6 large/US extra-large eggs

140 g/5 oz/⅔ cup cottage cheese

20 g/¾ oz/¼ cup grated Italian hard cheese

40 g/1½ oz/scant ½ cup grated extra-mature cheddar

½ tsp garlic granules

½ tsp onion granules

1 tsp fine sea salt

¼ tsp pepper

1   Preheat the air fryer or oven to 180°C fan/200°C/400°F/gas mark 6.

2   Place the broccoli florets into a microwave-safe bowl, along with a splash of water. Cover the bowl and microwave the broccoli for 3 minutes, or until tender. For a hob-/stovetop-based alternative, you can boil or steam the broccoli. Drain the broccoli, transfer the florets to a chopping board and chop them into small pieces.

3   Crack the eggs into a large mixing bowl and beat vigorously until no streaks of yolk remain. Add the chopped broccoli, cottage cheese, grated cheeses, garlic granules, onion granules, salt and pepper. Give everything a good mix, making sure the ingredients are evenly distributed throughout the egg mixture.

4   Spoon the mixture evenly amongst eight of the muffin holes in your prepared tray. They'll puff up a little when baked, so don't fill them right to the top.

5   Place the muffin tray into the oven or air fryer and cook for about 22 minutes, or until the eggs are set and the tops are golden. Let them cool slightly before popping them out of the tray.

Substitutions:

● **No broccoli?** Don't worry, pretty much any veggies go! ● **Dairy-free?** Use dairy-free cheese alternatives.

Future you:

🖂 Cool and place in an airtight container, storing in the fridge for up to 6 days.
❄ Cool and freeze for up to 2 months.
🌢 Thaw in the fridge overnight, or on low power in the microwave.
🔥 Enjoy at room temperature, or microwave for 20 seconds.

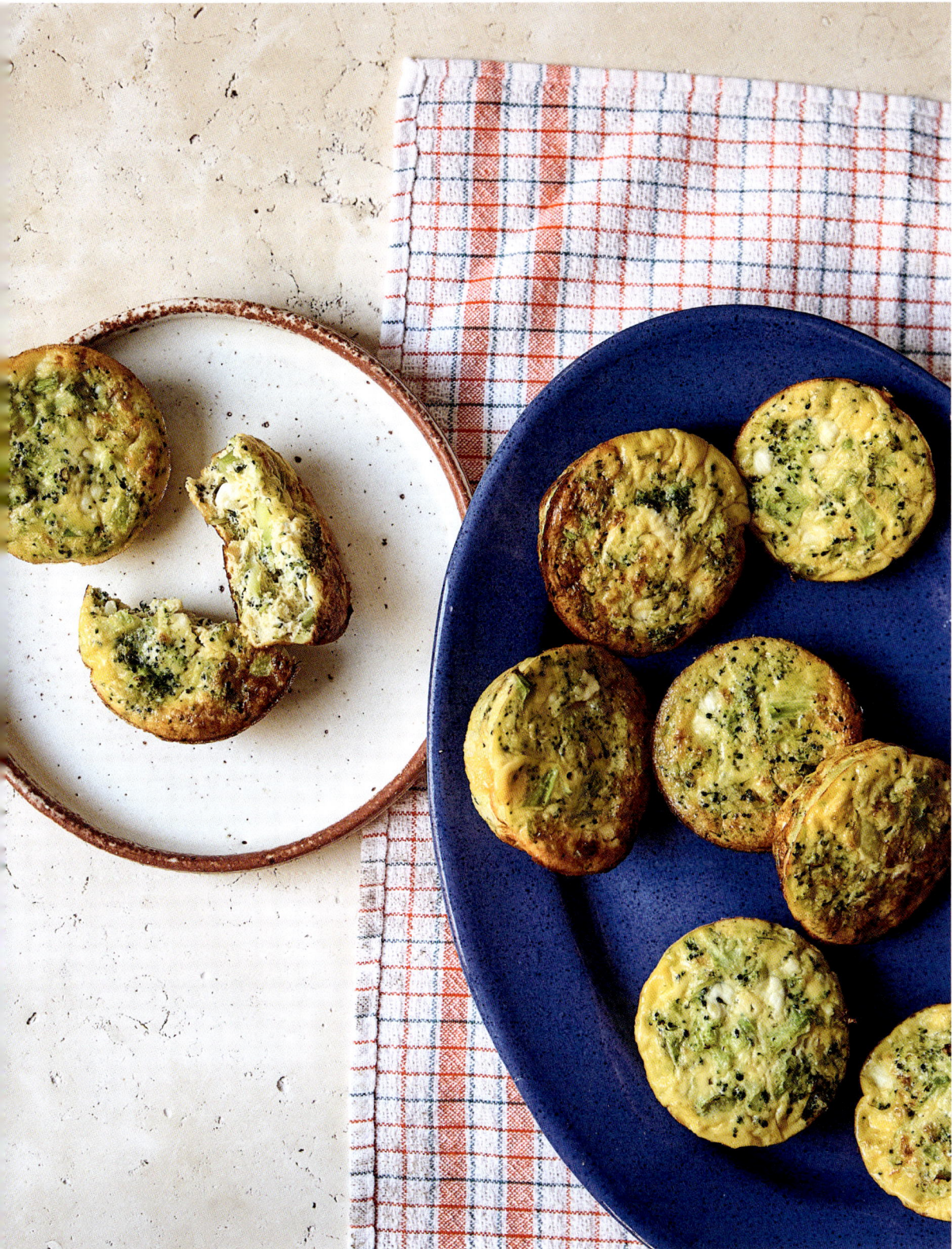

Zingy Mixed Bean Salad + Tortilla Chips

V
VE
DF
GF/O

This 'salad' is a revelation. So simple, yet an absolute explosion of flavour. It can happily be used as a dip, on toast, in wraps, in salads, in rice bowls or as a side dish when entertaining, bringing zing and a hit of protein and fibre. And if you can't be bothered to make your own tortilla chips, I get it. Just grab a pack of your favourite lightly salted tortilla chips and get scoopin'.

1 x 400-g/14-oz can black-eyed beans/black-eyed peas, drained

1 x 400-g/14-oz can black beans, drained

1 red (bell) pepper, finely diced

1 yellow (bell) pepper, finely diced

1 green (bell) pepper, finely diced

2 salad tomatoes, de-seeded and diced

150 g/5½ oz/1 cup sweetcorn/corn

50 g/1¾ oz pickled jalapeño slices, finely diced

1 tbsp roughly chopped parsley

1 tbsp roughly chopped coriander/cilantro

For the dressing

2 tbsp extra virgin olive oil

1 tbsp red wine vinegar

1 garlic clove, minced

½ tsp dried marjoram

1 tsp dried oregano

salt and pepper

For the tortilla chips

10 corn tortillas

olive oil spray

1 Preheat the air fryer or oven to 200°C fan/220°C/425°F/gas mark 7.

2 To make the bean salad, tip the black-eyed beans, black beans, peppers, tomatoes, sweetcorn, jalapeños, parsley and coriander into a large mixing bowl. Toss everything together until well combined.

3 In a small jar, combine the dressing ingredients. Secure the lid and shake vigorously until well combined and emulsified. Pour the dressing over the bean salad and toss again until everything is fully coated.

4 To make the tortilla chips, slice the tortillas into triangles and place them on a baking tray in a single layer. Spray the triangles with oil on both sides, then cook for around 5 minutes, or until they go golden and crispy. Make sure to keep an eye on them as they cook, as they can overbrown quickly.

5 Serve the bean salad with the tortilla chips on the side.

Substitutions:

● **No black beans or black-eyed beans?** Almost any beans will go! Red kidney, cannellini, chickpeas/garbanzo beans... you name it. ● **Gluten-free?** Use gluten-free tortillas.

Future you:

🥡 Store the bean salad in an airtight container in the fridge for up to 7 days. Store the tortilla chips in an airtight container at room temperature for up to 2 weeks.

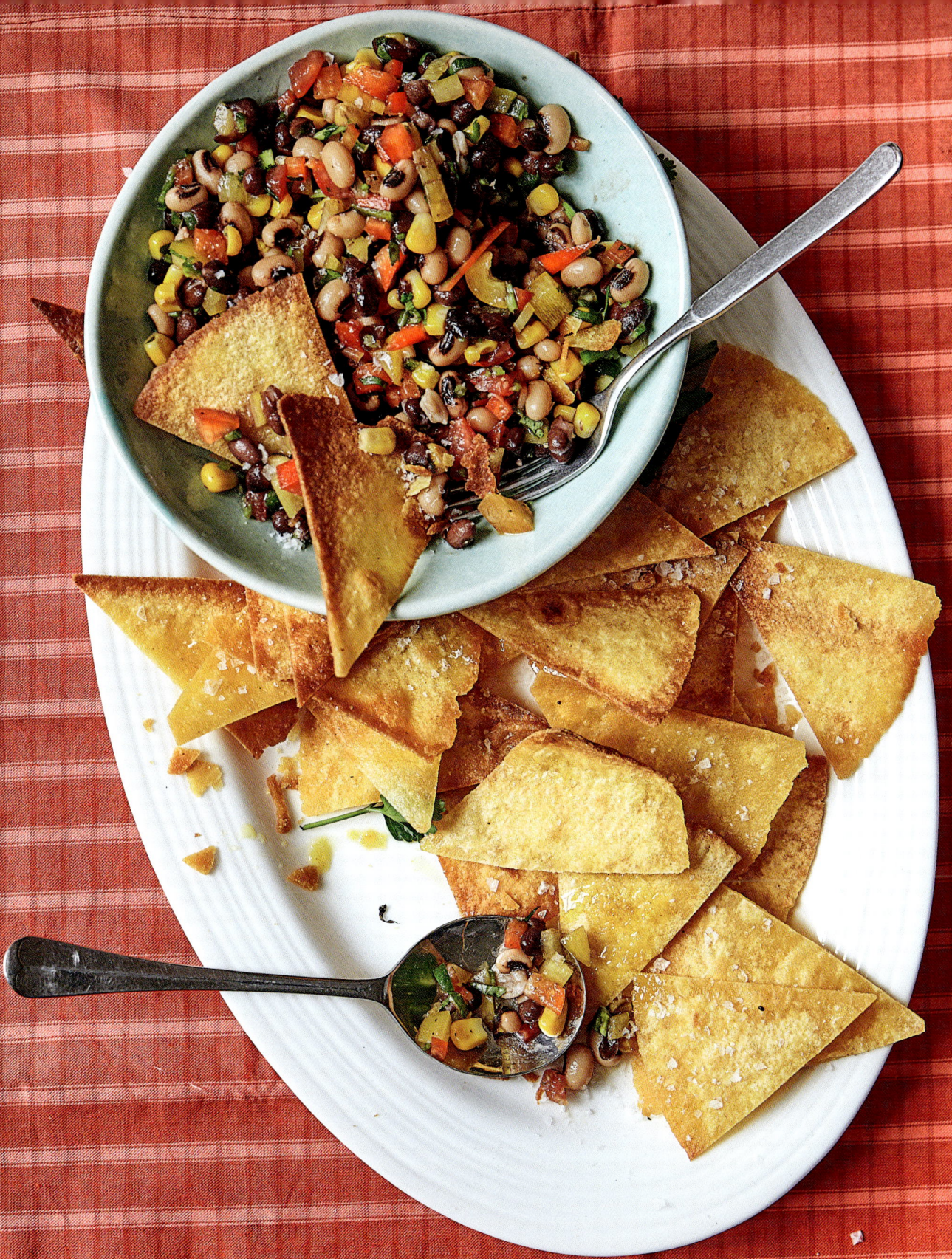

Makes 8 | Prep 15 minutes | Cook 10 minutes

Sweetcorn + Courgette Fritters with a Garlic Dip

V
DF/O
GF/O

I have such vivid memories of making these with my mum when I was younger; I think it was mostly a desperate attempt on her part to get me to eat more vegetables – but credit where it's due, it worked! Over the years, the recipe has definitely had a bit of a glow-up, now featuring courgette, fresh herbs and a little kick of spice. And let's not forget the garlicky yogurt dip that takes eating them to a whole new level of deliciousness.

- 70 g/2½ oz/generous ½ cup wholemeal/whole-wheat flour
- 1 tsp baking powder
- 1 tsp smoked paprika
- ½ tsp garlic granules
- ½ tsp onion granules
- ½ tsp crushed chilli flakes/hot red pepper flakes
- 1 tsp fine sea salt
- ¼ tsp pepper
- 1 medium egg
- 100 ml/3½ fl oz/6½ tbsp milk
- 150 g/5½ oz/1 cup sweetcorn/corn
- 100 g/3½ oz courgette/zucchini, coarsely grated
- 2 spring onions/scallions, thinly sliced
- 1 tbsp roughly chopped coriander/cilantro
- olive oil, for cooking

For the dip

- 50 g/1¾ oz/scant ¼ cup plain yogurt
- 1 garlic clove, minced
- juice of 1 lemon
- 1 tsp honey or maple syrup
- salt and pepper

1 In a large mixing bowl, whisk together the flour, baking powder, paprika, garlic granules, onion granules, chilli flakes, salt and pepper. Make a well in the middle, then crack the egg into it. As you begin to whisk again, pour in the milk gradually, until the mixture comes together into a smooth batter. Stir in the sweetcorn, grated courgette, spring onion and coriander.

2 Heat 2 tablespoons of olive oil in a frying pan/skillet over medium–high heat until it starts to shimmer. Drop heaped spoonfuls of batter into the pan, aiming for about 8 fritters total, and cook in batches if necessary to avoid overcrowding. Cook each fritter for 2–3 minutes per side, or until golden brown and crispy around the edges. Once cooked, transfer the fritters to a plate lined with paper towels to soak up any excess oil. Add more oil to the pan if needed, and repeat the process with the remaining batter.

3 While the fritters are cooking, prepare the garlicky yogurt dip. In a small bowl, mix together the yogurt, garlic, lemon juice and honey or maple syrup. Season to taste and serve the dip alongside the fritters.

Substitutions:

● **No courgette?** Replace the courgette with an extra 100 g/3½ oz sweetcorn. ● **Gluten-free?** Swap the wholemeal flour for buckwheat flour.

Future you:

- Cool and place in an airtight container, storing in the fridge for up to 5 days.
- Cool and freeze for up to 2 months.
- Thaw in the fridge overnight, or on low power in the microwave.
- Enjoy chilled, reheat in air fryer or oven for 10 minutes, or microwave for 30 seconds.

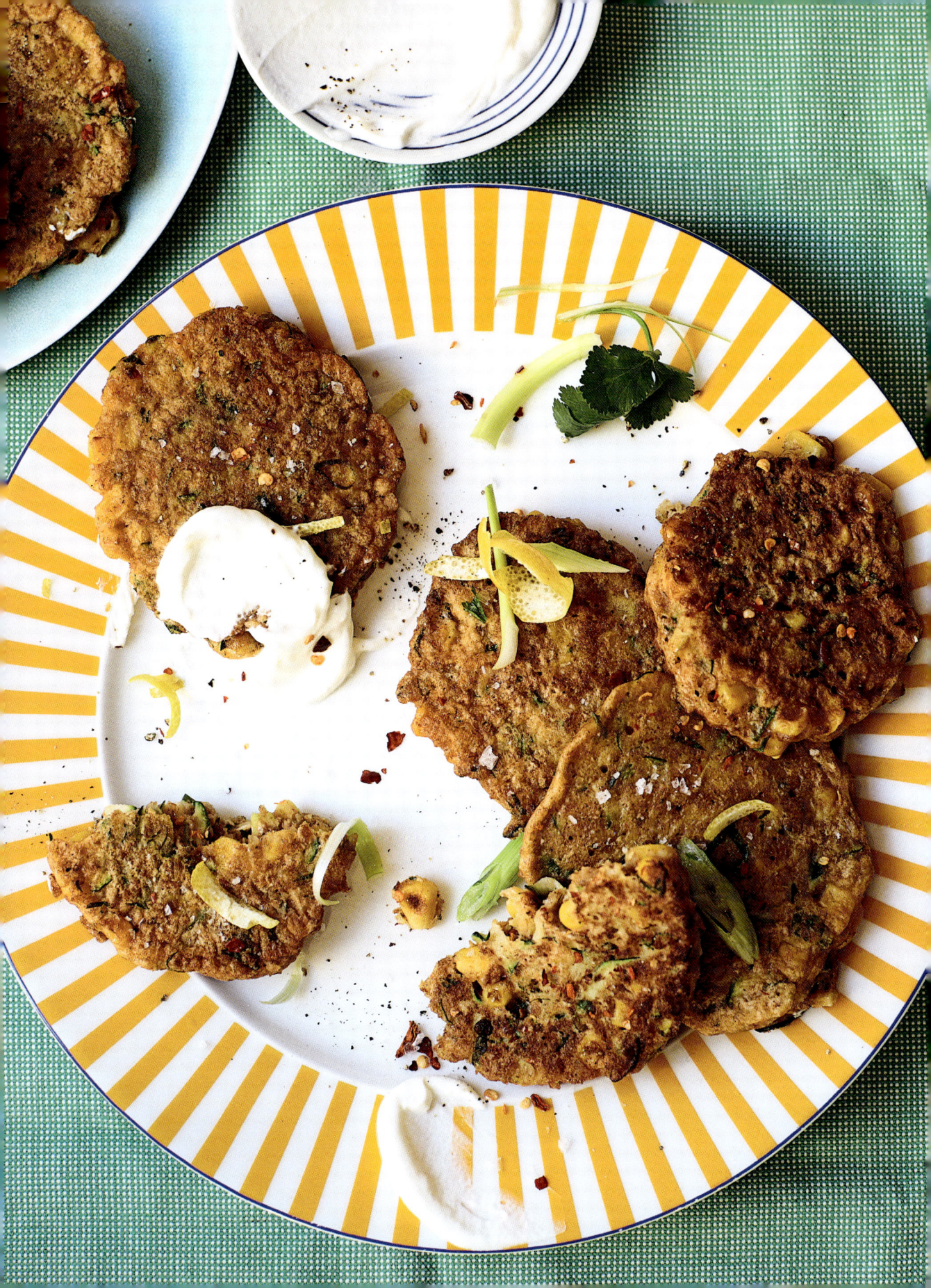

Chia Jam

V
VE/O
DF/O
GF/O

One for my fellow jam on toast lovers! If you didn't already know how easy it was to make your own jam at home, now you do. There's really no need for the heaps of sugar put in store-bought jars; just berries, maple syrup and chia seeds will do the trick. Even better, you can use pretty much any berries you like, and adjust the sweetness to your liking by adding more or less maple syrup. I like to slather mine on toast, loaded with yogurt, nut butter and seeds – but you do you.

400 g/14 oz/2⅔ cups fresh or frozen berries (I use raspberries)

1½ tbsp chia seeds

2 tbsp maple syrup

To serve

4–8 slices bread, toasted (I like sourdough)

yogurt

nut butter

a sprinkle of hemp seeds

1 You can make the jam in the microwave, or on the hob/stovetop. I prefer to do it on the hob because it tends to thicken up better, but I'll let you decide. If using the hob, place a saucepan over medium heat and add the berries. Cook, stirring occasionally, for a few minutes until the berries break down and bubble. Once the berries are hot and softened, use a fork or masher to crush them to your desired texture.

2 Next, add the chia seeds and maple syrup, and stir to combine. Take the pan off the heat and let the jam cool in the pan for a few minutes to thicken further.

3 Enjoy the jam however you like, but my favourite way is spreading it on toast, along with some yogurt, a good drizzle of your favourite nut butter and a sprinkle of hemp seeds.

Substitutions:

● **No raspberries?** Try blueberries, blackberries, strawberries or cherries instead. ● **Gluten-free?** Use gluten-free bread.

Future you:

☕ Place in an airtight container, storing in the fridge for up to 7 days.
❄ Cool and freeze for up to 3 months.
💧 Thaw in the fridge overnight, or at room temperature for a few hours.

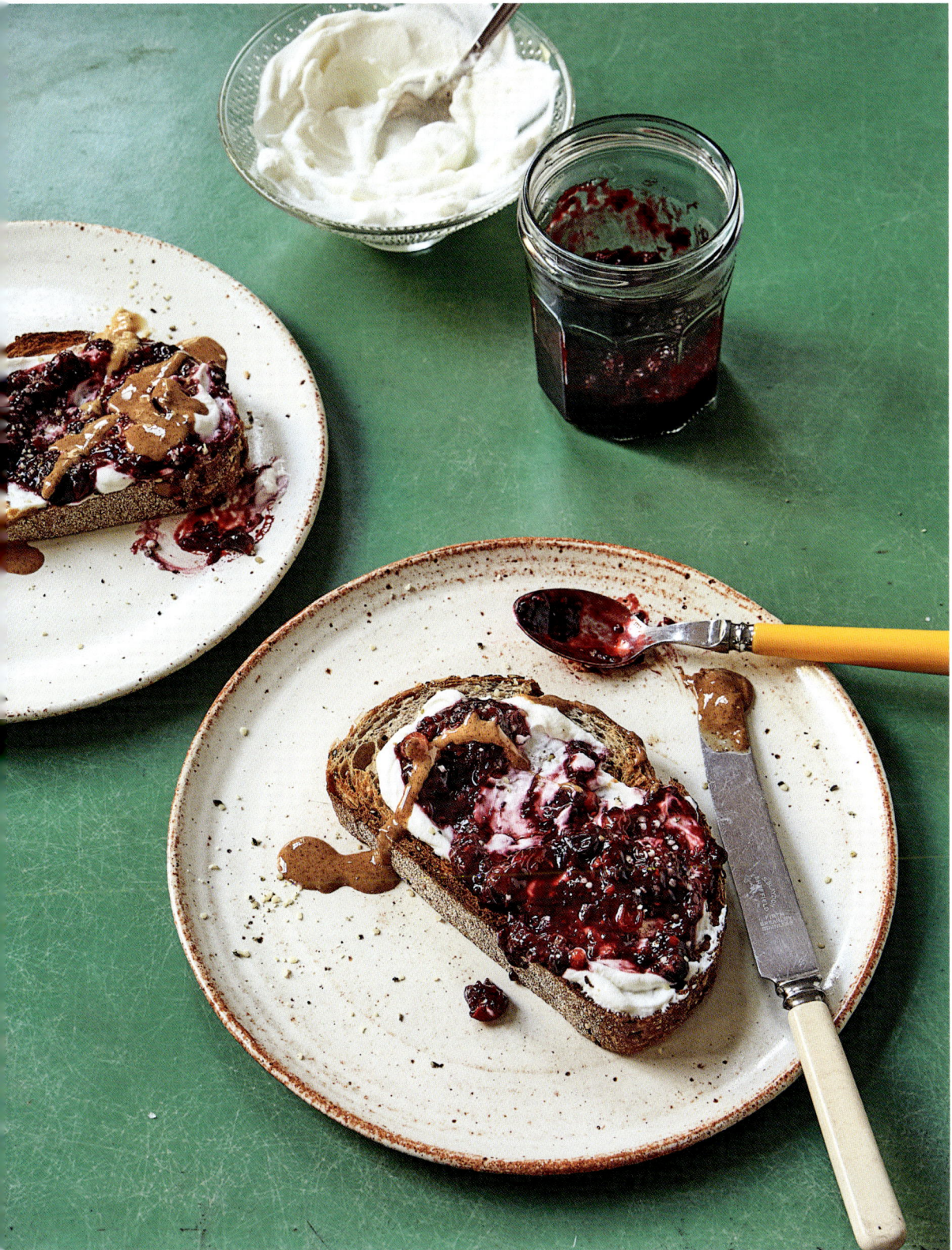

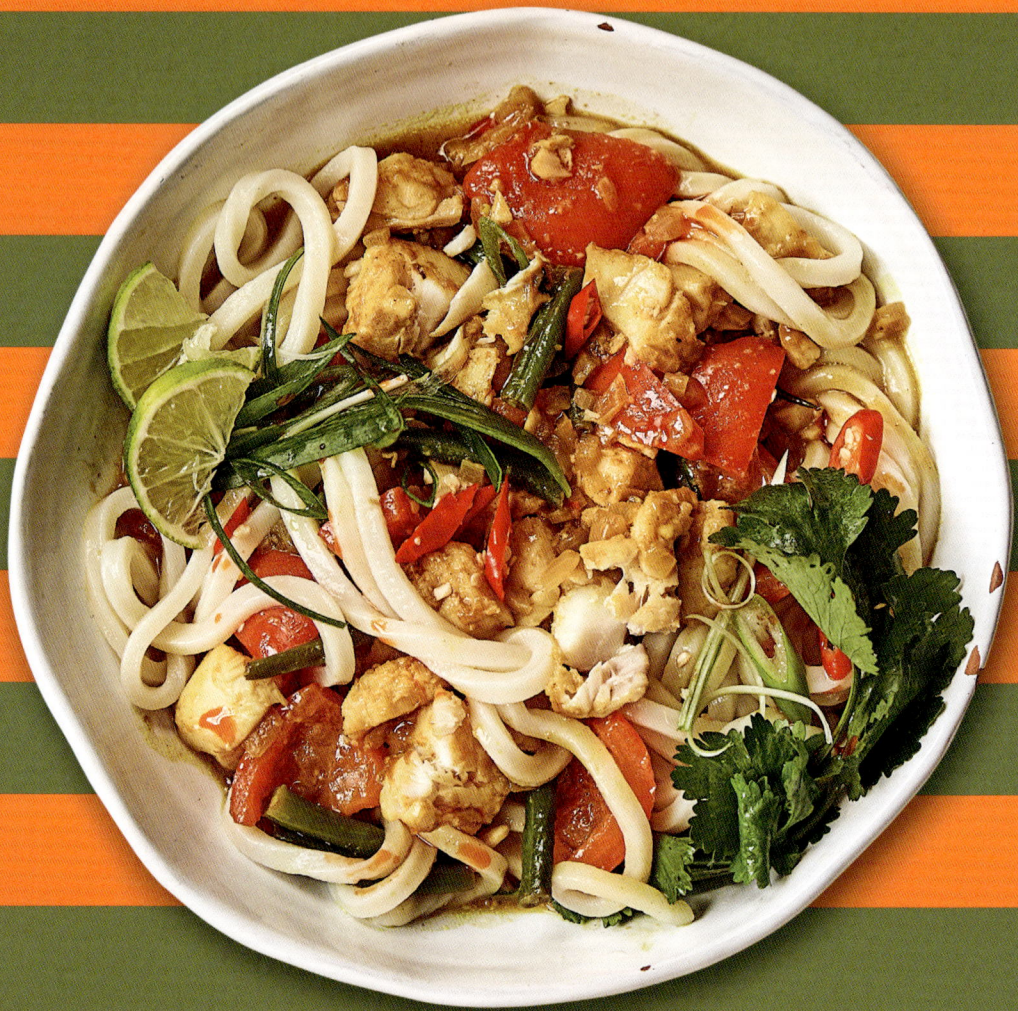

Dinners in Under 30

No Time to Cook? No Problem

We all have busy days, and it's almost a given that by the end of them we crave something quick and easy. But that shouldn't have to condemn us to another monotonous stir-fry for the third night in a row. Instead, here are some of my favourite flavour-packed recipes that can be whipped up in 30 minutes or less; perfect regulars to add some variety to your weeknight rotation.

Salmon Tacos + Mango Jalapeño Salsa

(V/O)
(VE/O)
(DF/O)
(GF/O)

The mango jalapeño salsa is a star and so good you'll probably just want to eat it straight from the bowl. It pairs perfectly with the buttery salmon, bringing freshness and comfort while all coming together faster than you can say 'where's my margarita?' Serve them pre-assembled or as a DIY-style spread in the middle of the table.

baking sheet, lined (if using an oven)

air fryer basket, lined (if using an air fryer)

4 salmon fillets

1 tsp ground cumin

1 tsp smoked paprika

½ tsp dried oregano

½ tsp garlic granules

½ tsp onion granules

8 mini tortillas

1 large ripe avocado, mashed

salt and pepper

olive oil spray, for cooking

crumbled feta, to serve

yogurt, to serve (optional)

For the salsa

1 ripe mango, diced (about 200 g/ 7 oz diced flesh)

1 red (bell) pepper, finely diced

1 small tomato, finely diced

¼ red onion, finely diced

1 tbsp sliced jalapeños, finely chopped

1 tbsp finely chopped coriander/cilantro

juice of ½ lime

1   Preheat the air fryer or oven to 200°C fan/220°C/425°F/gas mark 7.

2   Pat the salmon fillets dry with a paper towel and place them on the prepared baking sheet or in the lined air fryer basket. In a bowl, mix together the cumin, paprika, oregano, garlic granules, onion granules and a pinch each of salt and pepper. Lightly spray the salmon with oil, then sprinkle the seasoning over the fillets, making sure to coat the sides.

3   Place the salmon in the air fryer or oven, cooking for 15 minutes in the air fryer, or 20 minutes in the oven, until the exterior is golden and the flesh flakes easily with a fork.

4   While the salmon cooks, prepare the mango salsa by combining the mango, red pepper, tomato, onion, jalapeños and coriander in a bowl. Squeeze in the lime juice, stir everything together, and season to taste.

5   To warm the tortillas, heat a dry frying pan/skillet over medium heat. Place each tortilla in the pan, cooking for about a minute on each side until the first side starts to puff up and lightly char, then flip it over. Alternatively, you can microwave the tortillas on full power for about 30 seconds to save time, though the pan method adds more flavour.

6   Once everything is ready, assemble the tacos by spreading the mashed avocado across each tortilla, followed by a portion of the cooked salmon. Top with a generous spoonful of the mango salsa, a sprinkle of feta and some yogurt, if using, and serve immediately.

Substitutions:

● **Vegetarian?** Swap the salmon for tofu or your favourite meat-free protein alternative. ● **Vegan?** Follow the vegetarian advice above and use dairy-free feta and yogurt. ● **No mango?** Try pineapple instead. ● **Gluten-free?** Use gluten-free taco shells. ● **Dairy-free?** Use dairy-free feta and yogurt.

Future you:

🗺 Cool and place in an airtight container, storing in the fridge for up to 3 days.
🔥 Cooked salmon is always best on the day it's made, so I would recommend to enjoy it chilled. If you do want to reheat it, place on a baking sheet in the oven on a low heat (around 140°C fan/160°C/325°F/gas mark 3) until warmed through.

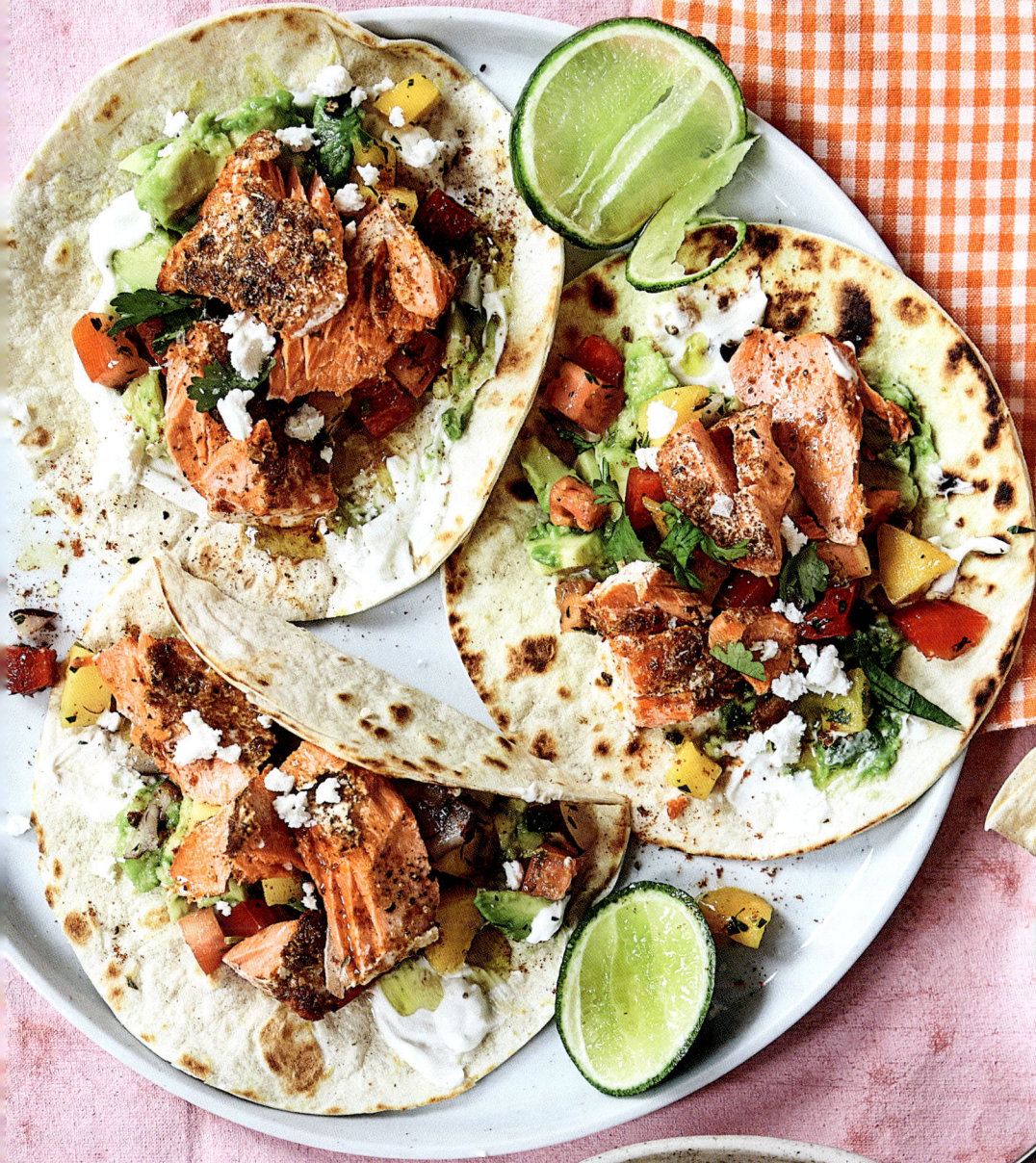

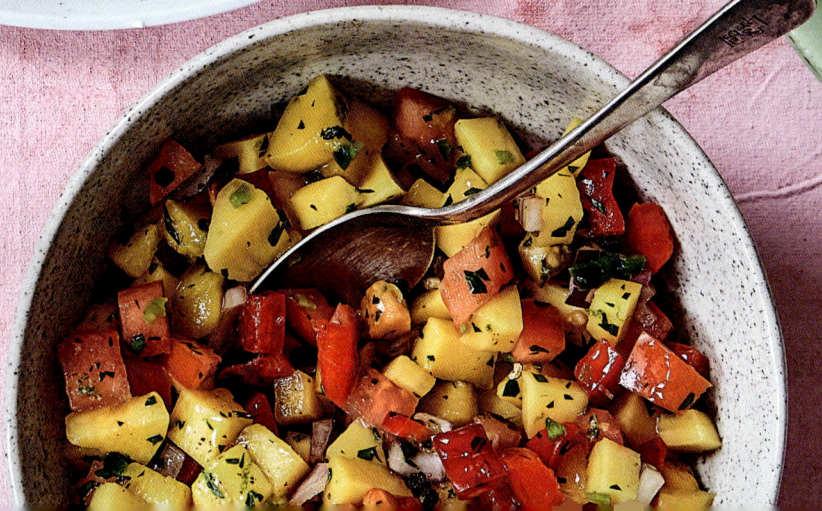

Glazed Lemon Tofu, Sticky Rice + Broccoli

V
VE
DF
GF/O

Sticky doesn't usually scream 'healthy', right? Well, I've ditched the usual appearance of sugar from the ingredients list and created this gorgeous takeaway-style sticky lemon tofu without any refined sugar that you'll absolutely love. Now the sticky limit does not exist.

baking sheet, lined (if using an oven)

air fryer basket, lined (if using an air fryer)

1 x 300-g/10½-oz block extra-firm tofu

1 tbsp cornflour/cornstarch

200 g/7 oz Tenderstem broccoli

1–2 x 250-g/9-oz pouches cooked sticky rice

2 spring onions/scallions, thinly sliced

a sprinkle of sesame seeds, plus extra to garnish

1 red chilli/chile, de-seeded and thinly sliced

salt and pepper

olive oil, for cooking

For the lemon glaze

1 thumb-sized piece ginger, grated

2 garlic cloves, minced

2 tbsp soy sauce

grated zest and juice of 1 lemon

1 tbsp maple syrup

1 tsp cornflour/cornstarch

1   Preheat the air fryer or oven to 200°C fan/220°C/425°F/gas mark 7.

2   Press out any water from the block of tofu (this will vary depending on the brand you use), then slice it into triangles or cubes. Transfer these pieces to a large mixing bowl, along with the cornflour and a good pinch each of salt and pepper. Mix until each piece of tofu is coated.

3   If using an oven, spread the tofu out on the lined baking sheet, drizzle with oil and bake for 20 minutes. If using an air fryer, add the tofu to the basket, drizzle with oil and cook for 15 minutes. When there are 10 minutes left, add the broccoli stalks and florets to the baking sheet or basket, drizzle with more oil, sprinkle with a little salt and let everything cook together for the remaining time.

4   While the tofu and broccoli cook, make the lemon glaze by combining the ginger, garlic, soy sauce, lemon zest, lemon juice, maple syrup, cornflour and 2 tablespoons of water in a small jar. Secure the lid and shake until well combined.

5   Heat the rice in the microwave according to the packet instructions, usually about 2 minutes per pouch.

6   Once the tofu is ready, heat a frying pan/skillet over low–medium heat and pour in the lemon glaze. Once it starts to bubble and thicken, take it off the heat. Add the tofu, most of the spring onion (saving some for garnish), sesame seeds and chilli, and stir to coat in the sticky glaze.

7   Divide the rice between bowls, add the sticky tofu and roasted broccoli on top. Finish with the spring onion and a sprinkle of sesame seeds.

Substitutions:

● **Gluten-free?** Use tamari instead of soy sauce. ● **No lemon?** Try this recipe with an orange instead; it's also delicious!

Future you:

🥡 Cool and place in an airtight container, storing in the fridge for up to 3 days.
❄ Cool and freeze for up to 2 months.
🌢 Thaw in the fridge overnight, or at room temperature for a few hours.
🔥 Reheat in the microwave for 2–3 minutes until piping hot. Cooked rice must only be reheated once.

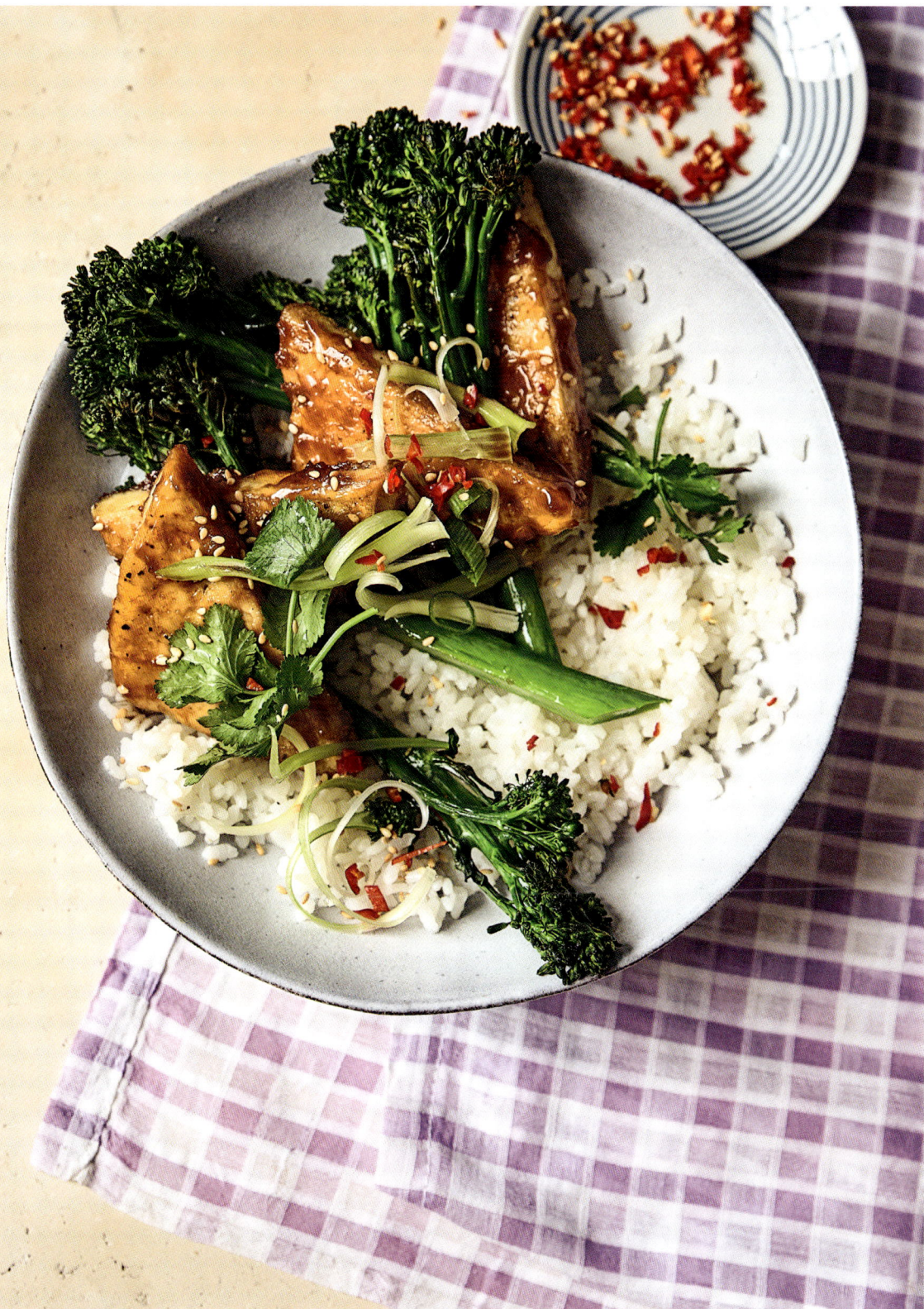

Sticky Soy Salmon Skewers + Noodle Salad

V/O
VE/O
DF
GF/O

Who's the real winner when healthy eating looks this good? We have cubes of salmon generously slathered in a sticky soy sauce, cooked on skewers until caramelized to perfection. You'll want to get your hands on the thickest pieces of salmon you can find, so you can keep the pieces chunky. I've served the skewers up with a vibrant noodle salad, but if you're in a pinch, a pouch of rice is a fab quick alternative.

8 small skewers

500 g/1 lb 2 oz (4 fillets) salmon, preferably skinless

2 tbsp dark soy sauce

grated zest and juice of 1 lime

1 tbsp honey

1 tsp miso paste

1 tbsp sesame oil

1 garlic clove, minced

sesame seeds, to garnish

lime wedges or slices, to serve

For the noodle salad

1 red (bell) pepper, thinly sliced

¼ white or red cabbage, shredded

1 carrot, julienned

1 red chilli/chile, de-seeded and finely chopped

2 spring onions/scallions, thinly sliced

1 tbsp roughly chopped coriander/cilantro, plus extra to serve

200 g/7 oz noodles of your choice

For the salad dressing

2 tbsp light soy sauce

1 tbsp tahini or natural peanut butter

1 tsp sesame oil

1 tsp rice vinegar

1 Preheat the air fryer or oven (using the grill/broiler setting) to 200°C fan/220°C/425°F/gas mark 7.

2 Cut the salmon into even bite-sized chunks and place them in a bowl. Add the soy sauce, lime zest and juice, honey, miso, sesame oil and garlic, and mix well to coat. Set aside for a few minutes to marinate; I like to use this time to prepare the veggies for the noodle salad.

3 Thread the marinated salmon onto the skewers, then pop them into the air fryer or grill. Cook for 10 minutes, flipping halfway if grilling.

4 While the salmon is cooking, cook the noodles according to the packet instructions. Once done, run them under cold water to cool.

5 To assemble the noodle salad, toss together the pepper, cabbage, carrot, chilli, spring onions, coriander and the cooled noodles in a large bowl.

6 In a separate bowl or small jar, whisk together the dressing ingredients until glossy and smooth. Tip the dressing over the salad and toss to coat.

7 Divide the noodle salad among 4 bowls and top each with 2 salmon skewers. I like to garnish the dish with a sprinkle of sesame seeds and some extra coriander, and serve with a wedge or slices of lime.

Substitutions:

● **Vegetarian?** Sub 450 g/1 lb extra-firm tofu in place of the salmon. ● **Vegan?** Sub 450 g/1 lb extra-firm tofu in place of the salmon. Use maple syrup instead of honey. ● **Gluten-free?** Use tamari instead of soy sauce and gluten-free noodles and miso paste.

Future you:

Cool and store in the fridge for up to 3 days.
Reheat the noodles by adding 1 tbsp of water and microwave for 1 minute; for the salmon, reheat slowly in the oven at 140°C fan/160°C/325°F/gas mark 3.

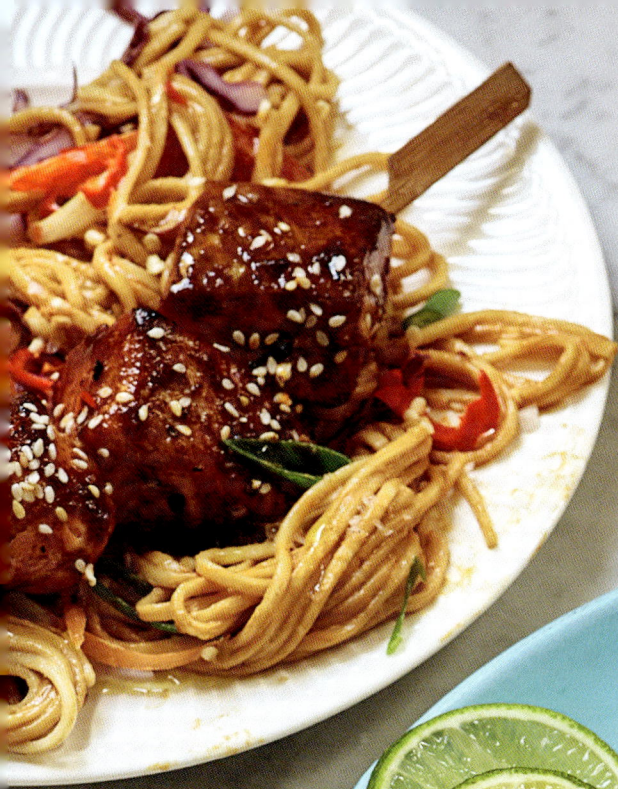

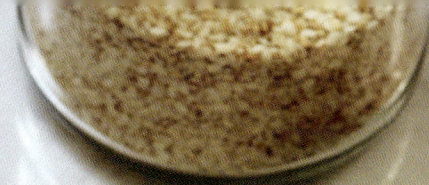

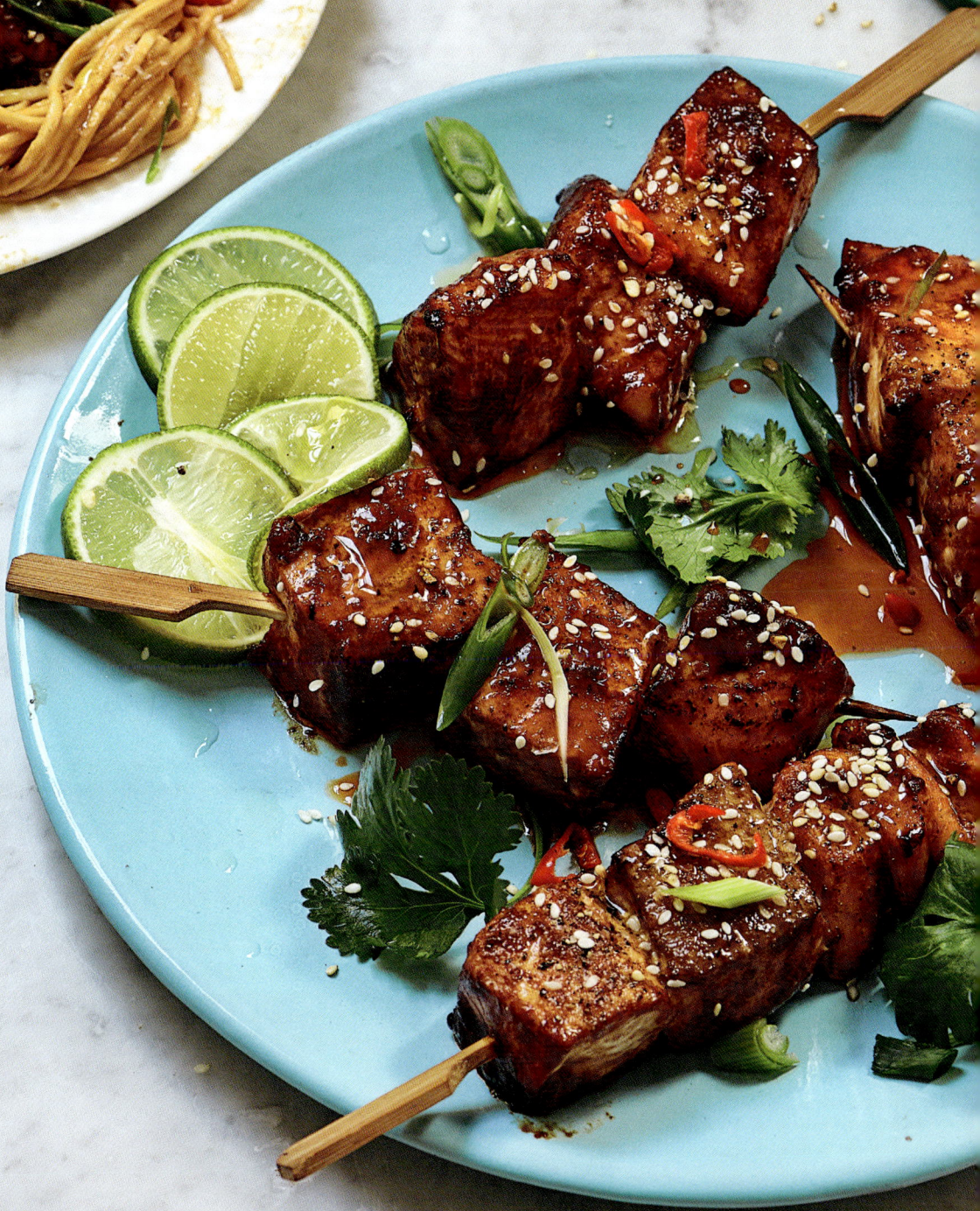

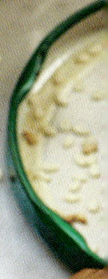

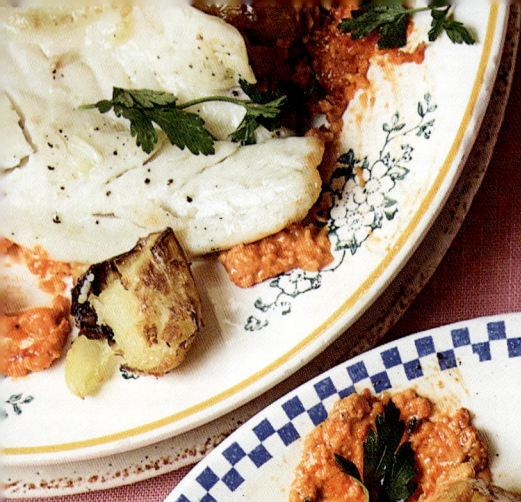

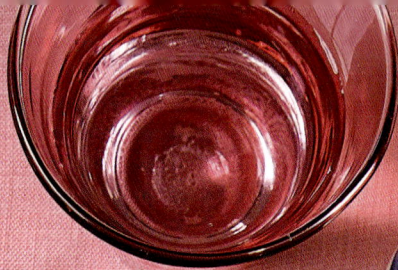

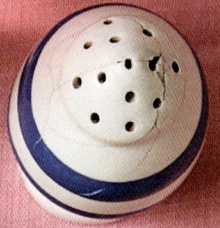

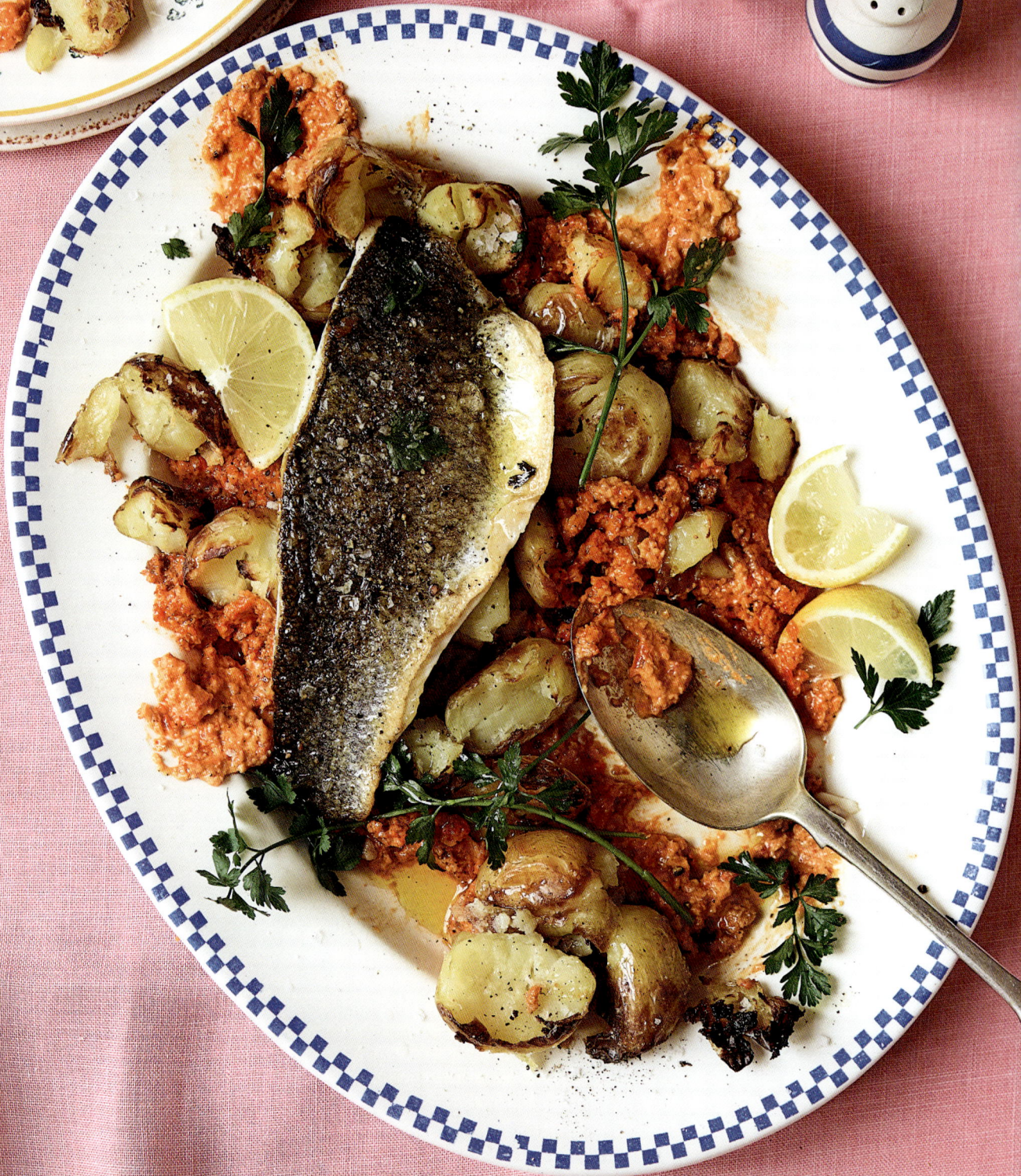

Pan-fried Sea Bass with Smashed Potatoes + Romesco

V/O
VE/O
DF
GF/O
N

Romesco sauce is a brilliant sauce made with roasted red peppers, rich tomato, toasted almonds and crunchy bread, and it's pure magic. Here, it accompanies gorgeously crispy smashed potatoes and fresh, skin-on fish, pan-fried to perfection. A meal that feels really special and impressive, but is actually a breeze to bring together.

baking sheet, lined

400 g/14 oz baby potatoes

3 tbsp olive oil

2 sea bass fillets

salt and pepper

chopped parsley, to garnish

squeeze of lemon juice, to serve

For the romesco

125 g/4 oz jarred roasted red peppers

½ tbsp tomato purée/paste

30 g/1 oz/generous ⅓ cup toasted flaked/slivered almonds

1 small slice of sourdough bread, toasted

1 garlic clove

30 ml/1 fl oz/2 tbsp extra virgin olive oil

1   Place the potatoes in a large microwave-safe bowl with a splash of water. Cover tightly with cling film/plastic wrap and pierce a small hole in the centre for steam to escape. Microwave on full power for 10 minutes until knife-tender. Alternatively, you can boil the potatoes.

2   Preheat the oven to 200°C fan/220°C/425°F/gas mark 7 on the grill/broiler setting.

3   Spread the potatoes on the prepared baking sheet and use the bottom of a glass or potato masher to gently flatten. Brush with 2 tablespoons of olive oil, and season with a pinch each of salt and pepper. Grill/broil for 20 minutes, or until golden and crisp around the edges.

4   Meanwhile, make the romesco sauce. In a food processor, combine the roasted red peppers, tomato purée, flaked almonds, toasted bread, garlic and olive oil. Season, then blend for 1–2 minutes. The consistency will depend on your processor – more powerful ones make it thinner, less powerful ones keep it thicker. Adjust as desired.

5   Finally, heat the remaining 1 tablespoon of olive oil in a frying pan/skillet over medium–high heat. Pat the fish dry, season lightly and place skin-side down in the pan. Cook for 2 minutes, then flip and cook for another 2 minutes until the fish is cooked through.

6   To serve, spread a thick layer of romesco sauce on each plate or a platter to create a base. Top with the potatoes, then the fish. Garnish with fresh parsley and finish with a good squeeze of lemon juice.

Substitutions:

● **No sea bass?** Use any other skin-on fish. ● **Vegan or vegetarian?** Sub the sea bass for your favourite meat-free protein alternative. ● **Gluten-free?** Use gluten-free bread. ● **Nut free?** Sub the almonds for sunflower seeds

Future you:

🍲 Cool and place in an airtight container, storing in the fridge for up to 3 days.
❄ Cool and freeze the romesco sauce for up to 2 months.
💧 Thaw in the fridge overnight, or at room temperature for a few hours.
🔥 Reheat the sea bass slowly on a low heat (around 140°C fan/160°C/325°F/gas mark 3) in the oven. The same for the potatoes. The romesco sauce is best enjoyed at room temperature.

Pulled Chipotle Chicken Burrito Bowl

(V/O)
(VE/O)
(DF)
(GF)

If you haven't tried steaming your chicken, you really should, and this recipe is your chance. Steaming locks in incredible moisture and helps the chicken shred effortlessly. Then, every glorious bit of that shredded chicken gets slathered in a smoky, spicy chipotle sauce and piled into a bowl with all the burrito fillings we love – but better – because you're in charge of what goes in and how much. It's equally delicious warm and cold – plus the fact that no two bites are the same will keep you coming back for more.

2 x 150-g/5½-oz skinless chicken breasts

1 ripe avocado

squeeze of lime juice

½ tbsp chipotle paste

1 tbsp tomato purée/paste

½ tsp smoked paprika

½ tsp honey or maple syrup

1–2 x 250-g/9-oz pouch(es) microwave brown rice, or 150 g/ 5½ oz brown rice cooked according to packet instructions

1 Little Gem/Boston lettuce, roughly chopped

50 g/1¾ oz/⅓ cup sweetcorn/corn

1 x 400-g/14-oz can black beans, drained

salt and pepper

olive oil, for cooking

For the salsa

1 tomato, finely diced

½ red onion, finely diced

a handful of roughly chopped coriander/cilantro

juice of ½ lime

1   Heat 1 tablespoon of olive oil in a lidded frying pan/skillet over medium-high heat. Sear the chicken breasts for 3 minutes per side until they brown. Add water to about 2.5 cm/1-in depth, pop the lid on, and steam the chicken for 10 minutes, or until fully cooked through.

2   While the chicken is steaming, prepare the salsa by combining the tomato, onion, coriander and lime juice in a bowl. Set aside.

3   Scoop out the flesh of the avocado and mash it in a bowl with a fork, adding a squeeze of fresh lime juice. Season to taste, then set aside.

4   Once the chicken is cooked, transfer it to a chopping board. Shred the chicken either by using two forks, or by placing it in a mixing bowl and using a hand mixer. The latter method is much quicker, but does lead to more washing up – I'll leave the choice with you. Add the chipotle paste, tomato purée, paprika, honey and a pinch each of salt and pepper to the shredded chicken, and toss until it's evenly coated with the sauce.

5   Heat the rice in the microwave according to the packet instructions, usually about 2 minutes per pouch.

6   Assemble your bowls, starting with rice, then add the chipotle chicken, mashed avocado, lettuce, sweetcorn, black beans and the salsa.

Substitutions:

● **Vegan or vegetarian?** Sub the chicken for tofu, or your favourite meat-free protein alternative.

Future you:

🥡 Cool and place in an airtight container, storing in the fridge for up to 3 days.
❄ Cool and freeze the pulled chicken for up to 2 months.
💧 Thaw in the fridge overnight, or at room temperature for a few hours.
🔥 Enjoy chilled, or heat in the microwave for 1–2 minutes until piping hot. Cooked rice must only be reheated once.

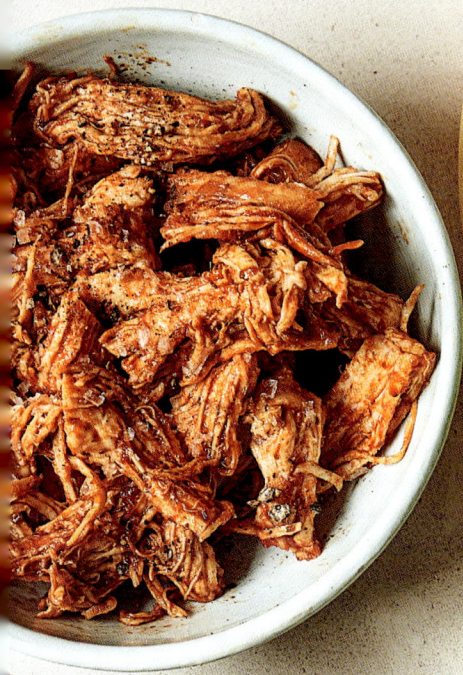

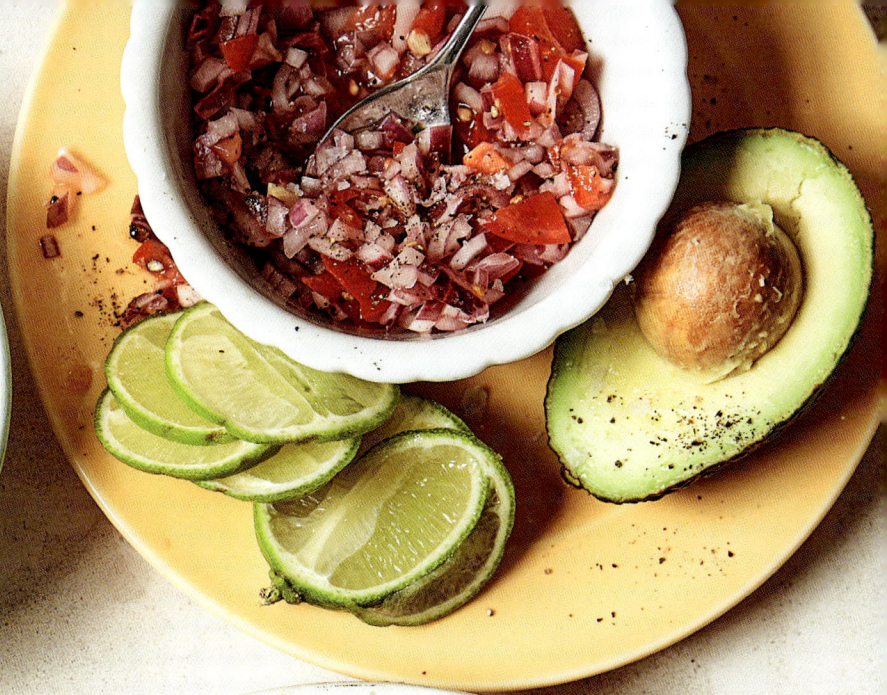

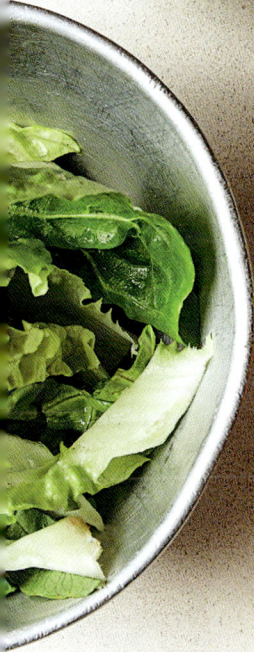

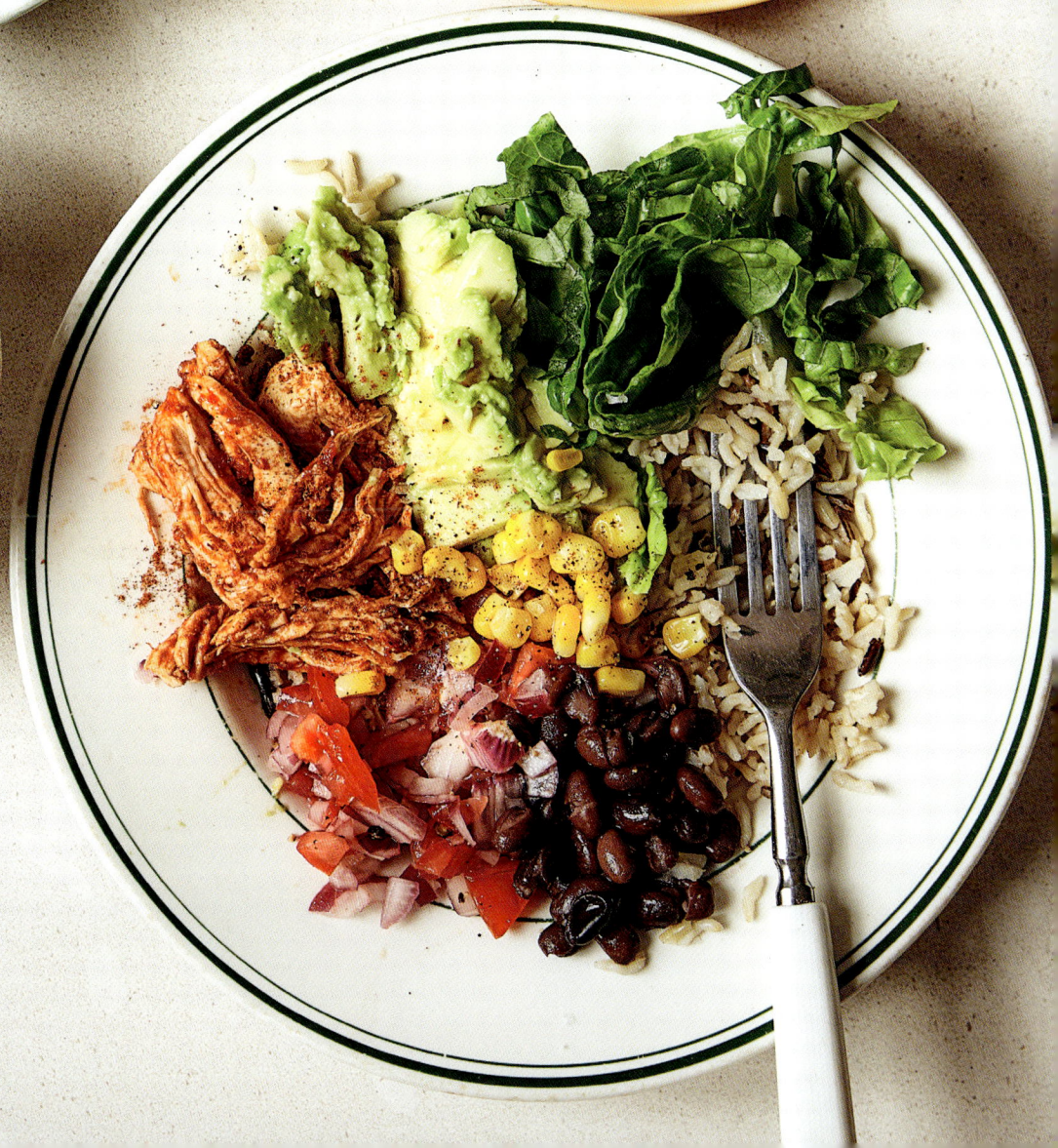

Creamy Red Pepper Cajun Pasta

(V)
(VE)
(DF)
(GF/O)

This recipe is one to bookmark for when you're craving a big bowl of comforting, creamy pasta. Yet again, featuring silken tofu – the secret ingredient to create a luscious sauce that satisfies every comfort-food craving while boosting the protein intake. I've used silken tofu in several pasta sauces in my time, but this creamy Cajun-spiced variation really is up there as one of my favourites. I know you'll love it too, so grab a bowl, and tuck in.

1 x 300-g/10½-oz block silken tofu

1 onion, finely diced

1 red (bell) pepper, cut into thin strips

2 garlic cloves, minced

200 g/7 oz cherry tomatoes, halved

250 g/9 oz pasta (I like radiatori here)

500 ml/18 fl oz/2 cups vegetable stock

50 g/1¾ oz/scant 1 cup spinach

olive oil, for cooking

chopped parsley, to garnish

For the Cajun seasoning

2 tsp smoked paprika

1 tsp dried oregano

1 tsp dried thyme

½ tsp cayenne pepper

1 tsp fine sea salt

¼ tsp black pepper

1   First up, the Cajun seasoning. In a small bowl, combine the paprika, oregano, thyme, cayenne pepper, salt and pepper.

2   In a blender, combine the silken tofu and half of the Cajun seasoning. Blend for 1 minute, or until you have a completely smooth, velvety consistency. Set aside.

3   Place a deep lidded frying pan/skillet over medium heat and add a good drizzle of olive oil. Once hot, sauté the onion for 3 minutes, before adding the pepper and cooking for a further 2 minutes until it begins to soften. Stir in the tomatoes and the remaining Cajun seasoning, letting everything cook for another couple of minutes until well coated and fragrant.

4   Add the dried pasta to the pan, then pour in the blended tofu mixture and stock. Stir to combine, ensuring the sauce evenly coats the pasta. Cover the pan with a lid and let everything simmer for 8–10 minutes, or until the pasta is almost cooked through.

5   Remove the lid from the pan and gently fold in the spinach, stirring until it wilts and blends into the sauce. Once the spinach is wilted, remove the pan from the heat.

6   Garnish with some fresh parsley and serve immediately.

Substitutions:

● **No silken tofu?** If you have a powerful blender, use firm tofu instead and add a splash of water to loosen.
● **Gluten-free?** Use gluten-free pasta.

Future you:

🍱 Cool and place in an airtight container, storing in the fridge for up to 4 days.
❄ Cool and freeze for up to 2 months.
🌢 Thaw in the fridge overnight, or at room temperature for a few hours.
🔥 Reheat in the microwave for 2–3 minutes, stirring halfway, until piping hot.

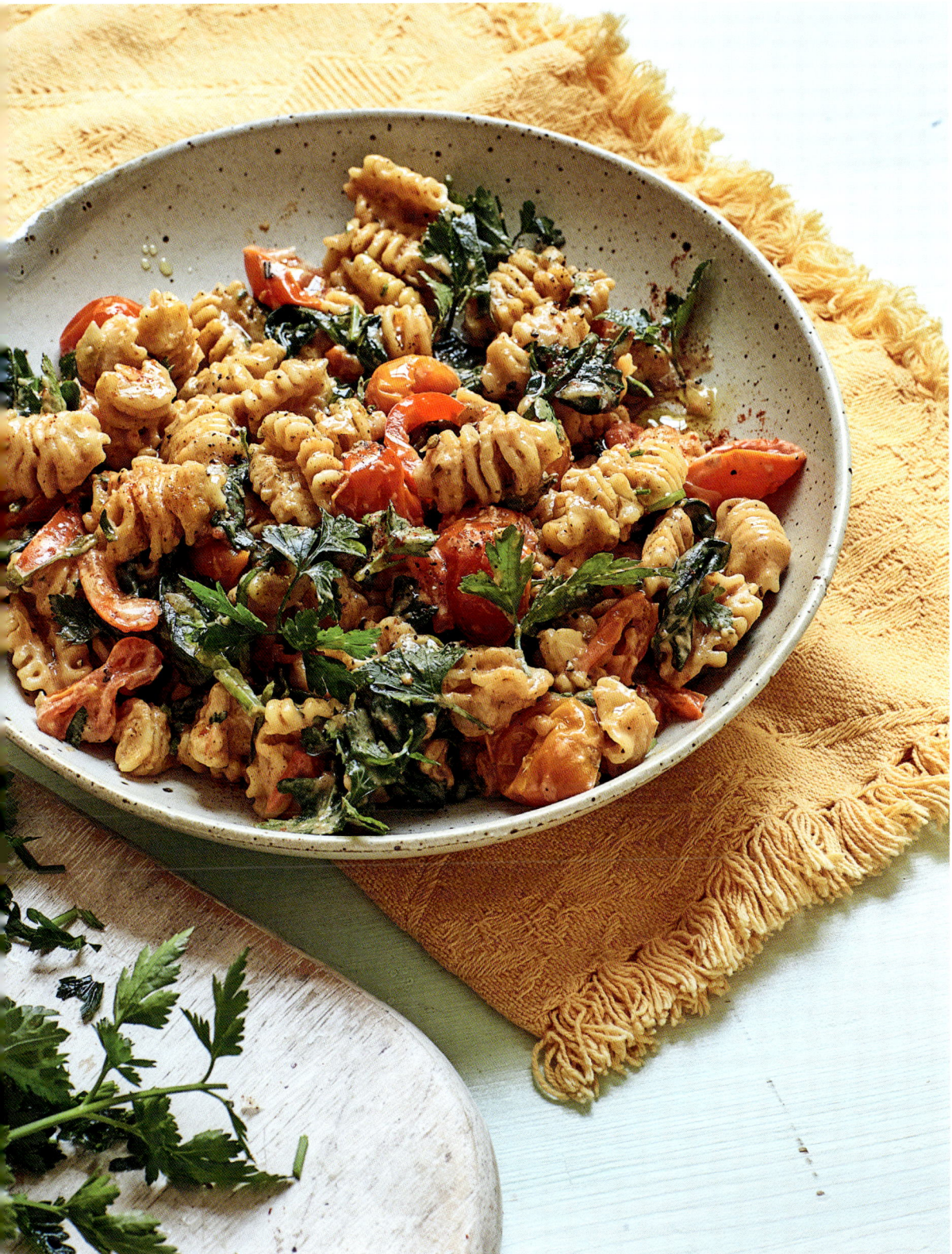

Lightly Dusted Spiced Fish + Chips

(DF/O)
(GF/O)

If I had to describe the dusting on this fish, honestly the first thing that comes to mind is KFC. Not in a bad, greasy way, but because it has that same salty, sweet, smoky combination, brought to life as the coating crisps in the pan. Chippy meets chicken shop. How's that for a fakeaway!

large baking sheet, lined (if using an oven)

air fryer basket, lined (if using an air fryer)

For the chips

400 g/14 oz Maris Piper or Yukon Gold (or equivalent) potatoes, cut into batons

1 tsp dried thyme

1 tsp salt

olive oil, for cooking

For the fish

1 egg

40 g/1½ oz/scant ⅓ cup wholemeal/whole-wheat flour

1 tsp smoked paprika

½ tsp dried thyme

½ tsp dried oregano

½ tsp garlic granules

½ tsp onion granules

2 large basa fillets (defrosted if using frozen)

salt and pepper

For the minted peas

200 g/7 oz/1½ cups frozen peas

a handful of chopped mint

1 tbsp low-fat crème fraîche or sour cream

juice of ½ lemon

Substitutions:

● **Dairy-free?** Use dairy-free yogurt instead of the crème fraîche.
● **Gluten-free?** Use gluten-free flour.

1 Preheat the air fryer or oven to 200°C fan/220°C/425°F/gas mark 7.

2 If using an air fryer, pop the potato batons into the basket with a drizzle of olive oil, the thyme and salt. Cook for 25 minutes. If using an oven, spread the potato batons evenly on the prepared baking sheet. Drizzle with oil, season with the thyme and salt, and bake for 30 minutes, turning halfway through to ensure even cooking.

3 Set up two shallow bowls for your fish dredging station. In the first bowl, crack the egg and beat until no streaks of yolk remain. In the second bowl, combine the flour, paprika, thyme, oregano, garlic granules, onion granules and a generous pinch each of salt and pepper.

4 Dip the fish into the beaten egg, ensuring both sides are coated, then transfer to the flour mixture, pressing gently to adhere. Shake off any excess flour. Repeat with the other fish fillet.

5 Heat 2 tablespoons of olive oil in a frying pan/skillet over medium heat. Once the oil is hot and shimmering, carefully place the coated fish into the pan and cook for about 3 minutes on each side, or until the coating is golden and crisp and the fish is cooked through.

6 While the fish is cooking, prepare the minted peas. In a microwave-safe bowl, microwave the peas on full power until tender, usually around 2 minutes, then transfer them to a bowl. Add the mint, crème fraîche and lemon juice, and use a potato masher to crush everything together until slightly chunky.

7 Serve the crispy fish with the golden chips, crushed minted peas and lemon wedges.

Future you:

🍲 Cool and place in an airtight container, storing in the fridge for up to 3 days.
🔥 Reheat the fish and chips at 180°C fan/200°C/400°F/gas mark 6 in the oven or air fryer for 10–15 minutes, or until hot all the way through.

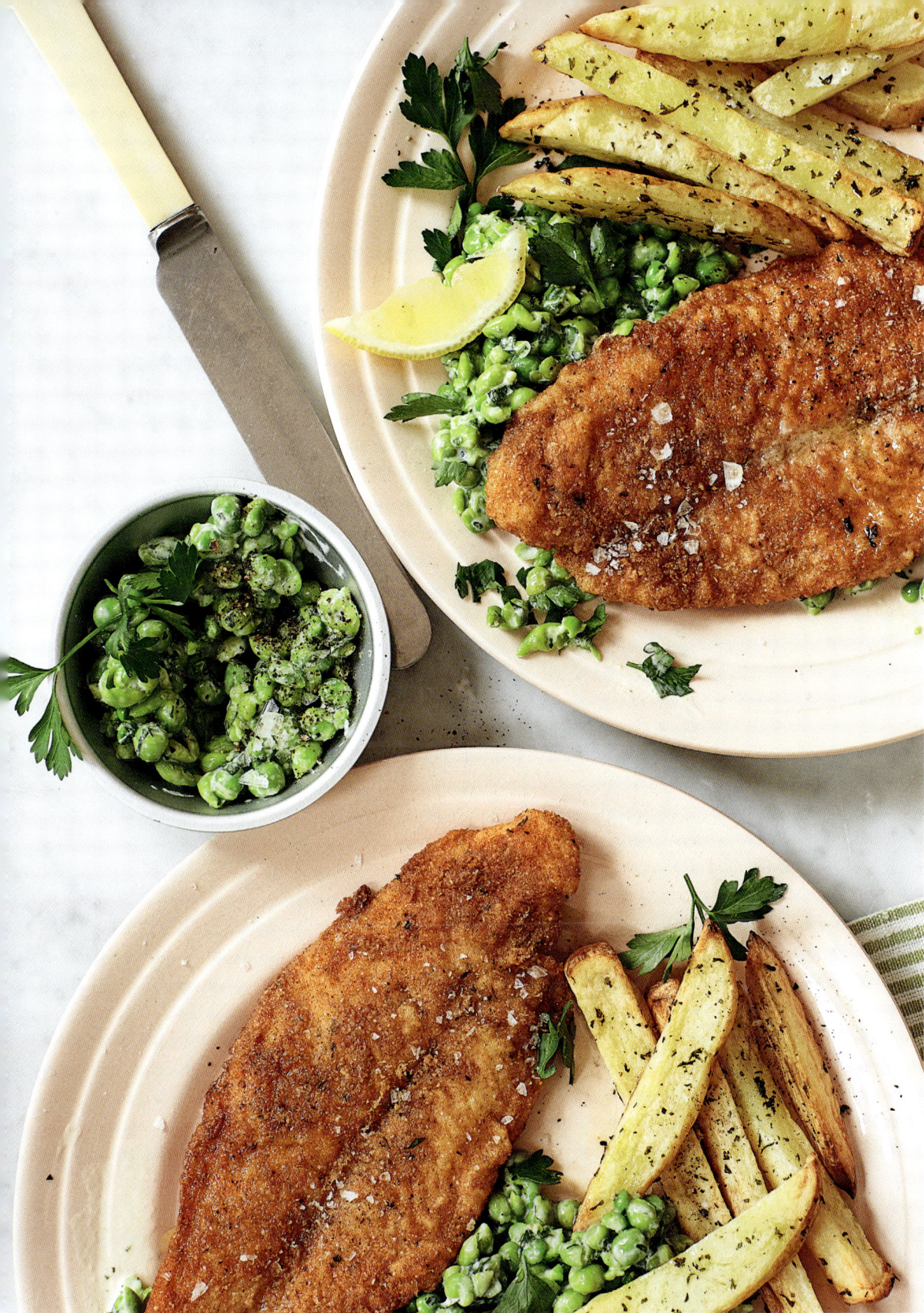

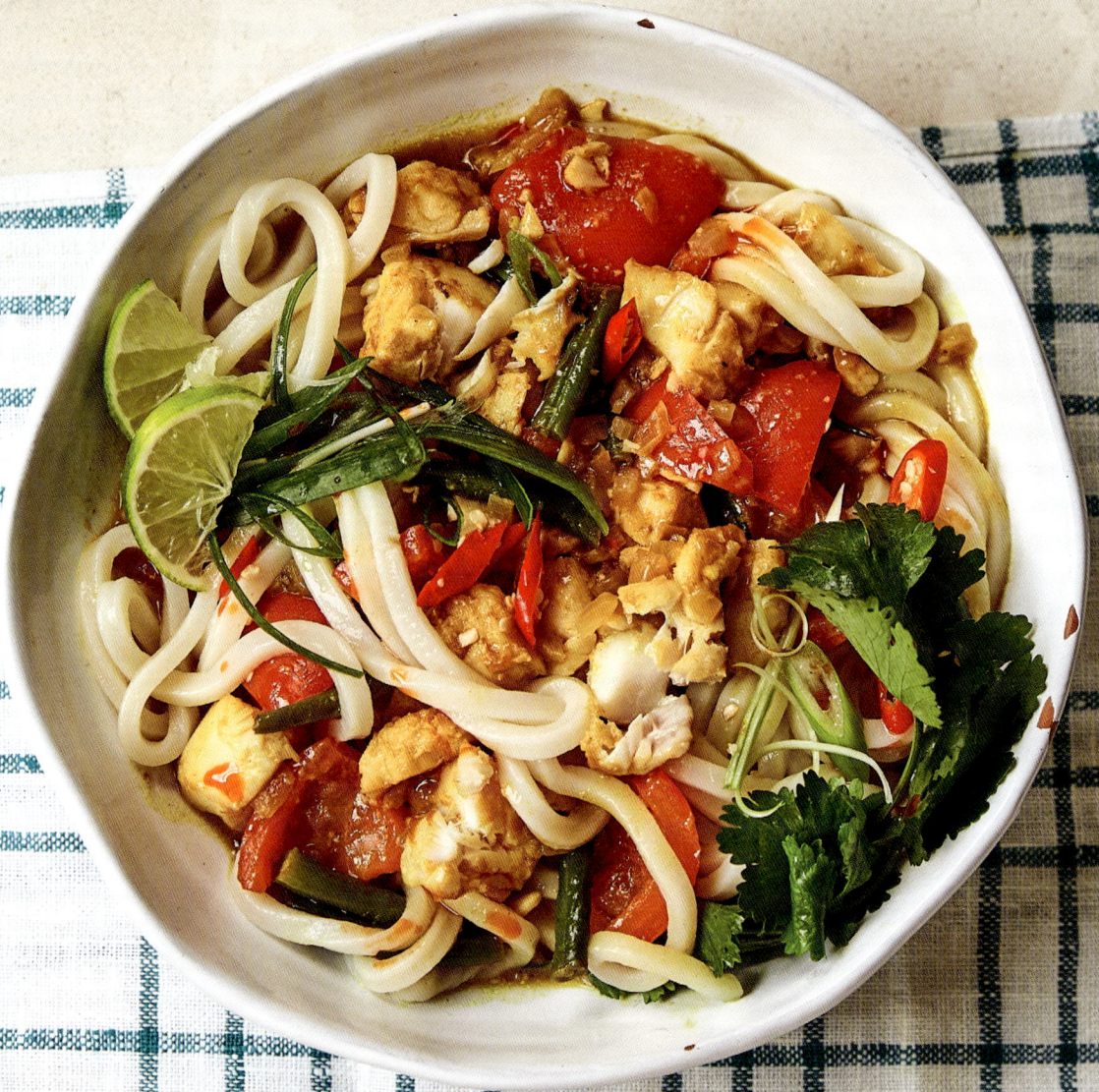

Cod Coconut Curry + Udon Noodles

(V/O) (VE/O) (DF) (GF/O)

Simple yet luxurious, this creamy cod curry is a perfect weeknight dinner that will be on your table in under 25 minutes. Inspired by a mix of Asian influences, it bursts with aromatic flavours, a little chilli kick and tender veggies, making it one that's sure to please everyone at the table. While rice is perhaps the instinctive pairing, there's a real joy in slurping up thick, chewy udon noodles coated in rich curry sauce – so that's the route we're taking here.

1 onion, finely diced

2 garlic cloves, minced

1 thumb-sized piece ginger, grated

1 red (bell) pepper, cut into chunks

50 g/1¾ oz fine green beans, cut into thirds

½ tsp ground cumin

½ tsp ground coriander

¼ tsp ground turmeric

1 small red chilli/chile, de-seeded and finely diced (optional)

1 x 400-g/14-oz can light coconut milk

½ tbsp fish sauce

1 tbsp soy sauce

juice of ½ lime

250 g/9 oz cod fillets, cut into bite-sized chunks

olive oil, for cooking

To serve

125 g/4 oz noodles of your choice

a handful of roughly chopped coriander/cilantro

lime wedges

1 Heat 1 tablespoon of olive oil in a deep frying pan/skillet over medium heat. Add the onion and sauté for about 3 minutes until it begins to soften. Stir in the garlic, ginger, pepper, green beans, ground cumin, ground coriander, turmeric and most of the red chilli if using (reserving some for garnishing). Cook for an additional 4 minutes until the vegetables are tender.

2 Give the can of coconut milk a good shake, then open it and pour it into the pan, followed by the fish sauce and soy sauce. Squeeze in the lime juice and give everything a good stir to combine. Add the chunks of fish to the pan and bring the mixture to the boil, then reduce the heat to a simmer. Let the curry simmer for 5 minutes, or until the fish is fully cooked through.

3 While the fish is cooking, bring a pot of water to the boil and cook the noodles according to the packet instructions.

4 Divide the curry between bowls and place the noodles alongside, allowing them to sink into the rich curry sauce. Garnish with the reserved red chilli and a sprinkle of fresh coriander, and serve with lime wedges.

Substitutions:

● **No cod?** Use any other 'meaty' white fish, such as haddock or basa. Or, try prawns. ● **Vegetarian or vegan?** Swap cod for tofu and omit the fish sauce. ● **Gluten-free?** Use gluten-free noodles. Use tamari instead of soy sauce.

Future you:

☐ Cool and place in an airtight container, storing in the fridge for up to 2 days.
❄ It is technically possible to freeze the curry for up to 2 months, but I would recommend against it as the fish is likely to become tough when reheating.
🔥 If you do want to reheat, do so in a pot over medium heat until piping hot.

Garlic Ginger Chicken + Smashed Cucumber Salad

(V/O)
(VE/O)
(DF)
(GF/O)

Sticky, sweet, zesty, and just a bit spicy – this one has it all. It leans heavily on store-cupboard items like rice vinegar, soy sauce and sesame oil, so once you're stocked up on those, you'll only need a handful of fresh ingredients to bring it to life. Plus, those same staples unlock so many other banging recipes like my Sticky Soy Salmon Skewers (see page 100) and my Asian-inspired Tempeh Burger (see page 123).

4 skinless, boneless chicken thighs

1 x 250-g/9-oz pouch cooked jasmine rice

salt and pepper

olive oil, for cooking

1 spring onion/scallion, thinly sliced, to garnish

For the glaze

1 thumb-sized piece ginger, grated

2 garlic cloves, minced

2 tbsp dark soy sauce

1 tsp sesame oil

1 tbsp maple syrup

1 tsp rice vinegar

1 tsp cornflour/cornstarch

For the cucumber salad

1 small cucumber

1 tsp sesame oil

1 tbsp light soy sauce

1 tsp rice vinegar

1 tsp maple syrup

2 tsp crispy chilli/chili oil

½ tsp sesame seeds

1 First up, the ginger glaze. Add the ginger, garlic, soy sauce, oil, maple syrup, vinegar, cornflour and 50 ml/1½ fl oz/3½ tablespoons of water to a jar or bowl. Mix or shake, until combined.

2 Heat 1 tablespoon of olive oil in a frying pan/skillet over medium–high heat. Season the chicken thighs, then lay them in the pan. Cook for 5 minutes on each side, or until browned and fully cooked through.

3 While the chicken is cooking, grab a chopping board and a bowl to prepare the cucumber salad. Slice the cucumber in half lengthways and place the halves flat-side down on the chopping board. Starting at one end, place a large knife flat against the cucumber and use your palm to crush until the skin breaks. Repeat along the rest of the cucumber, then chop it into rough chunks. In your bowl, mix together the sesame oil, soy sauce, rice vinegar, maple syrup and the crispy chilli oil. Add the cucumber chunks and toss until coated. Sprinkle with the sesame seeds and set aside to marinate until you're ready to serve.

4 Once your chicken is cooked, remove it from the pan and place it onto a clean plate or wooden board and cover with foil to keep warm. Then, reduce the heat, pour in the ginger glaze, and cook until it starts to bubble and thicken. Turn off the heat entirely, then return the chicken to the pan and coat each piece generously in the glaze.

5 Microwave the rice per the packet instructions and divide between 2 plates. Serve the glazed chicken thighs with the cucumber salad, drizzling any extra dressing over the rice, and garnish with the spring onion.

Substitutions:

● **Vegan or vegetarian?** Use cubed tofu in place of the chicken. ● **No rice vinegar?** Sub for fresh lime juice or mirin. ● **Gluten-free?** Use tamari instead of soy sauce.

Future you:

🍲 Cool and place in an airtight container, storing in the fridge for up to 3 days.
🔥 Remove the cucumber and microwave for 3 minutes to reheat. Ensure both the chicken and the rice are piping hot. Cooked rice must only be reheated once.

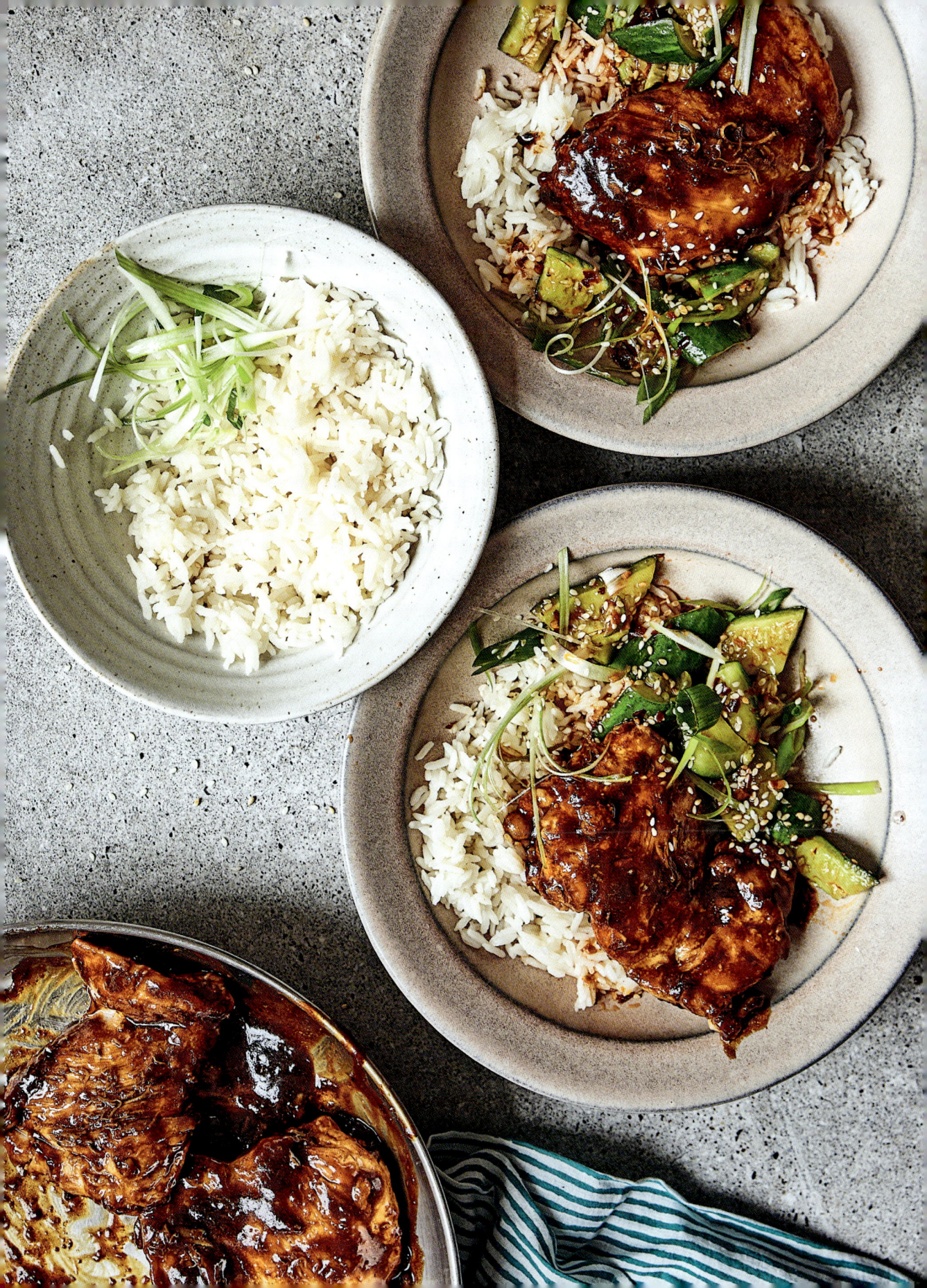

Tofu Curry + Cheat's Garlic Naan

(V)
(VE/O)
(DF/O)
(GF/O)

I make this curry when I'm craving something quick and comforting but don't want to compromise on flavour. It gets better over time, as everything melds together, making it ideal for doubling quantities to enjoy leftovers throughout the week.

baking sheet, lined (if using an oven)

air fryer basket, lined (if using an air fryer)

1 x 300-g/10½-oz block extra-firm tofu

1 tbsp cornflour/cornstarch

1 onion, finely diced

2 garlic cloves, minced

1 thumb-sized piece ginger, grated

½ tsp fennel seeds

1 tbsp tomato purée/paste

1 tsp ground turmeric

1 tsp ground cumin

1 tsp ground coriander

½ tsp hot chilli/chili powder

300 g/10½ oz passata/strained tomatoes

100 ml/3½ fl oz/6½ tbsp coconut milk

1 tbsp garam masala

50 g/1¾ oz/generous ⅓ cup petits pois (fresh or frozen)

60 g/2 oz/1 cup spinach

salt and pepper

olive oil, for cooking

plain yogurt, to serve

roughly chopped coriander/cilantro, to serve

For the naan

100 g/3½ oz/¾ cup self-raising/self-rising flour, plus extra for dusting

75 g/6 oz/⅓ cup low-fat plain yogurt

¼ tsp fine sea salt

1 tbsp olive oil

1 garlic clove, minced

1 Preheat the air fryer or oven to 200°C fan/220°C/425°F/gas mark 7.

2 Press out any water from the block of tofu, then tear into bite-sized chunks. Transfer to a large mixing bowl, along with the cornflour and a good pinch each of salt and pepper. Mix until each tofu chunk is coated.

3 If using an oven, spread out the tofu evenly on the prepared baking sheet. Drizzle with a little oil and bake for 20 minutes until golden and crisp. If using an air fryer, add the tofu to the basket, drizzle with oil and cook for 10 minutes until golden and crisp.

4 Heat 1 tablespoon of olive oil in a frying pan/skillet over medium heat. Add the onion, garlic, ginger and fennel seeds. Lower the heat and cook for 10 minutes, stirring every few minutes until softened.

5 While the onion mix is cooking, make the naan dough. Combine the flour, yogurt and salt in a bowl and mix until a rough dough forms. On a lightly floured surface, knead the dough before splitting into two portions. If the dough is too sticky, sprinkle on a little extra flour. Flatten each portion into a 5-mm/¼-in thick rectangle using your fingers or a rolling pin. Leave to rest while you continue with the curry.

6 Going back to the pan, add the tomato purée, ground turmeric, ground cumin, ground coriander and chilli powder to the softened onion mixture and cook for 1 minute. Stir in the passata and coconut milk, then add the garam masala, petits pois and spinach. Let this simmer for 5 minutes until the sauce thickens.

7 When the tofu is ready, add it to the curry. Turn the heat to low while you finish the naan.

8 Heat a drizzle of oil in a separate frying pan over medium–high heat. Place the naans (one at a time, if needed) into the pan and cook for 2 minutes on each side, or until golden and nicely puffed up. Combine the oil and garlic together in a bowl and brush over the warm naans.

9 Take the curry off the heat and serve with a dollop of yogurt and sprinkle of fresh coriander, with the garlic naan alongside.

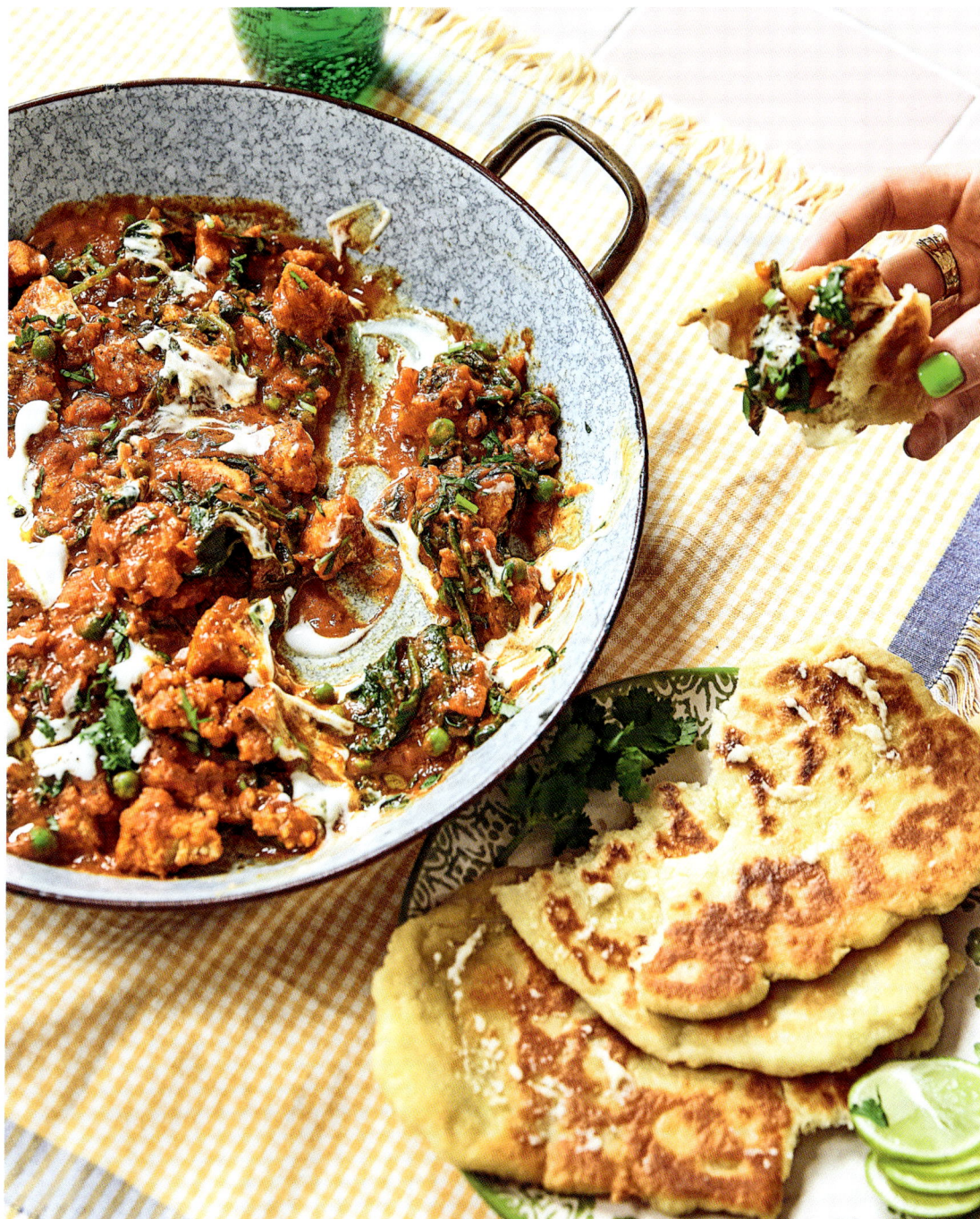

Substitutions:

● **No coconut milk?** Use single/light cream or soy cream instead.
● **No passata?** Use canned chopped tomatoes instead. ● **Gluten-free?** Serve with gluten-free naan.

Future you:

🍵 Cool and place in an airtight container, storing in the fridge for up to 3 days.
❄ Cool and freeze for up to 2 months.
💧 Thaw in the fridge overnight, or on low power in the microwave.
🔥 To reheat, microwave the curry for 15 seconds and the naan for 30 seconds.

Speedy Fishcakes + Herby Pea Salad

(DF)
(GF/O)

Fishcakes were my go-to meal at University – quick, easy and reliable. But an attempt to make them from scratch in my final year was a disaster, involving hours of prep and chilling. Who has time for that?! Since then, I've wanted to right the wrongs and create a homemade fishcake recipe that's speedy, but still packed with flavour, and these nail it.

350 g/12 oz floury potatoes

300 g/10½ oz fish pie mix (defrosted if using frozen)

2 spring onions/scallions, thinly sliced

1 tsp Dijon mustard

3 tbsp plain/all-purpose flour

1 egg, beaten

40 g/1½ oz/scant 1 cup panko breadcrumbs

salt and pepper

olive oil, for cooking

For the salad

60 g/2 oz/½ cup frozen peas

½ tbsp cider vinegar

1 tbsp extra virgin olive oil

1 small garlic clove, minced

50 g/1¾ oz watercress

1 tbsp roughly chopped parsley

1   Pierce the potatoes with a fork, then wrap them in a damp paper towel and microwave on full power for 3 minutes. Flip and microwave for another 3 minutes until knife-tender. Once done, run them under cold water until cool enough to handle.

2   While the potatoes are cooking, heat a drizzle of olive oil in a frying pan/skillet over medium heat. Add the fish and cook for 4–5 minutes, or until cooked through. Remove from the pan and set aside.

3   Mash the potatoes in a large bowl, keeping the skins on for extra nutrients (or scoop out the flesh if preferred). Add the fish, spring onions, mustard and 1 tablespoon of flour. Season and mix well. Divide into 4 portions and shape into patties with your hands.

4   Set up a station with three shallow dishes: one with the remaining flour, one with the beaten egg, and one with breadcrumbs. Coat each patty first in the flour, then in the egg, and finally in the breadcrumbs.

5   In a clean, large frying pan, heat 1–2 tablespoons of olive oil over medium heat. Cook the fishcakes for about 4 minutes on each side, until golden. While they cook, in a microwave-safe bowl, microwave the peas on full power for 2 minutes until tender. Drain and set aside.

6   In a small bowl, whisk together the vinegar, olive oil, garlic, salt and pepper to make the dressing. In your serving bowl, combine the watercress, peas, parsley and dressing, and toss to coat evenly.

7   Serve the fishcakes hot, alongside the herby pea salad.

Substitutions:

● **Gluten-free?** Use gluten-free flour and breadcrumbs. ● **No fish pie mix?** Use other skinless, boneless fish such as cod, haddock, hake, basa or salmon instead. ● **No Dijon mustard?** Use wholegrain or English mustard instead.

Future you:

🍱 Cool and place in an airtight container, storing in the fridge for up to 3 days.
❄ Cool and freeze the fishcakes for up to 2 months.
💧 Thaw in the fridge overnight, or at room temperature for a few hours.
🔥 Place the fishcakes on a baking sheet in a hot oven or air fryer (around 180°C fan/200°C/400°F/gas mark) for 10–15 minutes, or until hot all the way through.

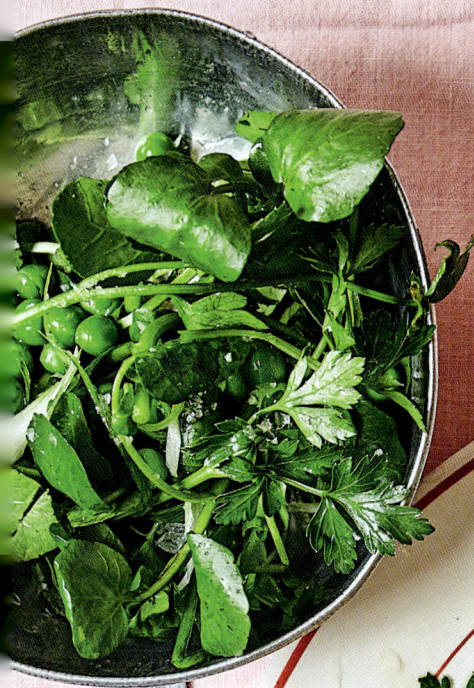

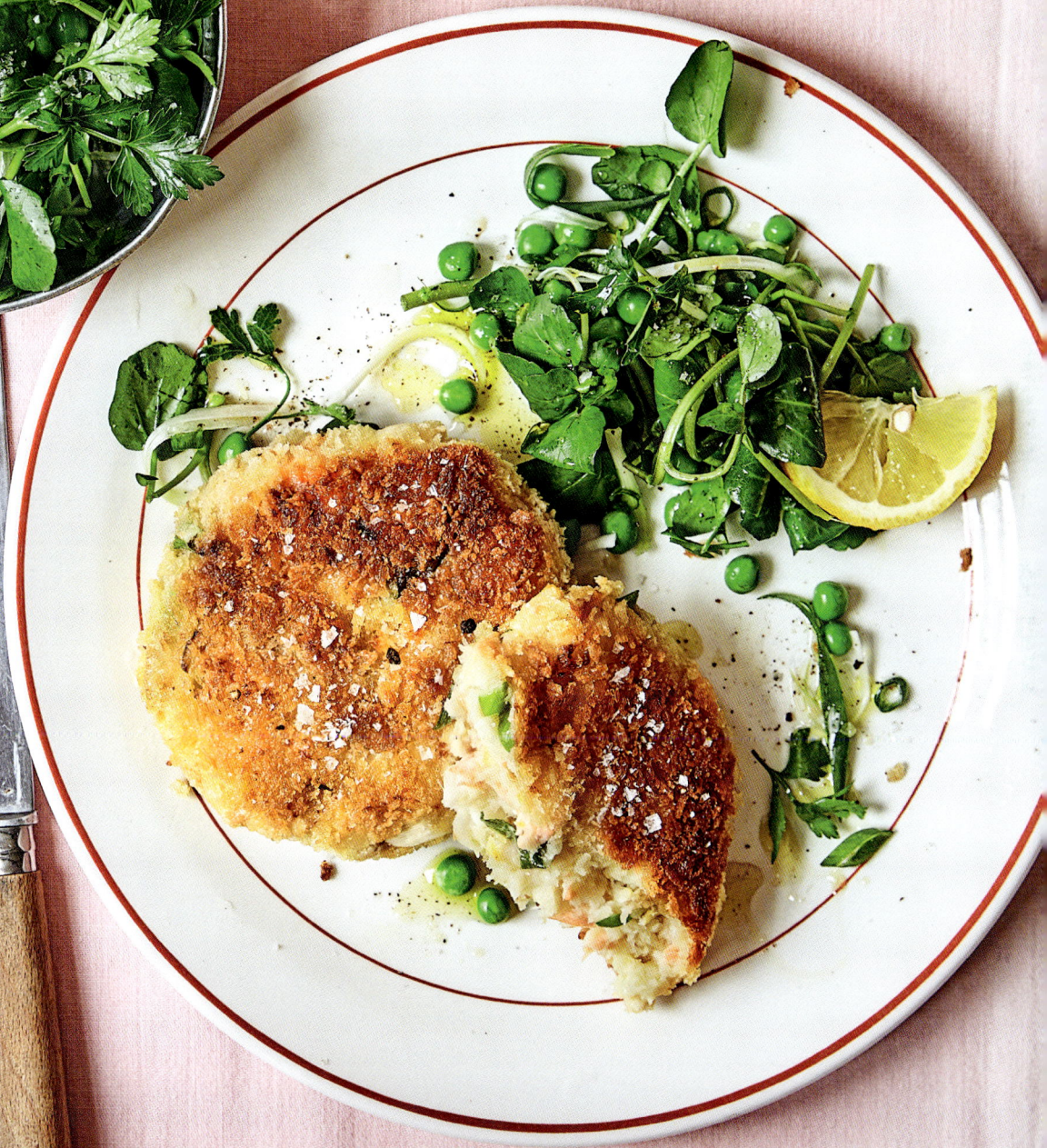

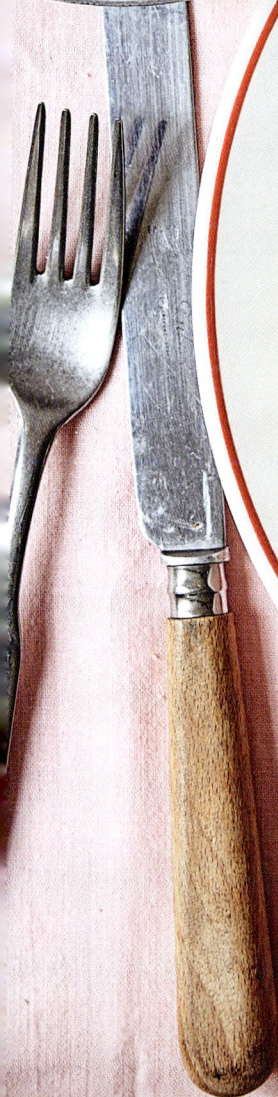

Tofu Kofta Flatbreads

V
VE/O
DF/O
GF/O

Bursting with Mediterranean flavours, this vibrant, high-protein meal is a refreshing addition to any weeknight dinner line-up. The tofu koftas, packed with fragrant herbs and bold spices, rival any meat version and make this healthy, meat-free recipe utterly de-lish.

½ cucumber, finely sliced

¼ red onion, finely sliced

1 tomato, finely sliced

3 flatbreads (see page 38 or use store-bought)

salt and pepper

pomegranate seeds (optional)

For the koftas

1 x 300-g/10½-oz block extra-firm smoked tofu

2 garlic cloves

2 sun-dried tomatoes

½ white onion

1 tsp ground cumin

½ tsp ground coriander

2 tbsp chopped parsley

2 tbsp chopped coriander/cilantro

1 tsp fine sea salt

¼ tsp black pepper

50 g/1¾ oz/generous ⅓ cup wholemeal flour

50 g/1¾ oz/1 generous cup panko breadcrumbs

For the feta yogurt

100 g/3½ oz/scant ½ cup thick yogurt

80 g/3 oz/⅔ cup crumbled feta

grated zest and juice of 1 small lemon

1 You can cook the koftas in the air fryer, or on the hob/stovetop. I prefer to do them in the air fryer as it's more hands-off, but I'll let you decide. If using the air fryer, preheat it now to 200°C/400°F.

2 Start by making the koftas. Press out any water from the block of tofu (this will vary depending on the brand you use), then place the tofu, along with all the other kofta ingredients, into a food processor. Pulse until the mixture is well combined, but still retains some texture.

3 Using your hands, portion out the mixture and shape it into 9 oval koftas.

4 If using an air fryer, place the koftas in the basket, spray with oil and cook for 15–20 minutes. If cooking on the hob, heat 1 tablespoon of olive oil over medium heat and cook the koftas for 8–10 minutes, turning them regularly. The koftas are done when the outside is golden and crisp and they feel firm to the touch.

5 While the koftas are cooking, prepare the feta yogurt. In a bowl or blender, mix together the yogurt, crumbled feta, lemon zest and lemon juice until well combined.

6 In another bowl, toss together the cucumber, onion and tomato, and season with a good pinch each of salt and pepper.

7 To assemble, smear each flatbread with a generous helping of feta yogurt, then top with the fresh salad and three koftas. Finish with a scatter of pomegranate seeds, if using.

Substitutions:

● **Dairy-free or vegan?** Use a dairy-free yogurt and feta alternative.
● **Gluten-free?** Swap the wholemeal flour for buckwheat flour. Serve on gluten-free flatbread.

Future you:

🥡 Cool and place in an airtight container, storing in the fridge for up to 3 days.
❄ Cool and freeze for up to 2 months.
💧 Thaw in the fridge overnight, or at room temperature for a few hours.
🔥 Enjoy cold, or warm in the microwave for 20–30 seconds.

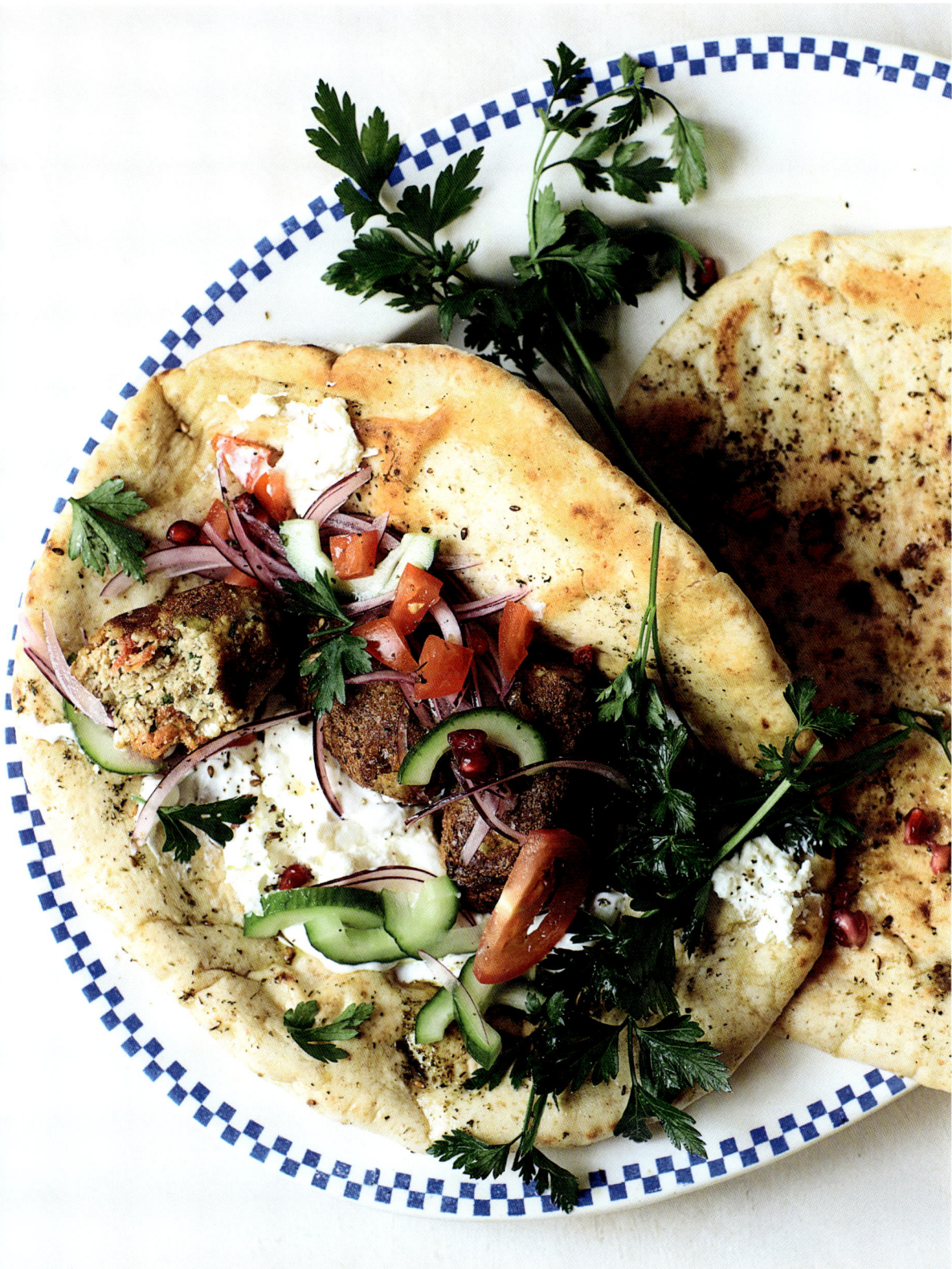

Baked Crunchy Tacos

(V)
(VE/O)
(DF/O)
(GF/O)

Imagine a fusion of a taco and a quesadilla, but without the hassle of monitoring them over a frying pan – instead, your oven (or air fryer) handles all the heavy lifting. Once baked, the tortillas get super crispy on the outside, while inside, the cheese melts and mingles into the filling for a flavour explosion. So fun to both make and eat, and a guaranteed hit.

baking sheet, lined (if using an oven)

air fryer basket, lined (if using an air fryer)

1 x 200-g/7-oz block tempeh

1 onion, finely diced

2 garlic cloves, minced

1 x 400-g/14-oz can black beans, drained

1 tsp smoked paprika

1 tsp ground cumin

3 tbsp tomato purée/paste

1 tsp chipotle paste

juice of 1 lime

½ tbsp maple syrup

1 tbsp roughly chopped coriander/cilantro

6 mini tortilla wraps

50 g/1¾ oz/generous ½ cup grated cheese (I like cheddar)

olive oil, for cooking

lime wedges, to serve

For the avocado dip

2 ripe avocados

juice of 1 lime

2 tbsp yogurt

2 tsp maple syrup

a pinch of salt

1   Preheat the oven or air fryer to 200°C fan/220°C/425°F/gas mark 7.

2   In a frying pan/skillet, heat 1 tablespoon of olive oil over medium heat. Crumble the block of tempeh into small pieces with your hands and add it to the pan, along with the diced onion and minced garlic. Cook the mix for about 5 minutes, or until the onion has softened.

3   Next, stir in the black beans, paprika, cumin, tomato purée, chipotle paste, lime juice and maple syrup. Mix well to combine and cook for a couple of minutes. Add the chopped coriander and stir again to distribute evenly. Remove the pan from the heat and set aside.

4   Now, it's taco assembly time. Brush 1 tablespoon of olive oil across a sheet of parchment paper and place the tortillas on top. Flip them over a couple of times to ensure both sides are coated with oil. Spoon some of the tempeh and black bean mixture onto one half of each tortilla, then top with a sprinkle of cheese. Fold the tortillas in half and press gently to seal. Repeat until all of the tacos are assembled.

5   If using an oven, arrange the tacos on the baking sheet and bake for 15 minutes. If using an air fryer, carefully place the tacos in the basket and cook for 10–12 minutes. In either case, flip the tacos halfway through the cooking time to ensure they crisp up evenly on both sides.

6   While the tacos are cooking, prepare the avocado dip. In a small blender, combine the avocados, lime juice, yogurt, maple syrup, salt and 1 tablespoon of water. Blend until smooth, adding more water if needed to reach your desired dip consistency.

7   Once the tacos are crispy and golden, serve them immediately alongside the creamy avocado dip.

Substitutions:

● **No tempeh?** Double up on the black beans. ● **Dairy-free or vegan?** Use dairy-free cheese and yogurt. ● **Gluten-free?** Use gluten-free tortillas.

Future you:

🥡 Cool and place in an airtight container, storing in the fridge for up to 4 days.
❄ Cool and freeze the taco filling for up to 3 months.
💧 Thaw in the fridge overnight, or in the microwave on low power.
🔥 Reheat in the air fryer or oven at 140°C fan/160°C/325°F/gas mark 3 for 10 minutes.

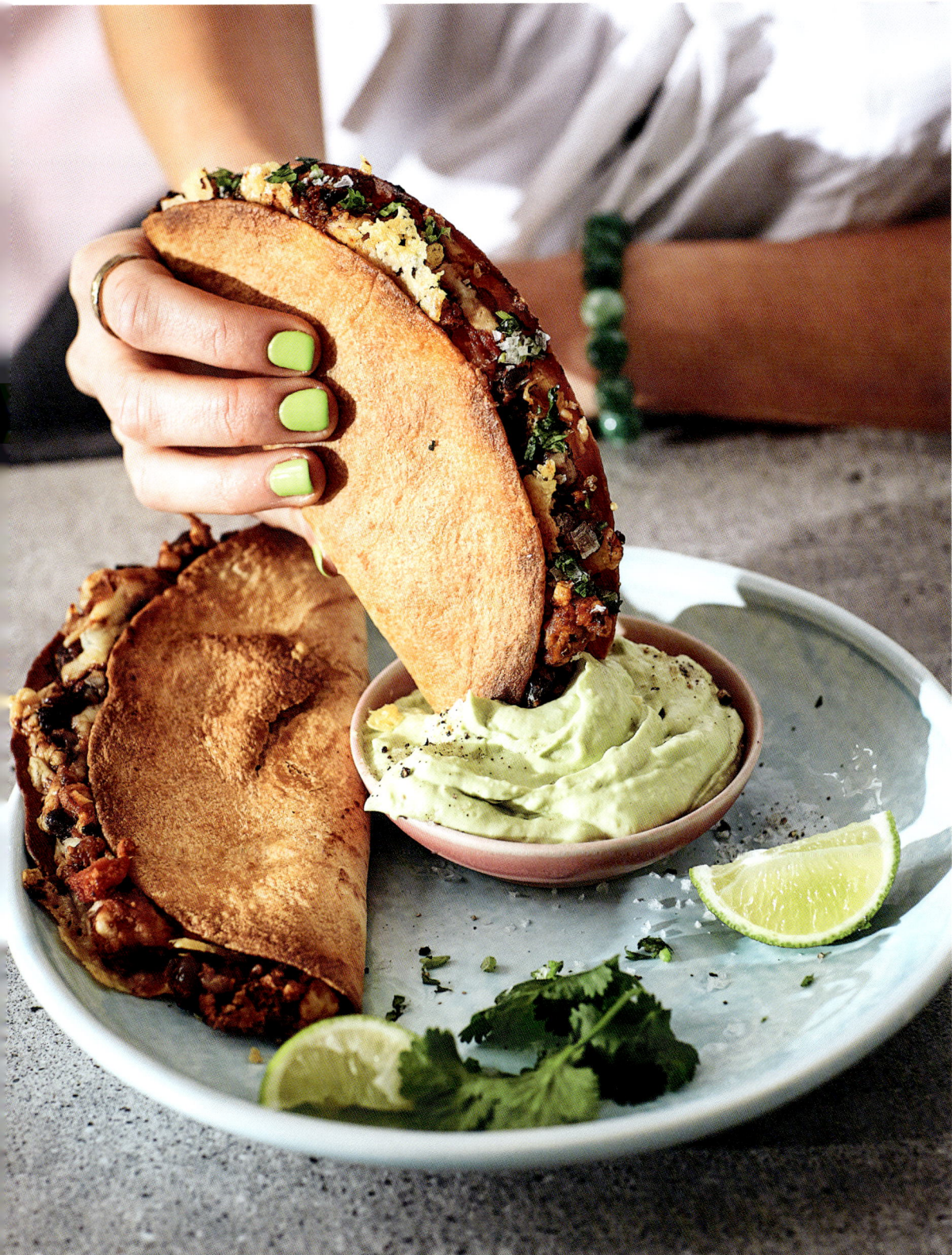

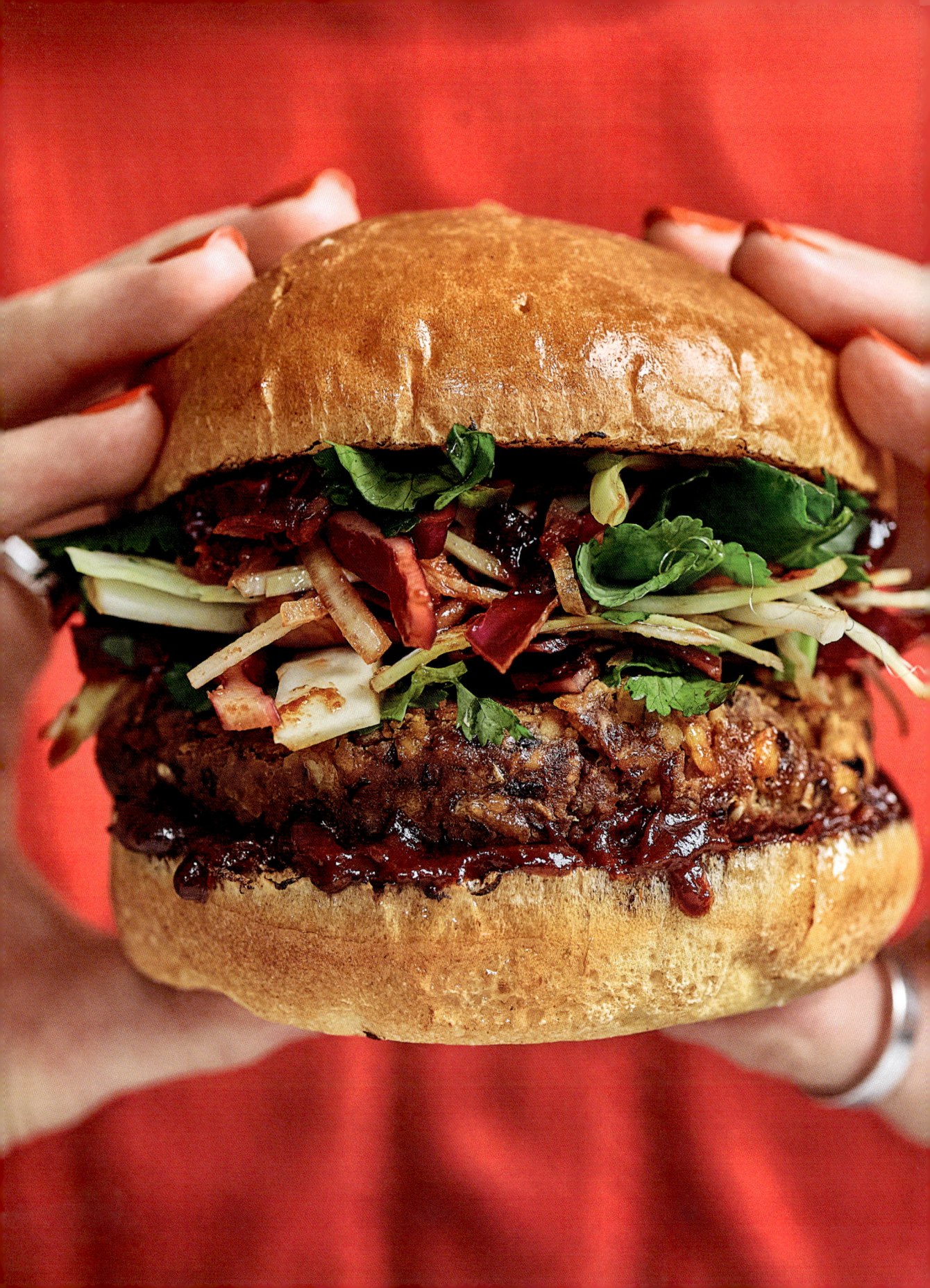

Asian-Inspired Tempeh Burger + Sesame Slaw

V
VE
DF
GF/O

This nails all the best burger qualities we crave: substantial, chunky and a good, satisfying handful when squeezed between a fluffy brioche bun. A zingy slaw brings the crunch, while a generous slather of spicy ketchup has just the right kick to wake everything up.

50 g/1¾ oz/½ cup rolled/old-fashioned oats

1 x 200-g/7-oz block tempeh

1 x 400-g/14-oz can black beans

2 garlic cloves

½ white onion

1 tbsp soy sauce

4 burger buns, lightly toasted

olive oil, for cooking

For the slaw

1 small carrot, grated

¼ red cabbage, shredded

½ white onion, thinly sliced

1 tbsp chopped coriander/cilantro

1 tsp sesame seeds

1 thumb-sized piece ginger, grated

2 garlic cloves, minced

2 tbsp soy sauce

1 tsp sesame oil

1 tbsp maple syrup

juice of 1 lime

For the spicy ketchup

2 tbsp tomato purée/paste

1 tbsp soy sauce

1 tbsp maple syrup

1 tsp crispy chilli/chili oil

Substitutions:

● **Gluten-free?** Use a gluten-free burger bun alternative. Use tamari instead of soy sauce.

1 Drain the black beans, then add to a food processor with the oats, tempeh, garlic, onion and soy sauce. Pulse until the mixture is well combined but still retains some texture – try to avoid over-processing, as you still want some bite. Shape the mixture into 4 even patties with your hands and place them on a sheet of parchment paper.

2 Heat 2 tablespoons of olive oil in a frying pan/skillet over medium heat. Gently place the patties into the pan and cook for about 6 minutes on each side until they're firm, browned and crispy all over.

3 While the patties are cooking, prepare the slaw. In a large mixing bowl, toss together the carrot, cabbage, onion, coriander and sesame seeds. In a smaller bowl, whisk together the ginger, garlic, soy sauce, sesame oil, maple syrup and lime juice. Pour the dressing over the slaw and toss until everything is evenly coated.

4 For the spicy ketchup, simply combine the tomato purée, soy sauce, maple syrup and crispy chilli oil in a small bowl, whisking together until smooth and glossy.

5 When all the components are ready, it's time to assemble the burgers. Start with a toasted bun, then spread a good dollop of spicy ketchup on the base, add the crispy patty and finish with a generous mound of sesame slaw. Serve alongside chips or a fresh salad – my smashed cucumber salad on page 112 is a tried-and-tested perfect pair!

Future you:

🍱 Cool and place in an airtight container, storing in the fridge for up to 4 days.
❄ Cool and freeze the burger patties for up to 2 months.
💧 Thaw in the fridge overnight, or at room temperature for a few hours.
🔥 Reheat by microwaving for 1–2 minutes, or in the air fryer or oven at 180°C fan/200°C/400°F/gas mark 6 for around 10 minutes until fully warmed through.

Salmon Poke Bowl

V/O
VE/O
DF
GF/O
N

During my time working in the City, I was no stranger to a poke bowl takeaway. They're colourful, wholesome, customizable, and delicious, but I wince to think how much I spent on them, especially after discovering how easy they are to make at home. Instead of the raw sushi-grade fish typically offered, my version stars a beautifully seasoned, cooked salmon fillet. Dare I say, I now prefer the flavour and textures even more this way.

baking sheet, lined (if using an oven)

air fryer basket, lined (if using an air fryer)

2 x 250-g/9-oz pouches cooked sticky rice

100 g/3½ oz/generous ⅔ cup shelled edamame beans

120 g/4 oz pineapple chunks

1 large carrot, shaved with a peeler

1 spring onion/scallion, thinly sliced

For the salmon

4 salmon fillets

grated zest and juice of ½ lemon

½ tsp garlic granules

½ tsp onion granules

½ tsp sesame seeds, plus extra to serve

salt and pepper

For the marinated beetroot

2 cooked beetroots/beets, cut into small cubes

1 tsp soy sauce

¼ tsp rice vinegar

½ tsp sesame oil

¼ tsp sesame seeds

For the dressing

2 tbsp soy sauce

1 tbsp natural peanut butter or tahini

1 tbsp honey

1 tsp sesame oil

juice of ½ lemon

1 Preheat the air fryer or oven to 200°C fan/220°C/425°F/gas mark 7.

2 Place the salmon fillets in a large bowl. Squeeze over the lemon juice, then add the lemon zest, garlic granules, onion granules, sesame seeds and a generous pinch each of salt and pepper. Gently toss to evenly coat the salmon with the seasoning.

3 Arrange the seasoned fillets in the air fryer basket or on the prepared baking sheet. Cook for 10–12 minutes, or until the salmon is cooked to your preference.

4 While the salmon is cooking, prepare the marinated beetroot. Add the beetroot to a small bowl and toss with the soy sauce, rice vinegar and sesame oil. Set aside to marinate.

5 Next, grab a small jar to make the dressing. Add in the soy sauce, peanut butter or tahini, honey, sesame oil and lemon juice. Seal with the lid and shake well until the mixture is smooth and combined.

6 Heat the rice in the microwave according to the packet instructions, usually about 2 minutes per pouch.

7 Once all the components are ready, assemble the bowls. Begin with a base of rice, then top with the cooked salmon and arrange the remaining ingredients around it. Generously drizzle the dressing over the top and scatter with sesame seeds.

Substitutions:

● **Vegetarian or vegan?** Swap the salmon for tofu, or your favourite meat-free protein alternative. ● **Gluten-free?** Use tamari instead of soy sauce.

Future you:

🥡 Cool and place in an airtight container, storing in the fridge for up to 3 days.

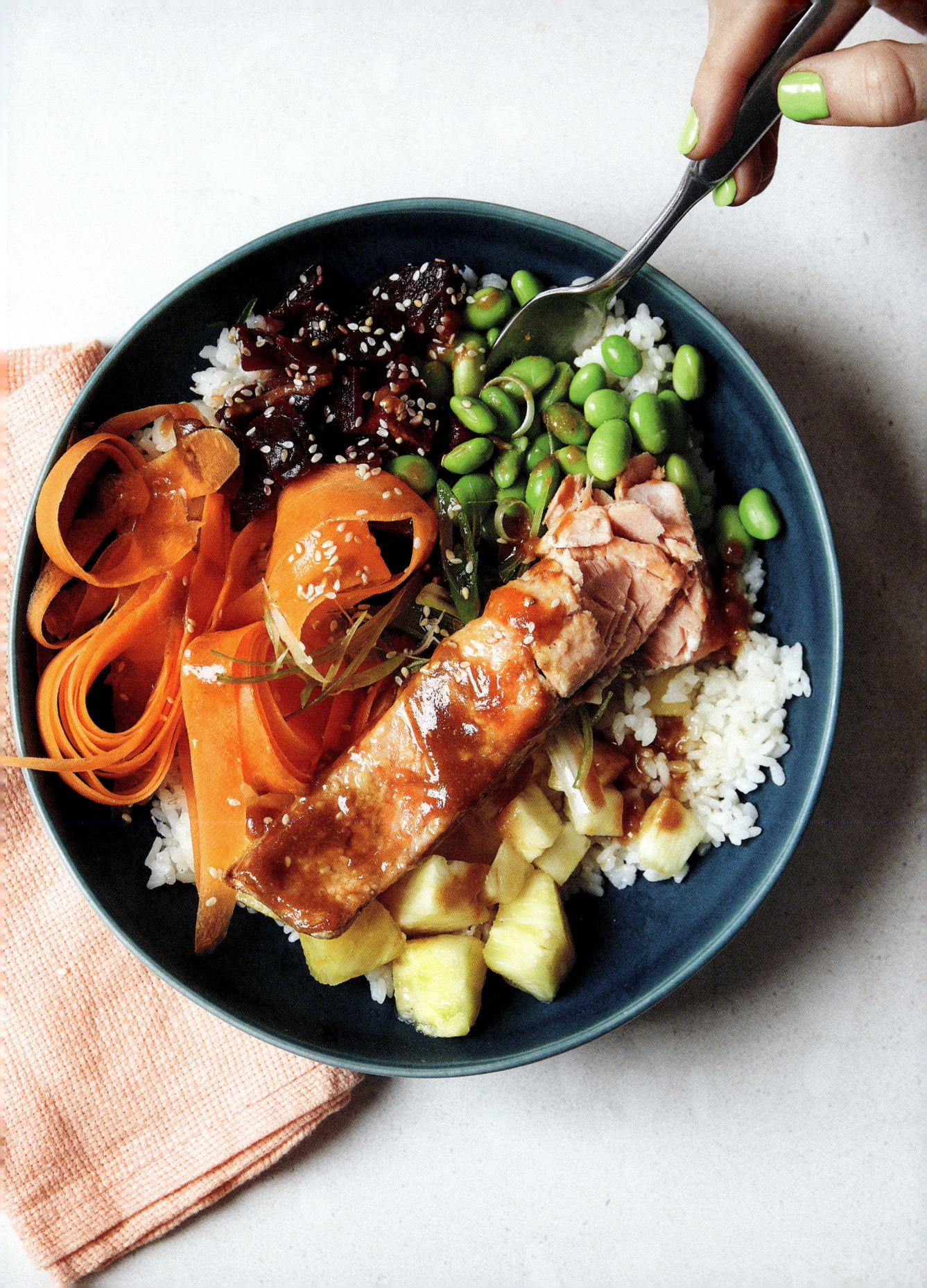

Chicken Schnitzel + Parmesan Salad

V/O
VE/O
DF/O
GF/O

This homemade chicken schnitzel is the ultimate quick weeknight dinner – comforting and delicious, but healthier than you'd expect. By pan-frying the chicken in olive oil (or air frying) instead of deep-frying, you still get that coveted golden, crispy perfection of traditional schnitzel, but without the heavy, greasy feel. It's a joy to make and eat.

2 x 140-g/5-oz skinless chicken breasts

2 heaped tbsp wholemeal/whole-wheat flour

1 egg

1 tsp Dijon mustard (optional)

50 g/1¾ oz/generous 1 cup panko breadcrumbs

½ tsp dried oregano

¼ tsp garlic granules

¼ tsp onion granules

salt and pepper

olive oil, for cooking, or olive oil spray

lemon wedges, to serve

For the salad

1 tbsp extra virgin olive oil

1 tbsp crème fraîche or sour cream

1 tsp wholegrain mustard

juice of ½ lemon

1 garlic clove, minced

1 tbsp finely chopped dill

1 romaine lettuce, roughly chopped

a handful of rocket/arugula

1 shallot, thinly sliced

15 g/½ oz/3 tbsp grated Parmesan

1   I would recommend pan-frying the schnitzels for the best, juicy results, but they will also work in an air fryer. If air frying, preheat now to 200°C/400°F.

2   Sandwich the chicken breasts between 2 pieces of parchment paper and smash them with a rolling pin to 5 mm–1 cm/¼–½-in thick, being careful not to tear through the chicken.

3   Set up your coating station with three shallow bowls. In bowl 1, add the flour. In bowl 2, crack in the egg and add the mustard (if using), then beat until no yolk remains. In the final bowl, combine the breadcrumbs with the oregano, garlic granules, onion granules and a good pinch each of salt and pepper.

4   Coat the chicken in the flour and shake off any excess. Then dip into the bowl with the egg, letting any excess drip off. Finally, press the chicken into the breadcrumbs until well coated. Repeat with the other chicken breast.

5   For pan-frying, heat 2 tablespoons of olive oil in a frying pan/skillet over medium–high heat until shimmering. Cook the schnitzels for 3 minutes on each side, or until the panko coating is golden and the chicken cooked. For air frying, spray the schnitzels with oil and cook for 10 minutes, or until the chicken is cooked through.

6   While the chicken cooks, make the salad. Add the oil, crème fraîche, mustard, lemon juice, garlic, dill, salt and pepper to a jar and shake to mix. Pour the dressing into your serving bowl and add the romaine, rocket and shallot. Toss to combine, then sprinkle with Parmesan.

7   Serve the chicken with the salad and a wedge of lemon.

Substitutions:

● **Vegetarian?** Swap the chicken for slices of tofu and use a vegetarian Italian hard cheese instead of Parmesan. ● **Vegan?** See vegetarian advice above. Swap the egg dip for dairy-free milk. Omit the crème fraîche and Parmesan. ● **Gluten-free?** Use gluten-free flour and breadcrumbs.

Future you:

🍱 Cool and place in an airtight container, storing in the fridge up to 3 days.

🔥 Pop the chicken in the oven or air fryer on a moderate heat (180°C fan/200°C/400°F/gas mark 6) for 10–15 minutes until piping hot in the middle.

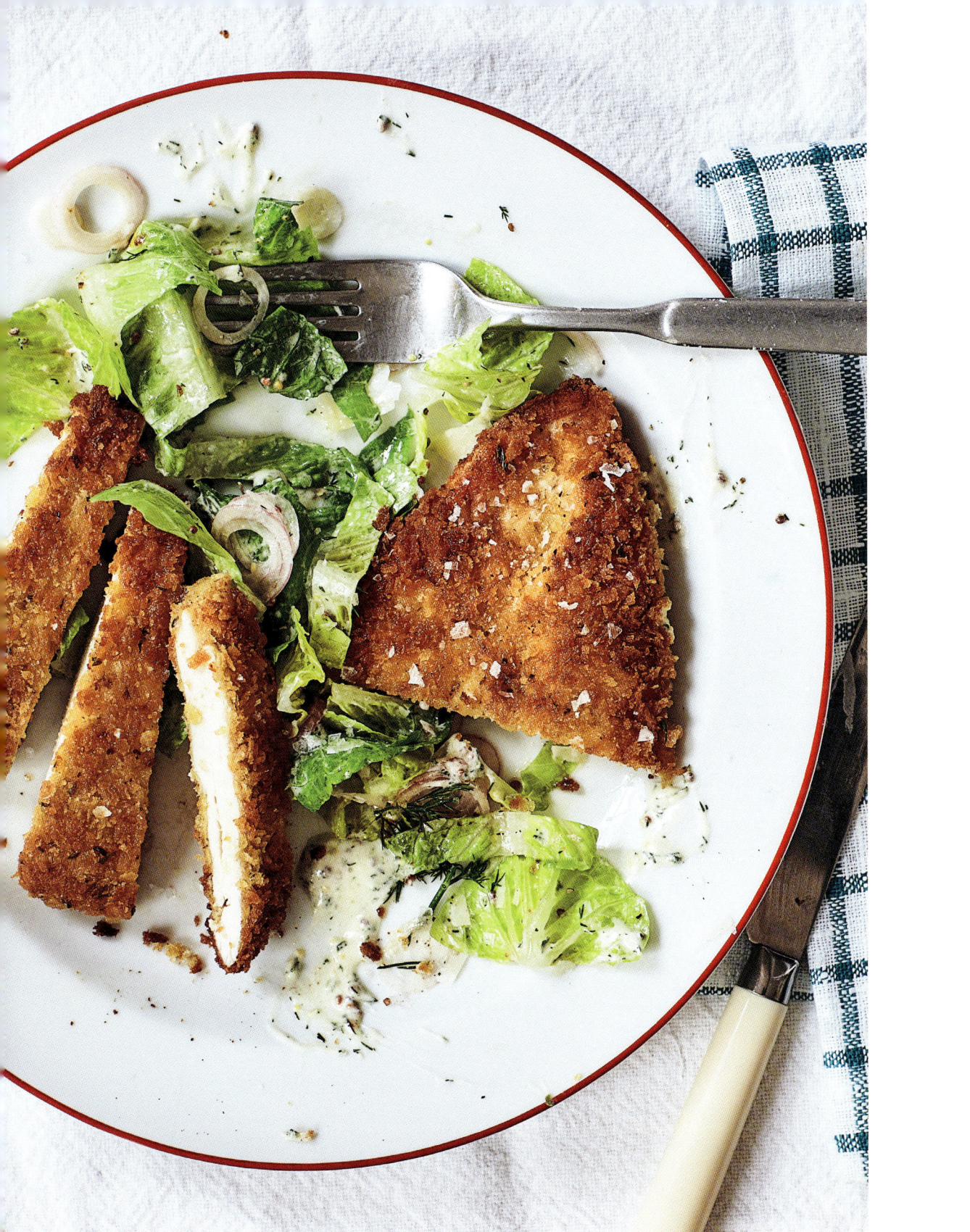

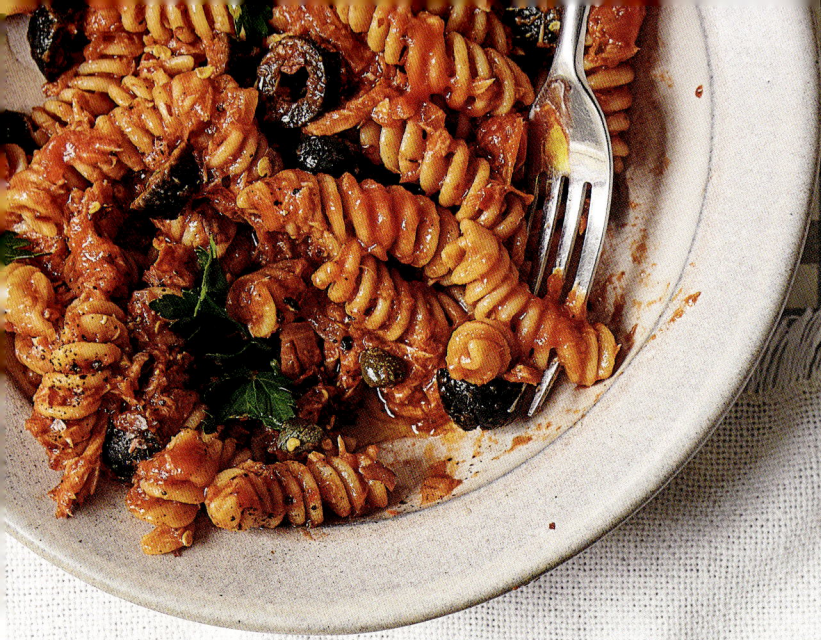

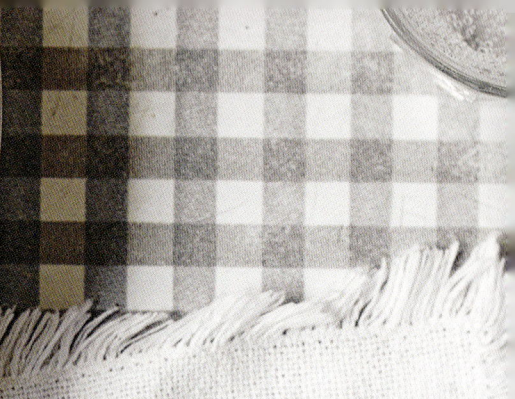

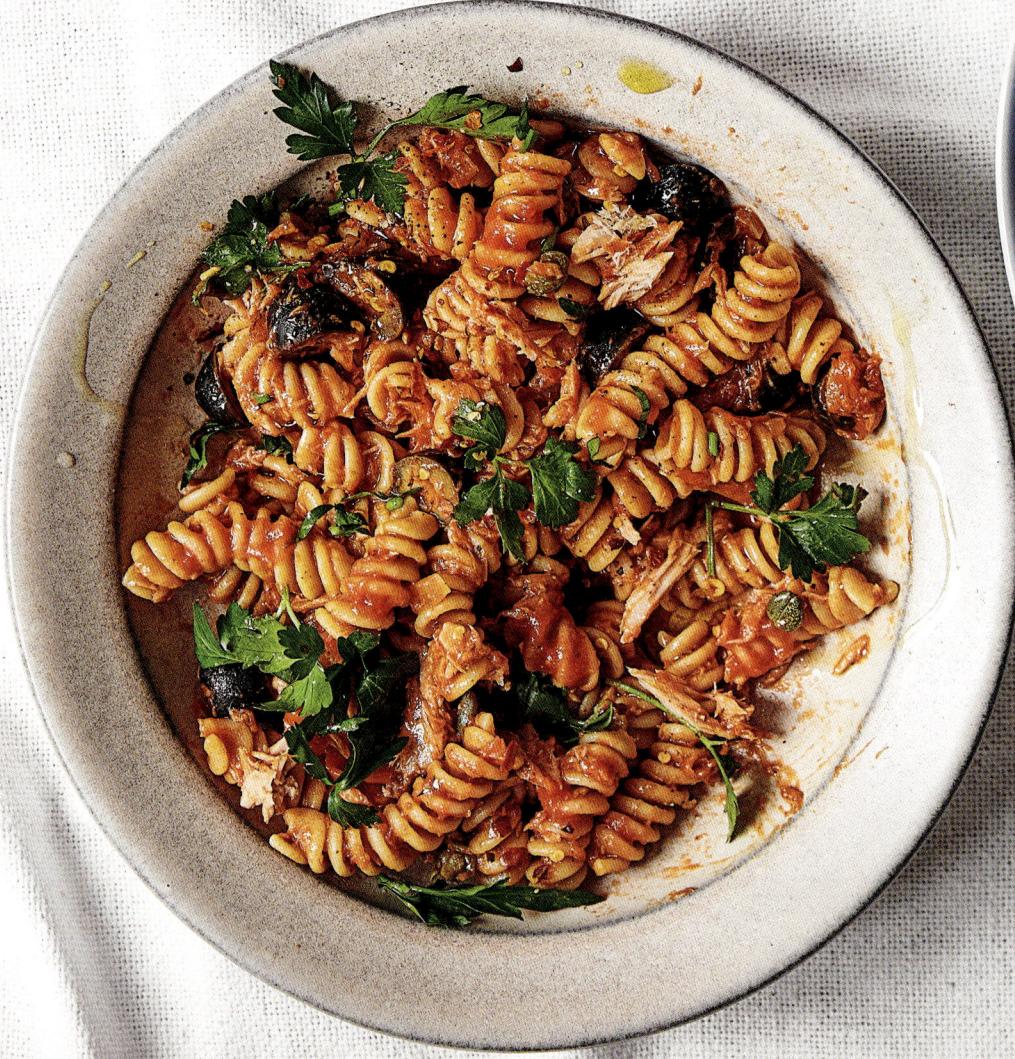

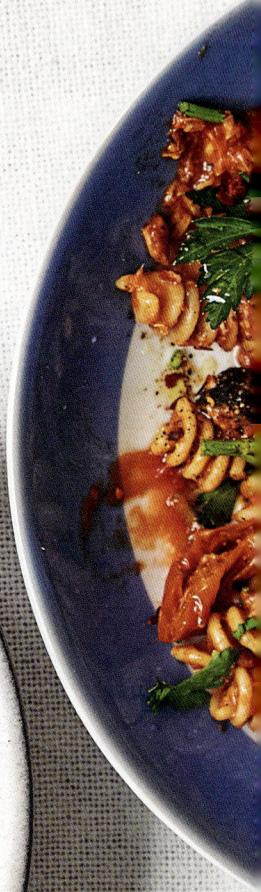

Spicy Tuna Pasta

V/O
VE/O
DF
GF/O

Like so many of my happy kitchen accidents, this was born from one of those night-before-the-food-shop cupboard raids. I started with a pack of pasta and got to work from there: a jar of sun-dried tomatoes – yum; herbs and spices, of course; ooh, a few forlorn olives that need using too; a seemingly endless jar of capers I've had for years; and a carton of passata for the base, perfect. But then came the question of protein. With half of the cupboard's contents now scattered across the kitchen, a can of tuna emerged like some kind of beacon from heaven. Sorted. And so, this happy accident came to life.

1 onion, finely diced
4 garlic cloves, minced
250 g/9 oz whole-wheat pasta, I like fusilli here
60 g/2 oz/scant ⅔ cup sun-dried tomatoes, roughly chopped
½–1 tsp crushed chilli flakes/hot red pepper flakes
1 tsp dried oregano
500 g/1 lb 2 oz passata/strained tomatoes
100 g/3½ oz/1 cup pitted black olives, halved
1 tbsp capers
2 x 145-g/5-oz cans tuna chunks
salt and pepper
chopped parsley, to garnish
olive oil, for cooking and to serve

1 In a large frying pan/skillet, heat 1 tablespoon of olive oil over medium heat. Sweat the onion for 5 minutes until completely softened, then add in the garlic and cook for a further minute.

2 Fill a large pot with boiling water and add a pinch of salt. Add your pasta and let it cook until al dente, following the packet instructions.

3 Going back to the pan, add in the sun-dried tomatoes, chilli flakes (saving some back to garnish) and oregano. Cook for 2 minutes, then pour in the passata, olives and capers. Give everything a good stir, season to taste with salt and pepper, then reduce the heat slightly and let the sauce simmer for a few more minutes until thickened.

4 Stir the tuna into the pan, breaking it up gently with your spatula until it is evenly distributed throughout the sauce. Turn the heat to low until the pasta is ready to add in.

5 Once your pasta is cooked, reserve a splash of the starchy pasta water before draining the rest. Add the cooked pasta to the pan with the sauce. Pour in a little of the reserved pasta water, adding more as needed to reach your desired sauce consistency. Toss everything together until the pasta is well coated with the tuna and sauce.

6 Dish out the pasta into bowls and garnish with parsley and extra chilli flakes. I like to serve it with a drizzle of good-quality olive oil.

Substitutions:

● **Vegan or vegetarian?** Omit the tuna entirely, or substitute for a meat-free protein alternative. ● **No passata?** Canned chopped tomatoes will also work, but make sure they are good quality. ● **Gluten-free?** Use a gluten-free pasta alternative.

Future you:

🍲 Cool and place in an airtight container, storing in the fridge for up to 5 days.
❄ Cool and freeze for up to 2 months.
💧 Thaw in the fridge overnight, or at room temperature for a few hours.
🔥 Enjoy cold, or reheat in the microwave for 2 minutes, stirring halfway.

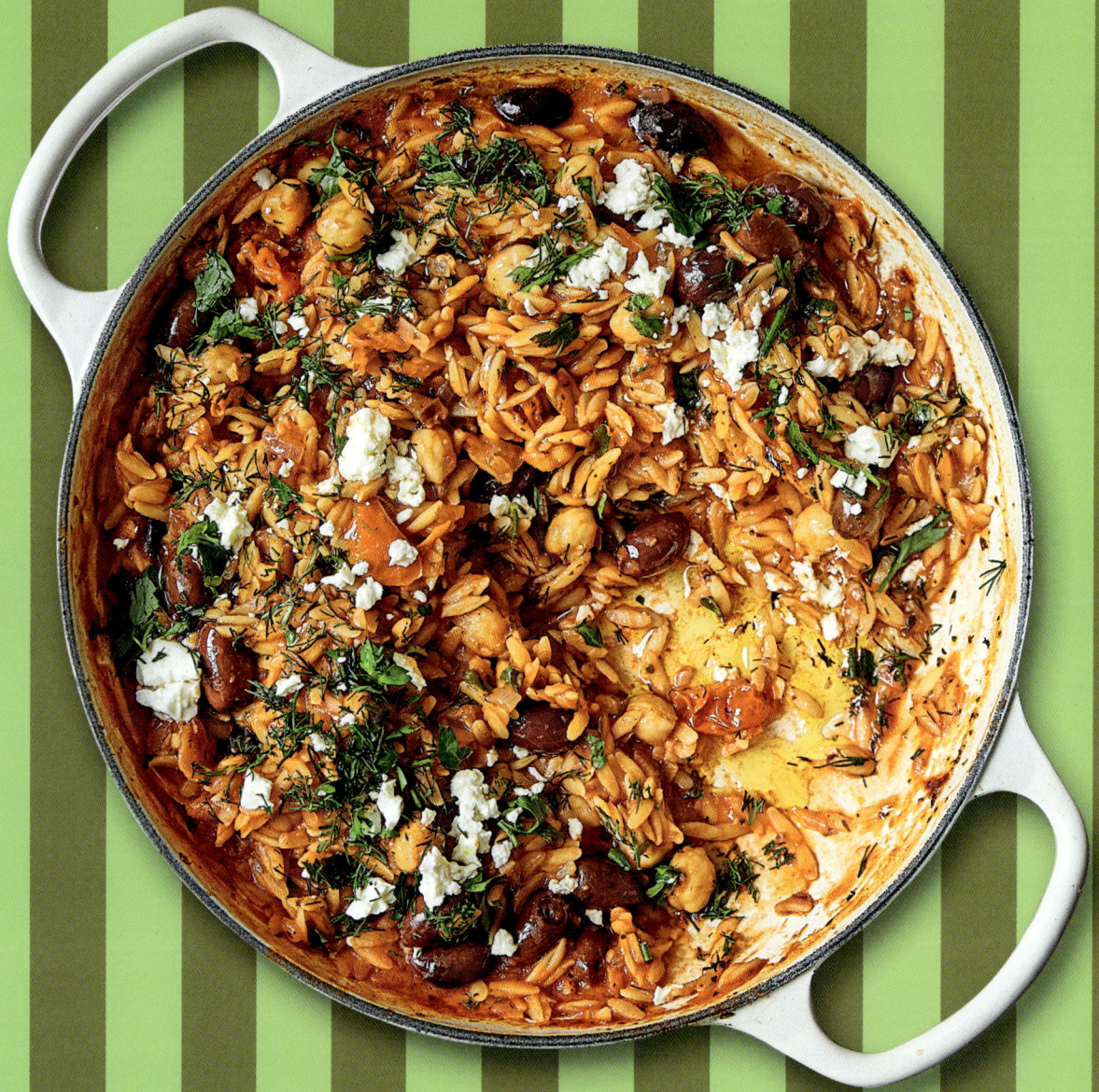

One-Pan Winners

Minimum Effort and Mess, Maximum Taste

One-pan meals aren't just about preventing faff in the kitchen and saving time on washing up (although we can all agree that's what we love about them the most!), they're also about maximizing flavour in minimal time. Often cooking all the ingredients together allows the flavours to mingle and develop throughout the process, creating dishes that are remarkably complex and super tasty.

Harissa Tofu + Chickpea Frying Pan Filo Pie

V
VE
DF
GF/O

Making a pie in a pan is my definition of 'working smart, not hard'. It's WOW enough for a dinner party, but easy enough for any weeknight. Plus, you can take this technique and let your imagination run wild. How about creamy chicken with puff pastry (take inspo from page 134) or tofu curry with shortcrust pastry (page 114)? The pie world is your oyster!

baking sheet, lined (if using an oven)

air fryer basket, lined (if using an air fryer)

1 x 450-g/1-lb block extra-firm tofu

1 tbsp cornflour/cornstarch

1 onion, finely diced

4 garlic cloves, minced

2 carrots, finely diced

1 tsp ground coriander

1 tsp ground cumin

2 tbsp rose harissa paste

2 x 400-g/14-oz cans chickpeas/garbanzo beans, drained

1 x 400-g/14-oz can chopped tomatoes

250 ml/9 fl oz/1 cup vegetable stock

50 g/1¾ oz/scant 1 cup spinach

30 g/1 oz/scant ¼ cup dried apricots, finely chopped

4 filo pastry sheets

1 tsp za'atar

salt and pepper

olive oil, for cooking and brushing

1   Preheat the air fryer or oven to 200°C fan/220°C/425°F/gas mark 7.

2   Press out any water from the tofu (this will vary depending on the brand you use), tear it into bite-sized chunks, and toss in a mixing bowl with the cornflour and a good pinch of salt and pepper until coated.

3   In a deep oven-proof frying pan/skillet, heat 1 tablespoon of olive oil over medium heat. Sauté the onion, garlic, and carrots for about 5 minutes, then add the coriander, cumin, harissa and chickpeas. Cook for a couple of minutes, then stir in the chopped tomatoes and vegetable stock. Season everything well with salt and pepper, bring to a boil, then reduce to a simmer. Gradually add the spinach, letting it wilt before adding more. Then, cover the pan and simmer for about 5 more minutes, stirring occasionally.

4   Add the cooked tofu and the chopped apricots to the pan. Give everything a good stir and add a splash of water if the mixture looks too thick. If you're using an air fryer, transfer the mixture to a pie dish that fits the basket.

5   Brush each filo sheet with a thin layer of oil, scrunch them up, and arrange to cover the filling completely. Sprinkle za'atar and a pinch of salt on top.

6   Place the frying pan, uncovered, into the oven for 10 minutes, or until the filo is golden and crispy. If air frying, cook for 8 minutes, until the pastry is crisp on top.

Substitutions:

● **No filo?** Use ready-rolled puff or shortcrust pastry instead. ● **No za'atar?** Use a mixture of dried oregano, dried thyme and sesame seeds instead. ● **Gluten-free?** Use gluten-free pastry instead.

Future you:

🍱 Cool and place in an airtight container, storing in the fridge for up to 4 days.
❄ Freeze the pie filling (not the filo) for up to 2 months.
💧 Thaw in the fridge overnight, or in the microwave on low power.
🔥 Reheat in a preheated oven or air fryer at 180°C fan/200°C/400°F/gas mark 6 for 5–10 minutes until hot and crispy.

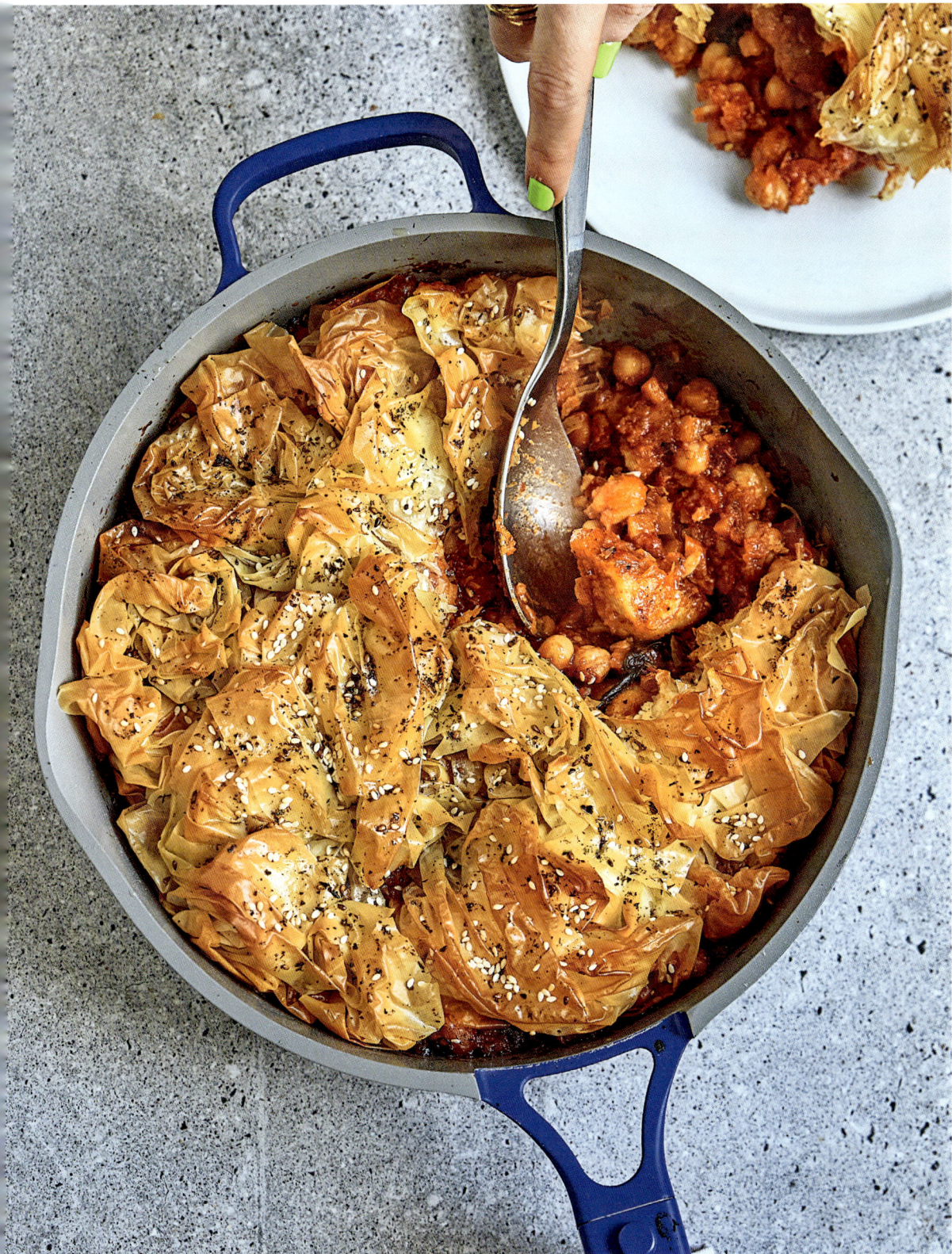

Creamy Mushroom + Tarragon Tagliatelle with Chicken

(V/O)
(DF/O)
(GF/O)

This one's inspired by a favourite dinner that my dad used to cook for me (and still does!). It's informally known in our family as "creamy chicken" – a stroganoff of sorts that I've reimagined here as a saucy pasta dish. It's probably the meal I've eaten most in my life, and I still vividly remember sitting in the kitchen at 18, notebook in hand, furiously scribbling down Dad's step-by-step instructions to make his infamous recipe, determined to take it with me to University. Naturally, I made it over and over again – broken up with the odd pesto pasta, of course – during those first few months away. So, to me, this dish has always felt like home, and I'm so happy to share a piece of that comfort with you here.

2 x 180-g/6-oz skinless chicken breasts
1 onion, finely diced
2 garlic cloves, minced
200 g/7 oz chestnut mushrooms, thinly sliced
1 tbsp plain/all-purpose flour
500 ml/18 fl oz/2 cups chicken stock
150 g/5½ oz/¾ cup crème fraîche or sour cream
1 heaped tsp wholegrain mustard
a handful of roughly chopped tarragon, plus extra to serve
juice of ½ lemon (optional)
500 g/1 lb 2 oz fresh tagliatelle
salt and pepper
olive oil, for cooking
grated Italian hard cheese, to serve
any side salad, to serve

1 Using a sharp knife, butterfly the chicken breasts by slicing them in half horizontally, taking care not to cut all the way through, so you can open them up like a book. Season both sides with salt and pepper.

2 Heat 2 tablespoons of olive oil in a large, deep frying pan/skillet over medium–high heat. Cook the chicken for 4–5 minutes on each side, or until they have colour and are cooked through. Transfer the chicken to a clean plate or wooden board, and cover with foil to keep warm.

3 Lower the heat to medium and give the pan another drizzle of oil if needed. Add the onion and garlic, and cook for around 3 minutes until softened. Then turn the heat up slightly and add the mushrooms. Cook for another 3 minutes until the mushrooms release their moisture and start to brown. Sprinkle in the flour and stir briefly until it dissolves.

4 Deglaze the pan by pouring in the chicken stock, using a wooden spoon to scrape up any browned bits from the bottom. Stir in the crème fraîche, mustard, tarragon and a generous amount of black pepper. Reduce the heat to medium–low and simmer for a couple of minutes until the sauce thickens. If you're a citrus fan like me, add a squeeze of lemon juice now, too.

5 Add the fresh pasta to the pan. Grab some tongs and carefully lift the pasta over itself until every strand is coated in the sauce. Let that cook for 4 minutes, stirring occasionally until the pasta is al dente.

6 Remove the pan from the heat, slice the chicken into strips, and place the chicken on top of the pasta. Garnish everything with fresh tarragon and a good amount of grated cheese, and serve alongside your favourite side salad.

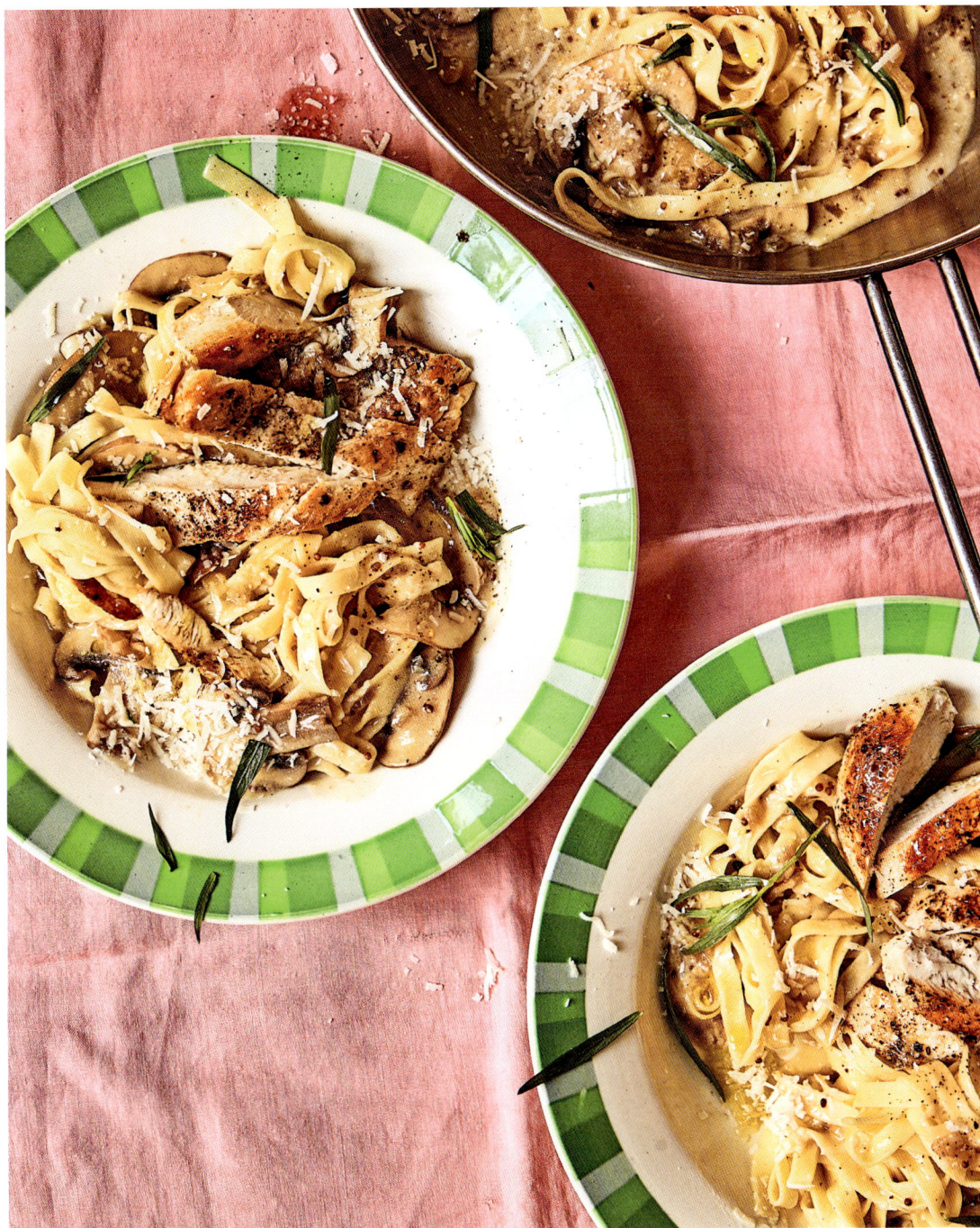

Substitutions:

● **Dairy-free?** Use a dairy-free cream alternative. Soy cream works great. Omit the cheese. ● **Vegetarian?** Use tofu instead of chicken (cook everything in the same way) and vegetable stock instead of chicken stock. ● **Gluten-free?** Use gluten-free pasta (best to boil separately). ● **No fresh tarragon?** Dried tarragon also works, or parsley is lovely, too.

Future you:

🥡 Cool and place in an airtight container, storing in the fridge for up to 3 days.

🔥 Add a splash of water if needed and warm up in the microwave for 2–3 minutes until piping hot.

Citrusy Chicken Rice with Fennel

(V/O)
(VE/O)
(DF/O)
(GF)

My hack for one-pan rice dishes is to look out for 'easy cook' rice at the supermarket. It's rice that's been part-cooked, then dried after milling, meaning it's ready in around 10-15 minutes; about half the time of regular rice. It's also less starchy, so you get perfectly fluffy grains every time with no need to wash them first. Work smart, not hard, remember?

640 g/1 lb 7 oz skinless, boneless chicken thighs

grated zest and juice of 1 lemon

juice of ½ orange

1 tbsp Dijon mustard

1 garlic clove, minced

1 tsp dried thyme

1 fennel bulb (reserve the fronds for the garnish), stalks removed and bulb cut into wedges

1 onion, finely diced

2 garlic cloves, minced

a handful of pitted green olives, halved

salt and pepper

olive oil, for cooking

For the rice

250 g/9 oz easy-cook basmati rice

600 ml/1 pint/2½ cups chicken stock

juice of ½ orange

juice of ½ lemon

a handful of roughly chopped parsley

20 g/¾ oz/scant ¼ cup crumbled feta, to serve

1 Pat the chicken dry with a paper towel, then place in a mixing bowl. Add the lemon zest, lemon juice, orange juice, mustard, garlic, thyme and a good pinch each of salt and pepper. Toss the chicken to coat it evenly in the marinade.

2 Heat 2 tablespoons of olive oil in a large lidded frying pan/skillet over medium–high heat. Once the oil is hot, carefully add in the chicken thighs, along with any residual marinade juices. Cook the thighs for 4–5 minutes on each side until they are nicely browned and about 90 per cent cooked through. Remove the chicken from the pan and set aside.

3 In the same pan, re-oiling if necessary, sauté the fennel before adding the onion and garlic, cooking for 3 minutes until softened.

4 Stir through the olives and rice until the rice becomes well coated with the oil. Then pour in the stock, along with the orange and lemon juices, and season. Bring the mixture to the boil, then reduce the heat and simmer for 8 minutes, stirring occasionally to prevent sticking.

5 After the initial 8 minutes of cooking time, the rice should be more than halfway cooked. Now, you can stir in the parsley. If the mixture starts to look too dry at this point, add an additional 100 ml/3½ fl oz/6½ tablespoons of water from the kettle. Nestle the chicken thighs back into the pan, cover and cook for another 5 minutes, or until the liquid is absorbed, the rice is tender, and the chicken is fully cooked through.

6 Top with crumbled feta and garnish with the reserved fennel fronds.

Substitutions:

● **Vegetarian?** Swap the chicken for tofu, or your favourite meat-free protein alternative, and replace the chicken stock with vegetable stock. ● **Vegan?** Follow the vegetarian advice above and omit the feta. ● **Dairy-free?** Omit the feta.

Future you:

🍲 Cool and place in an airtight container, storing in the fridge for up to 3 days.
❄ Cool and freeze for up to 1 month.
💧 Thaw in the fridge overnight.
🔥 Microwave for 2–3 minutes, stirring halfway through, until piping hot. Cooked rice must only be reheated once.

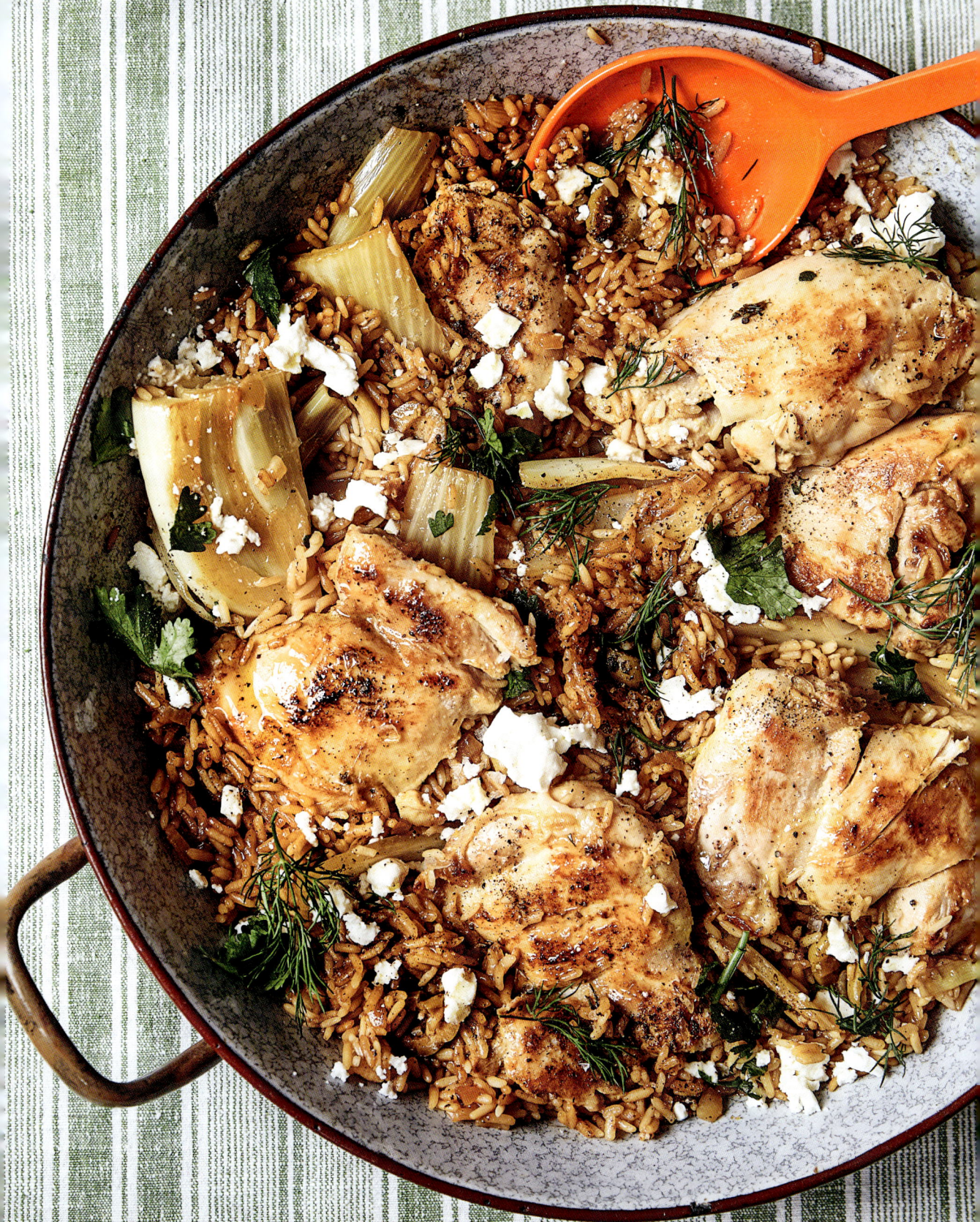

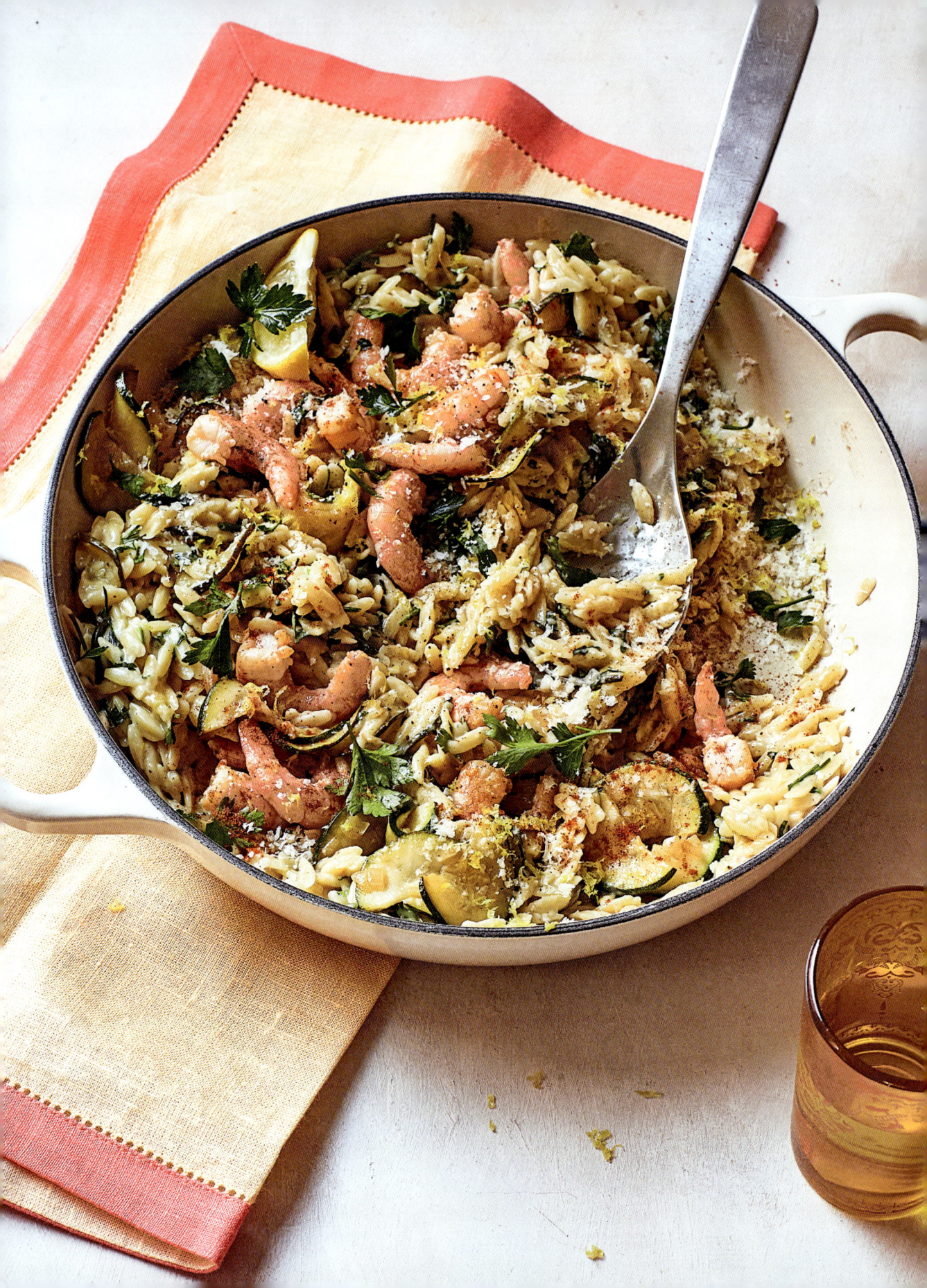

Garlic + Parmesan Prawn Orzotto

(DF/O)
(GF/O)

I've dubbed this orzotto because, you guessed it, it's like a risotto, but made with orzo pasta instead of rice, which is not only easier but, in my humble opinion, tastier too. The orzo cooks right in the garlicky stock, soaking up all the deliciousness accumulated in the pan.

400 g/14 oz raw king prawns/jumbo shrimp

4 garlic cloves, minced

1 onion, finely diced

1 courgette/zucchini, sliced thinly into half moons

250 g/9 oz orzo

1 litre/34 fl oz/4 cups vegetable stock

1 heaped tbsp low-fat crème fraîche or sour cream

1 tbsp roughly chopped parsley, plus extra to serve

juice of ½ lemon

1 tbsp grated Italian hard cheese, plus extra to serve

salt and pepper

olive oil, for cooking

lemon wedges, to serve

1　Heat 1 tablespoon of olive oil in a lidded frying pan/skillet over medium–high heat. Season the prawns with salt, pepper and 1 minced garlic clove. Add the prawns to the pan and fry them for 2 minutes on each side, or until just cooked through and beautifully charred on the outside. Remove from the pan and set aside.

2　Into the same pan, re-oiling if necessary, add the onion, remaining minced garlic cloves and the courgette moons. Cook over medium heat for 5 minutes until the courgette has softened.

3　Tip in the orzo, give everything a good stir to coat the pasta in the mixture, then pour in three-quarters of the stock. Use the back of your spoon to scrape up any browned bits from the bottom of the pan. Bring it to the boil, then cover and reduce the heat to a simmer for 6-10 minutes, according to your orzo's packet instructions. Remove the lid and give the pasta a stir every few minutes to ensure the orzo doesn't stick to the bottom of the pan. If and when the mixture starts to look a little dry, add in the remainder of the stock.

4　After the 6-10 minutes have passed, remove the lid and raise the heat. Cook, uncovered, for a final few minutes, stirring frequently, until the liquid is mostly absorbed and the orzo al dente.

5　Take the pan off the heat and stir through the crème fraîche, parsley, lemon juice and grated cheese. Season to taste with salt and pepper. Return the prawns to the pan and stir them in.

6　Serve the orzo with a sprinkle of parsley and grated cheese and a lemon wedge on the side.

Substitutions:

● **No prawns?** Sub for 2 chicken breasts, cut into small chunks (method stays the same). ● **Dairy-free?** Use soy cream in place of the crème fraîche and omit the Italian hard cheese. ● **Gluten-free?** Use a gluten-free pasta alternative.

Future you:

☗ Cool and place in an airtight container, storing in the fridge for up to 3 days.
🔥 Reheat either in the microwave or on the hob/stovetop until piping hot. Add a splash of water if the mixture has become too thick.

Honey-Mustard Salmon Traybake

(V/O)
(VE/O)
(DF/O)

Once all the chopping is out of the way, all you need to do with this traybake is chuck it in a dish and let the oven (or air fryer) do the rest of the hard work. You can get back to your evening, only returning halfway through to coat everything in an easy honey-mustard glaze.

large deep roasting tin, lined (if using an oven)

air fryer basket, lined (if using an air fryer)

750 g/1 lb 10 oz baby potatoes

1 red onion, cut into chunks

1 large broccoli head, cut into florets

1 tsp garlic granules

4 salmon fillets

200 g/7 oz vine cherry tomatoes

25 g/1 oz/⅓ cup grated Italian hard cheese

juice of 1 lemon

salt and pepper

olive oil, for cooking

roughly chopped parsley, to garnish

For the glaze

1 tbsp wholegrain mustard

½ tbsp Dijon mustard

2 tbsp honey or maple syrup

1 Preheat the air fryer or oven to 210°C fan/230°C/450°F/gas mark 8.

2 Slice the potatoes in half, or quarter any larger ones to ensure they cook through evenly (the smaller they are, the quicker they'll cook). Put the potatoes in the prepared roasting tin or air fryer basket, along with the onion and broccoli. Drizzle over 2 tablespoons of olive oil and season with the garlic granules and a good pinch each of salt and pepper. Toss everything together to coat evenly, then place in the oven or air fryer for 15 minutes.

3 While the vegetables roast, prepare the glaze simply by mixing the mustards and honey or maple syrup together in a small bowl.

4 After the initial 15 minutes of roasting time, remove the tin from the oven or air fryer and pour most of the glaze over the vegetables, reserving a spoonful or so. Toss the vegetables to coat, re-arrange them in an even layer, then place the salmon fillets over the top and nestle the cherry tomatoes around them. Brush the salmon fillets with the reserved glaze and season with a pinch each of salt and pepper.

5 Return to the oven or air fryer and roast for a final 15 minutes, or until the salmon is cooked through and the glaze has caramelized.

6 Remove from the oven and sprinkle the cheese over the top. Finish with a good squeeze of lemon juice and garnish with chopped parsley.

Substitutions:

● **Vegetarian?** Sub the salmon for extra-firm tofu or your favourite meat-free protein alternative. ● **Vegan?** Follow vegetarian advice above. Omit the cheese. ● **Dairy-free?** Omit the cheese. ● **Not a fan of salmon?** Use any of the following 'meaty' fish instead: tuna, swordfish, halibut, basa or cod.

Future you:

🍲 Cool and place in an airtight container, storing in the fridge for up to 3 days.
🔥 Cooked salmon is always best eaten on the day it's made. However, if you do wish to reheat, place the salmon on a tray in the oven on a low heat (around 140°C fan/160°C/325°F/gas mark 3) until warmed through. The other components can be reheated in the oven too, or the microwave.

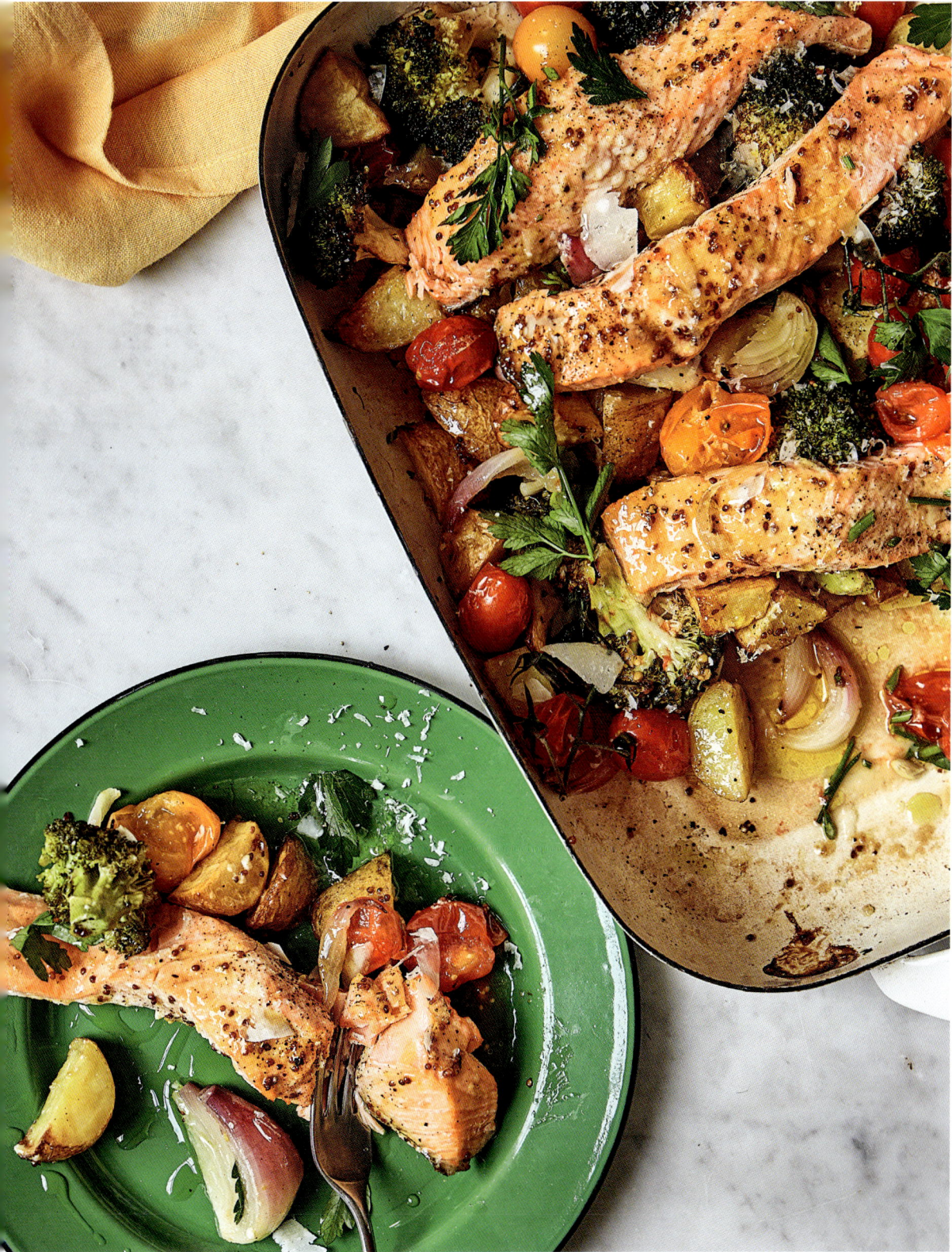

Smoky Harissa Beans + Cod

V/O
VE/O
DF/O
GF/O

Beans, especially butter beans, had a big moment last year, and like many others, I hopped on the trend and fell in love with using them in my cooking. Not only do they up the nutritional ante of any dish, but they add gorgeous texture and interest. That said, beans and cod are a little bland on their own, so they're the perfect pair for bold flavours like harissa, sun-dried tomatoes, olives and a splash of balsamic. Here, these big, punchy ingredients meld into a rich, tangy tomato sauce, while the cod steams gently in the same pan as everything deepens in flavour together. Just serve with a hunk of crusty bread to mop up every last bit of the sauce, and dive in.

½ onion, finely diced

2 garlic cloves, minced

1 red (bell) pepper, diced

125 g/4 oz cherry tomatoes, halved

50 g/1¾ oz/½ cup sun-dried tomatoes, roughly chopped

1 heaped tbsp rose harissa paste

1 tsp smoked paprika

1 tsp dried oregano

1 x 400-g/14-oz can plum tomatoes

1 x 400-g/14-oz can butter beans/ lima beans, drained

50 g/1¾ oz/½ cup pitted Kalamata olives

1 tbsp balsamic vinegar

2 skinless cod fillets

½ lemon, cut into slices

salt and pepper

olive oil, for cooking

a handful of roughly chopped dill

crusty bread, to serve

1 Heat 1 tablespoon of olive oil in a deep lidded frying pan/skillet over medium heat. Add the onion, garlic and pepper, and cook for 2–3 minutes until they begin to soften. Stir in the cherry tomatoes, sun-dried tomatoes, harissa paste, paprika and oregano, and let everything cook for another 3–4 minutes until the cherry tomato skins begin to break down.

2 Squash down the cherry tomatoes with the back of your spatula to release some of their juices, then tip in the can of plum tomatoes and add the drained butter beans, olives and balsamic vinegar. Use your spatula to break up the plum tomatoes a little, then season everything generously with salt and pepper. Bring the mixture to the boil, then reduce the heat and simmer for a couple of minutes until thickened.

3 Nestle the cod fillets into the pan, season them with salt and pepper, and lay 1 or 2 lemon slices on top of each fillet. Cover the pan with a lid and cook for 8–10 minutes, or until the cod is cooked all the way through and flakes easily with a fork.

4 Once the cod is cooked, sprinkle the fresh dill across the top and serve the dish alongside a generous chunk of crusty bread to mop up the sauce.

Substitutions:

● **Vegetarian or vegan?** Swap the cod for cubes of pan-fried smoked tofu. ● **No cod?** Use any other boneless fish such as haddock or basa. ● **Dairy-free?** Use a dairy-free feta alternative, or omit. ● **Gluten-free?** Serve with gluten-free bread.

Future you:

☐ Cool and place in an airtight container, storing in the fridge for up to 2 days.
🔥 Either pop the portion into the microwave for 2–3 minutes until piping hot, or warm through over low–medium heat the hob/stovetop.

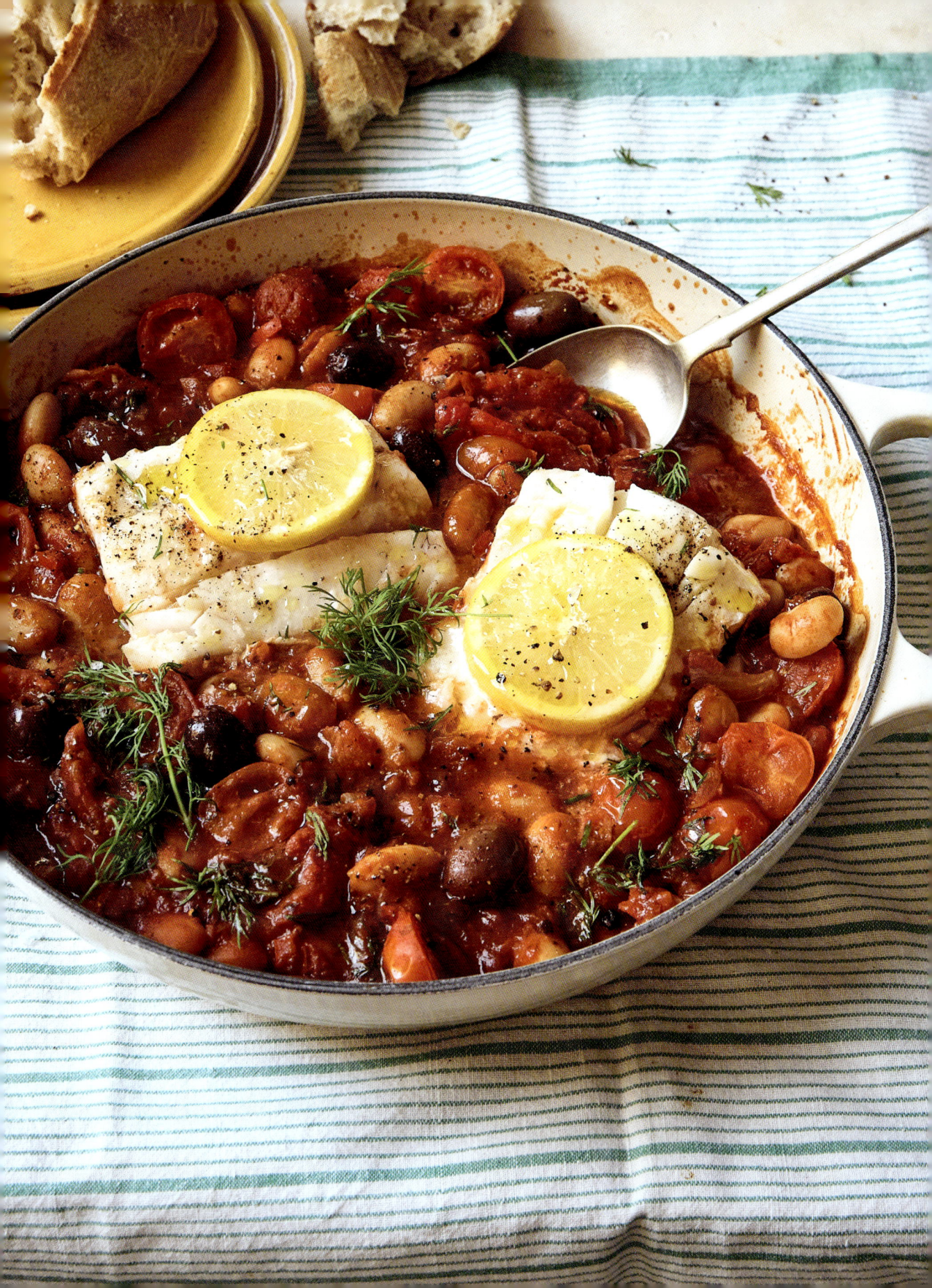

Green Goddess Gnocchi

(V)
(VE/O)
(DF/O)
(GF/O)

I'm all about speedy, low-effort meals that deliver big flavours, and this one does just that. It's vibrant, creamy, and dressed in a pesto-esque sauce that, alongside the burrata, feels effortlessly luxurious. Best of all, though, it's sneakily packed with good-for-you ingredients. Enjoy it as a hearty main, or pair it with a protein source for a satisfying side.

100 g/3½ oz/¾ cup frozen peas

50 g/1¾ oz/scant 1 cup spinach

2 spring onions/scallions

1 garlic clove

60 g/2 oz/½ cup crème fraîche or sour cream

20 g/¾ oz/¼ cup grated Italian hard cheese

15 g/½ oz basil (about half a bunch)

15 g/½ oz parsley (about half a bunch)

30 g/1 oz/scant ⅓ cup pitted green olives

juice of ½ lemon

500 g/1 lb 2 oz fresh gnocchi

1 burrata

salt and pepper

olive oil, for cooking

crispy chilli/chilli oil, to serve

For the breadcrumbs

30 g/1 oz/⅔ cup panko breadcrumbs

½ tsp garlic granules

½ tsp onion granules

½ tsp dried rosemary

1   Place the peas and spinach in a microwave-safe dish, cover and microwave for 2 minutes until the peas are tender and the spinach has wilted.

2   In a blender (not a food processor, as it won't achieve the same silky texture), combine the peas, spinach, spring onions, garlic, crème fraîche, cheese, basil, parsley, olives, lemon juice, a generous pinch of salt and pepper and 100 ml/6½ tablespoons water. Blend for 1–2 minutes, until completely smooth and vibrant green.

3   Heat a drizzle of olive oil in a frying pan/skillet over medium heat. Add the breadcrumbs, garlic granules, onion granules, dried rosemary and a good pinch each of salt and pepper. Toast the breadcrumbs for a couple of minutes, stirring frequently to ensure they turn golden and crisp without burning. Transfer to a bowl and set aside.

4   Lower the heat and add the gnocchi directly into the pan. Pour in the green sauce and stir to coat the gnocchi. Simmer for 4–5 minutes, stirring occasionally, until the gnocchi is cooked. If the sauce thickens up too much, add a splash of water to loosen.

5   Remove the pan from the heat and tear the burrata over the top, letting it melt into the sauce. Scatter three-quarters of the toasted breadcrumbs over the dish, and finally drizzle with chilli oil.

6   Place the pan in the middle of the table, along with the bowl of extra breadcrumbs for topping up as needed.

Substitutions:

● **Vegan or dairy-free?** Use dairy-free alternatives for burrata, Italian hard cheese and crème fraîche. ● **Gluten-free?** Ensure your gnocchi is gluten-free. ● **No burrata?** Omit, or substitute for regular mozzarella. ● **No gnocchi?** Use any fresh pasta as an alternative.

Future you:

🍲 Cool and place in an airtight container, storing in the fridge for up to 5 days.
❄ Cool and freeze for up to 2 months.
💧 Thaw in the fridge overnight, or at room temperature for a few hours.
🔥 Warm in the microwave for 2–3 minutes, stirring halfway, until piping hot.

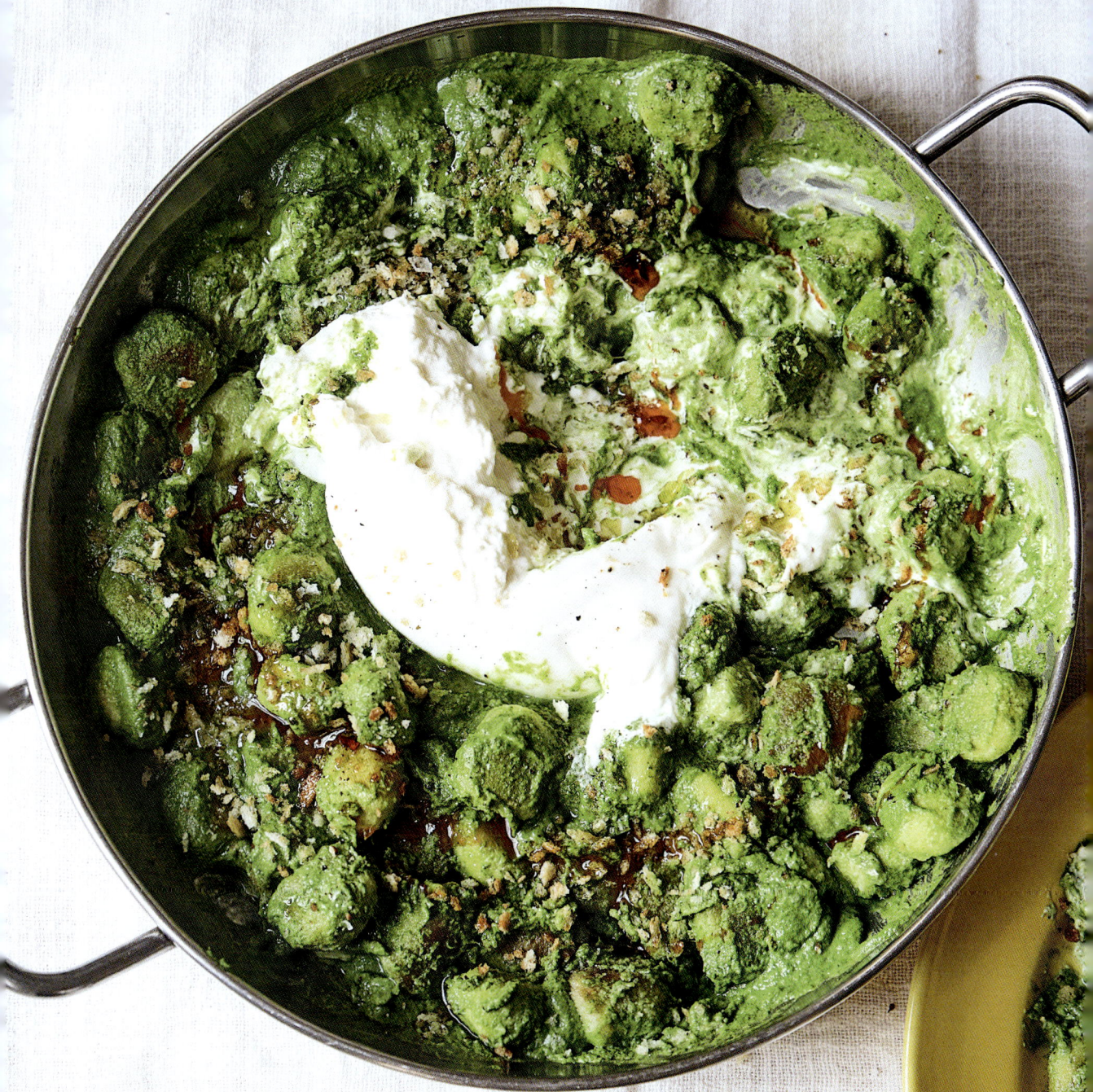

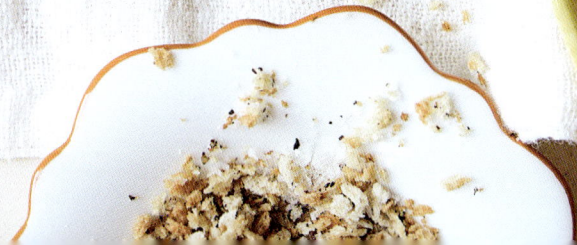

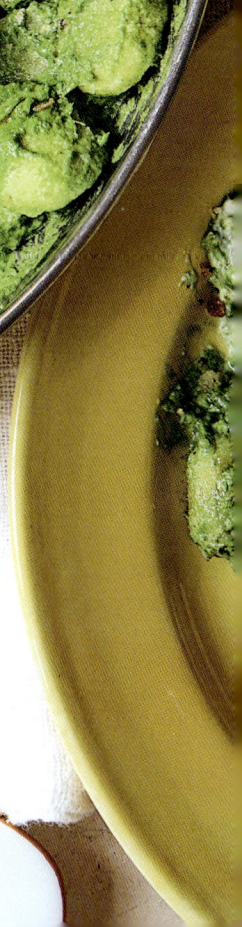

Thai Green Curry Rice

V/O
VE/O
DF
GF

There are two types of people in this world: those who like their curry and rice side-by-side, and those who stir it all together until every grain is drenched in saucy goodness. Some might say the latter is culinary blasphemy, but I say it's pure genius (any guesses which type I am?). This one-pan Thai green curry rice is for all the rule-breakers out there – and honestly, even the side-by-side folks are going to love it. The rice greedily soaks up every last drop of creamy, coconutty, spicy curry, turning each bite into a perfect one. It's comfort food at its finest, requiring minimal effort and delivering maximum satisfaction. No need for sides here, just grab a spoon and dive in.

2 large chicken breasts, cut into bite-sized chunks

1 onion, finely diced

1 red (bell) pepper, cut into thin strips

1 green (bell) pepper, cut into thin strips

2 tbsp Thai green curry paste

1 garlic clove, minced

1 thumb-sized piece ginger, grated

300 g/1⅔ cups easy-cook long-grain rice

1 x 400-g/14-oz can light coconut milk

350 ml/12 fl oz/1½ cups chicken stock

juice of 1 lime

1 tbsp roughly chopped coriander/cilantro

½ red chilli/chile, de-seeded and finely diced

salt and pepper

olive oil, for cooking

lime wedges, to serve (optional)

1　Heat a tablespoon of olive oil in a lidded frying pan/skillet over medium–high heat. Once hot, add the chicken and cook for about 4 minutes, or until browned and cooked through. Transfer the chicken to a clean plate and set aside.

2　Lower the heat to medium and re-oil the pan if necessary. Add the onion and cook for a couple of minutes, before increasing the heat slightly and adding the peppers. Sauté for another 2 minutes until the peppers begin to soften. Then, stir in the curry paste, garlic and ginger, and let everything cook for a further 2 minutes until lovely and fragrant.

3　Tip the rice into the pan and stir until each grain gets coated in the curry paste. Pour in the coconut milk and stock. Bring the mixture to the boil, then reduce the heat to a simmer. Season to taste with salt and pepper.

4　Cover the pan with a lid and let everything cook for around 15 minutes, stirring once midway, until the rice is tender and the liquid is absorbed. This will take longer if you use regular rice. A few minutes before the rice is done, return the chicken to the pan to warm it through.

5　Finish by stirring in a generous squeeze of lime juice, to taste, and the fresh coriander. Sprinkle the diced chilli on top and serve with lime wedges, if desired.

Substitutions:

● **Vegetarian or vegan?** Swap the chicken for tofu or your favourite meat-free protein alternative. Use vegetable stock instead of chicken stock.

Future you:

🍲 Cool and place in an airtight container, storing in the fridge for up to 3 days.
❄ Cool and freeze for up to 2 months.
💧 Thaw in the fridge overnight.
🔥 Microwave for 3 minutes, stirring halfway through, until piping hot. Cooked rice must only be reheated once.

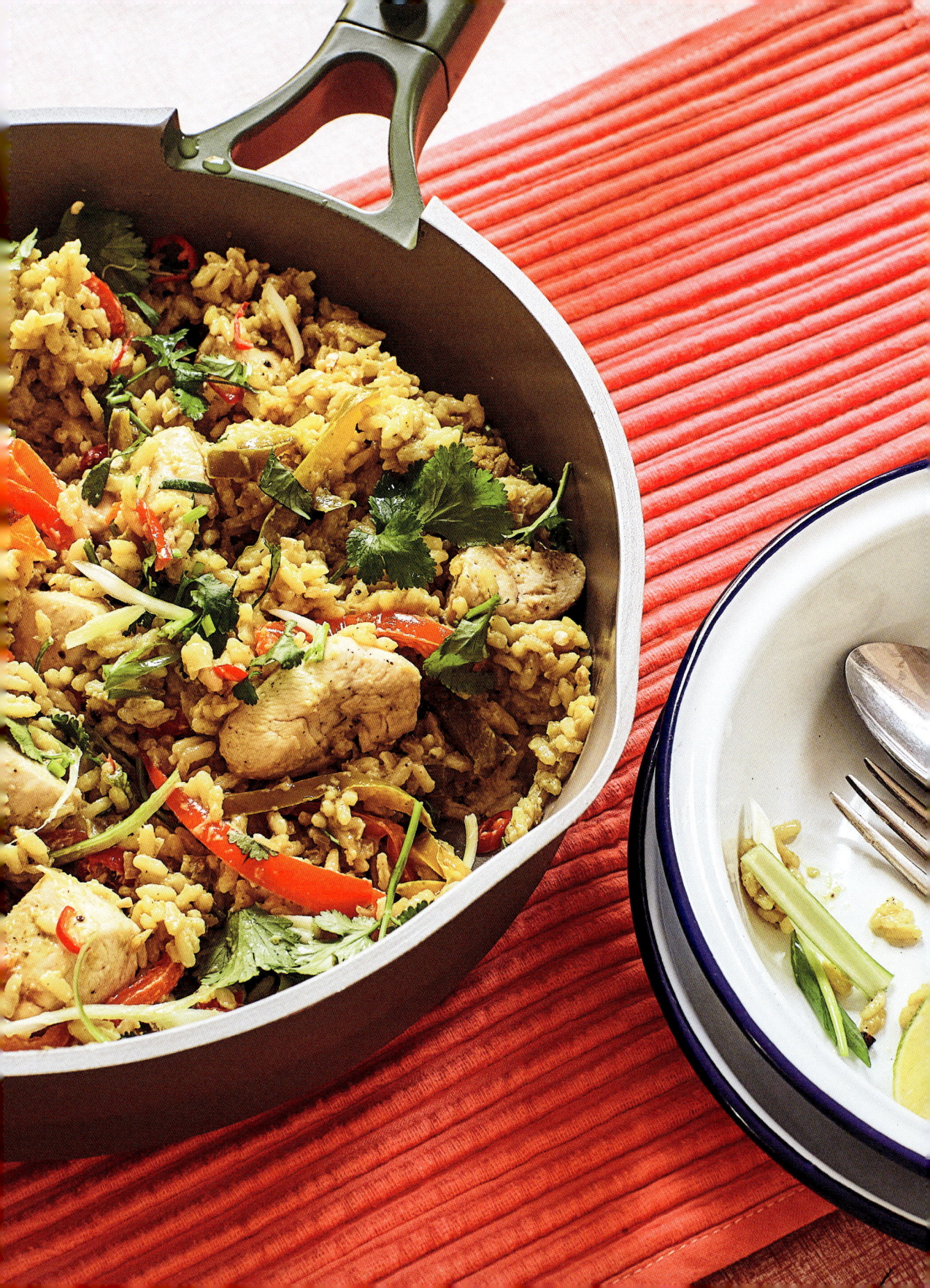

Red Lentil Dal + Rice

(V) (VE) (DF) (GF)

I went backpacking around India when I was 21, and ever since, I've been hooked on dal. For all the amazing food I ate there – from dosas to biryanis – it was this simple lentil curry that I craved the most, and still do. Dal (or dhal, daal) refers to dried, split pulses, but also to the comforting dish made by simmering them into a stew. In India, it's a dish everyone eats, no matter where you are or who you are. And while most regions have their own version, the essentials are the same: it's always packed with flavour, budget-friendly and loaded with plant protein and fibre. Following these principles, I've created this version with red lentils that comes together in just 30 minutes. It's creamy, rich and so satisfying, especially when served alongside some fluffy rice. A proper hug in a bowl.

1 large onion, finely diced

4 garlic cloves, minced

1 thumb-sized piece ginger, grated

1 tsp ground coriander

1 tsp ground cumin

1 tsp curry powder

300 g/10½ oz/1⅔ cups dried red split lentils, rinsed and drained

850 ml/1½ pints/3½ cups vegetable stock

200 ml/7 fl oz/scant 1 cup coconut milk

2 tbsp tomato purée/paste

a generous pinch of salt

2 x 250-g/9-oz pouches cooked basmati rice, or 300 g/10½ oz basmati rice cooked according to packet instructions

100 g/3½ oz/scant 2 cups spinach

juice of 1 lemon

1 tsp garam masala

olive oil, for cooking

roughly chopped coriander/cilantro, to garnish

crispy chilli/chili oil, to serve (optional)

Substitutions:

● **No red lentils?** Yellow split lentils work well.

1 Heat 1 tablespoon of olive oil in a large frying pan/skillet over medium heat. Add the onion, garlic and ginger, and cook for 5 minutes, stirring frequently to prevent burning, until they all soften and meld together. Sprinkle in the spices and toast for a further minute, allowing the flavours to bloom.

2 Add the lentils, followed by the stock, coconut milk and tomato purée. Give everything a good stir until well combined, then season with a generous pinch of salt. Bring the dal to the boil, then reduce the heat and simmer for around 15 minutes, or until the lentils are tender and creamy.

3 While the dal is simmering, heat the rice in the microwave according to the packet instructions, usually about 2 minutes per pouch.

4 Once the lentils are near the end of cooking, stir through the spinach, a handful at a time, until wilted. Then you can give everything a good squeeze of lemon juice and stir through the garam masala.

5 Serve the dal alongside your cooked rice, garnished with fresh coriander and a drizzle of chilli oil, if you like.

Future you:

☕ Cool and place in an airtight container, storing in the fridge for up to 3 days.
❄ Cool and freeze for up to 3 months.
💧 Thaw in the fridge overnight, or on low power in the microwave.
🔥 Warm in the microwave for 2–3 minutes, stirring halfway, until piping hot. Cooked rice must only be reheated once.

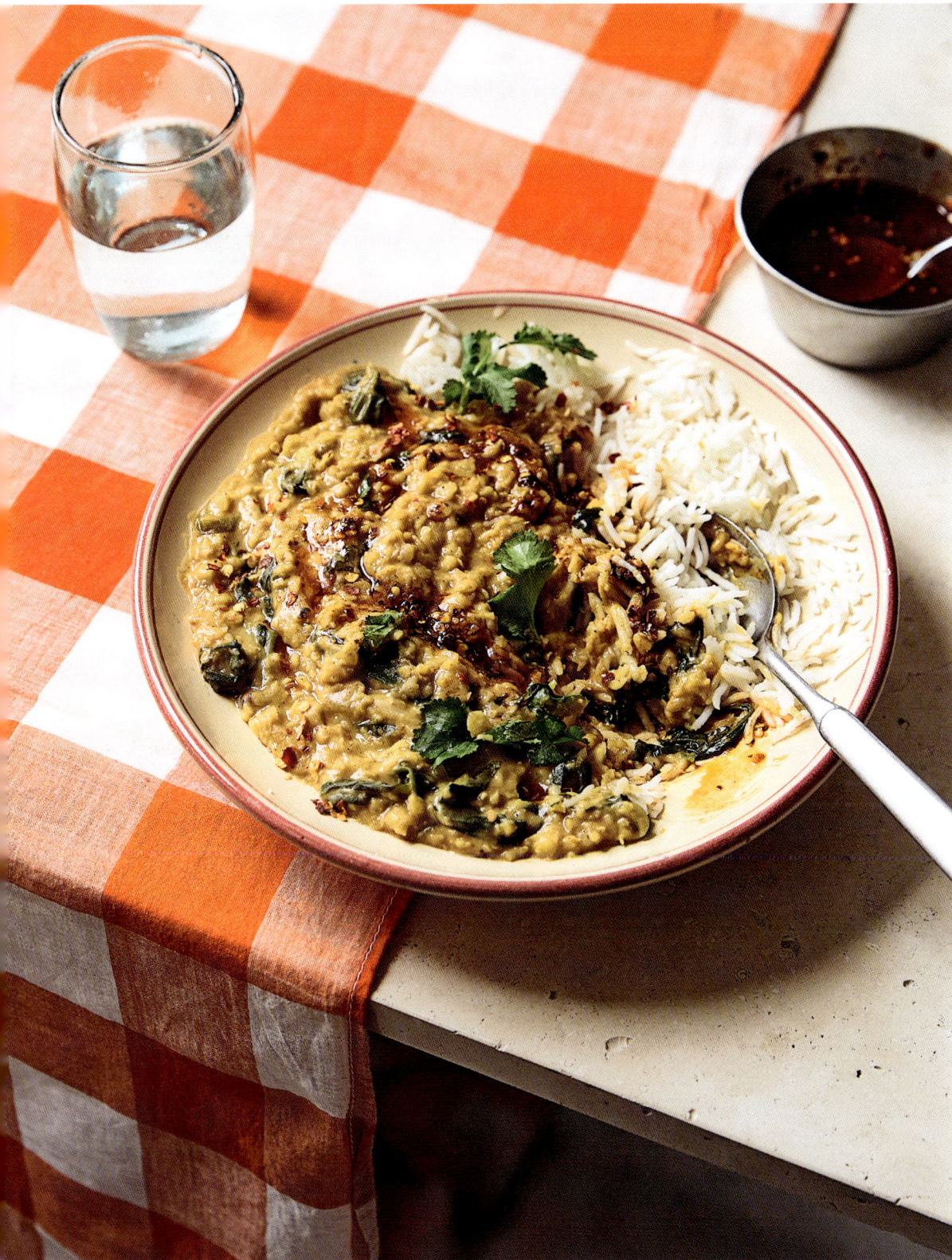

Peanut Butter Tofu Ramen + Soba Noodles

V
VE
DF
GF/O
N

Some traditional ramen recipes are complex to make, and of course they're delicious, but when I need something that's quick enough for a weeknight, yet still tastes like I've got my life together, this is the one. It's indulgent, comforting and the kind of meal you want to eat curled up on the sofa after a long day, not worrying about posture as you slurp away.

1 x 300-g/10½-oz block extra-firm tofu, cut into small cubes

1 tbsp dark soy sauce

1 tbsp maple syrup

1 tsp sesame oil

½ tsp garlic granules

½ tsp onion granules

1 tbsp cornflour/cornstarch

olive oil, for cooking

For the ramen broth

1 thumb-sized piece ginger, grated

2 garlic cloves, minced

1 tbsp miso paste

30 g/1 oz/2 tbsp natural peanut butter

1 tbsp soy sauce

500 ml/18 fl oz/2 cups vegetable stock

200 ml/7 fl oz/scant 1 cup milk

1 pak choi/bok choy, halved

125 g/4 oz soba noodles

To serve

a drizzle of crispy chilli/chili oil (optional)

1 spring onion/scallion, thinly sliced

a sprinkle of sesame seeds

lime wedges

Substitutions:

● **Gluten-free?** Use tamari instead of soy sauce. ● **No tofu?** Sub for tempeh or cooked chicken. ● **Nut-free?** Use tahini instead of peanut butter.

1 Place the cubed tofu in a food-safe container with a lid and add the soy sauce, maple syrup, sesame oil, garlic granules, onion granules and cornflour. Seal the box with the lid and shake well until the tofu is fully coated in the marinade. Optional step: if you have time, let the tofu sit to marinate for 15 minutes.

2 In a deep frying pan or wok, heat 1 tablespoon of olive oil over a medium heat. Add the marinated tofu and stir-fry for about 5 minutes until nicely caramelized on all sides. Remove the tofu from the pan and set it aside in a clean bowl.

3 Make the ramen broth in the same pan. Drizzle in a bit more oil if needed, and return the pan to medium heat. Add the ginger and garlic, cooking for 1 minute while continuously stirring to prevent burning. Then, add the miso paste, peanut butter and soy sauce, stirring vigorously to combine. Pour in 100 ml/3½ fl oz/6½ tablespoons of the stock and keep stirring until the miso paste and peanut butter are fully melted and incorporated.

4 Bring the mixture to the boil, then carefully pour in the remaining stock and the milk. Lower the heat and add the pak choi and noodles. Let everything simmer for 4–5 minutes, or until the noodles and pak choi are tender.

5 To serve, ladle the broth into bowls, then spoon in the noodles and pak choi. Top each bowl with the fried tofu, a drizzle of chilli oil (if using), sliced spring onion, sesame seeds and a wedge of lime.

Future you:

🍱 Cool and place in an airtight container, storing in the fridge for up to 2 days.
🔥 Microwave for 2 minutes, stirring halfway, until piping hot.

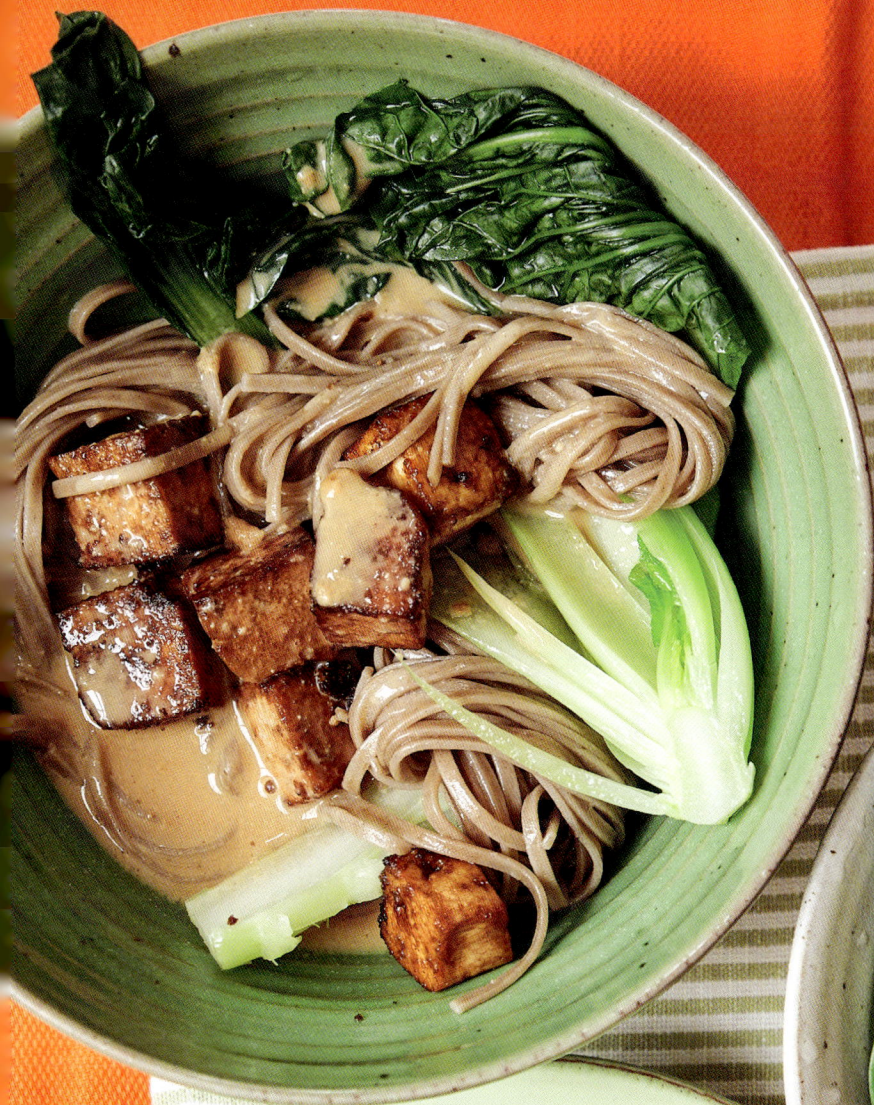

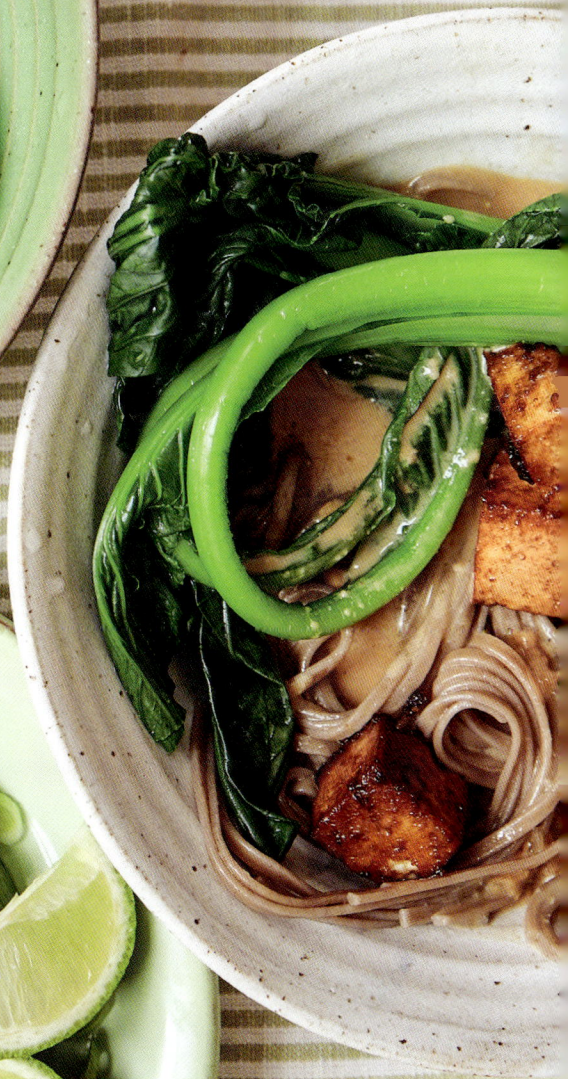

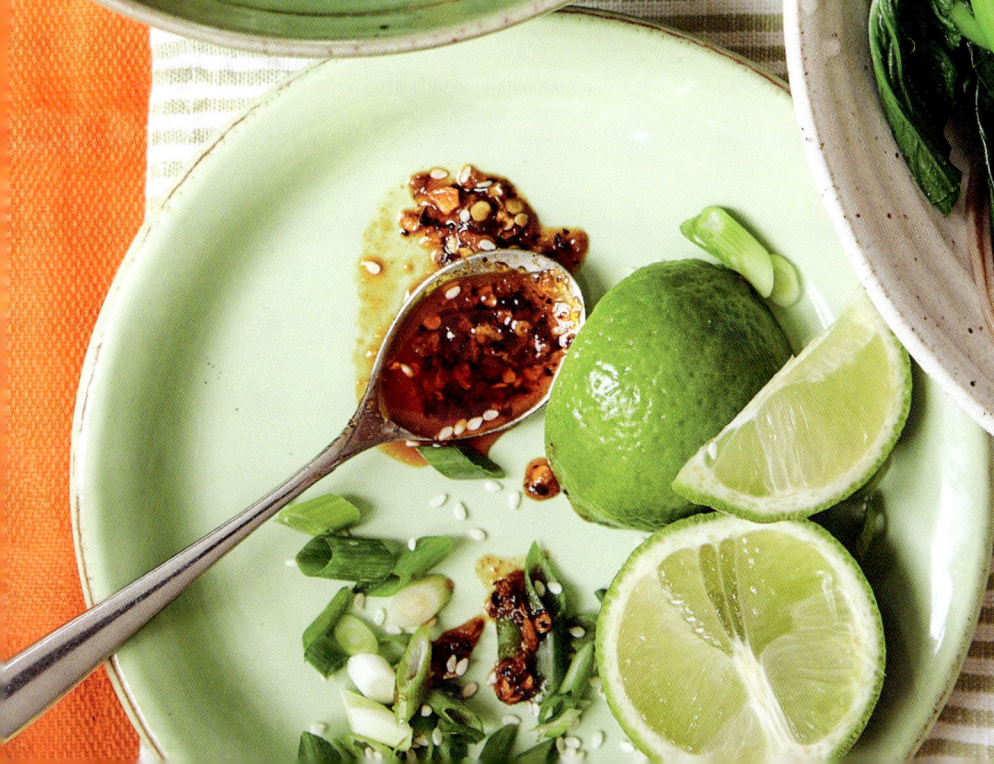

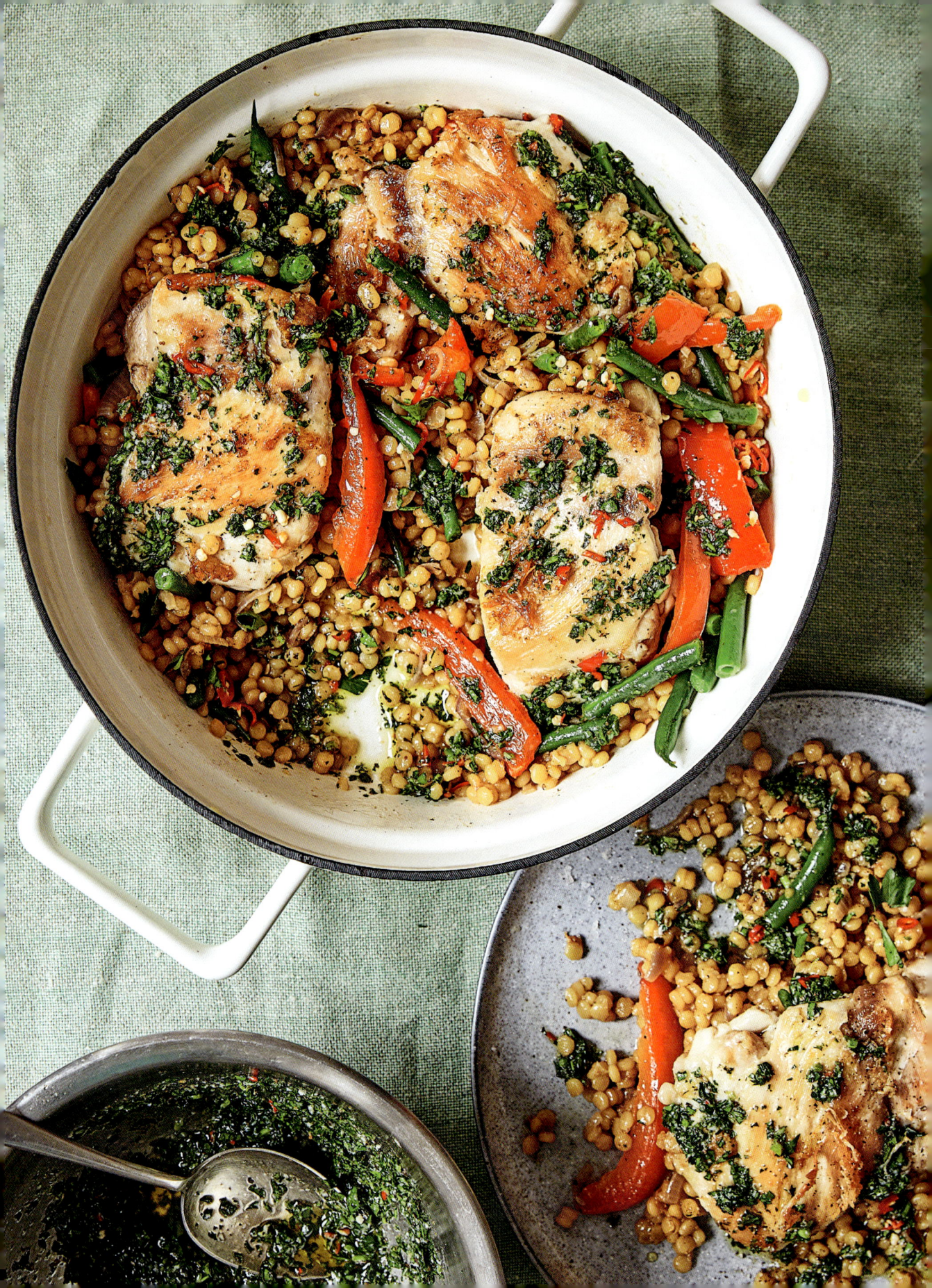

Vibrant Chimichurri Chicken Thighs + Giant Couscous

V/O
VE/O
DF
GF/O

Giant couscous is such a brilliant ingredient – it's actually a type of pasta, which is why it has a lovely, satisfying bite and soaks up all the goodness from the pan. The chimichurri dressing is the definition of maximum flavour with minimum effort, making the whole dish feel like a mini summer escape with its fresh, zingy notes, while still being ideal for colder days when you crave a bit of comfort and some faux sunshine. I think chicken thighs are a perfect pairing, but please feel free to swap in chicken breasts or go meat-free with a plant-based protein. Either way, it'll be glorious.

600 g/1 lb 5 oz skinless, boneless chicken thighs

1 red onion, thinly sliced

1 red (bell) pepper, thinly sliced

100 g/3½ oz fine green beans, cut in half

200 g/7 oz giant couscous

400 ml/14 fl oz/1¾ cups chicken stock

salt and pepper

olive oil, for cooking

For the chimichurri

3 tbsp extra virgin olive oil

1 tbsp any wine vinegar

2 tbsp finely chopped parsley

3 garlic cloves, minced

1 small red chilli/chile, de-seeded and finely chopped

1 tsp dried oregano

1 tsp fine sea salt

½ tsp pepper

1   Heat 1 tablespoon of olive oil in a deep lidded frying pan/skillet over medium–high heat. Add the chicken thighs, season them well with salt and pepper, and cook for about 5 minutes on each side until they gain some colour and are fully cooked through. Transfer the chicken to a clean plate, cover with foil and set aside to keep warm.

2   Return the same pan to medium heat, adding more oil if needed. Add the onion and pepper and sauté for about 2 minutes until they start to soften. Add the green beans and cook for an additional 4 minutes.

3   Tip in the couscous and briefly stir to coat the grains in the oil, then pour in the stock. Season to taste with salt and pepper. Reduce the heat to a simmer, cover and let the mixture bubble away for about 10 minutes, stirring halfway through, until the couscous is tender and the liquid is mostly absorbed.

4   While the couscous is cooking, whisk together the ingredients for the chimichurri in a small bowl until well combined.

5   Once the couscous is ready, nestle the chicken thighs back into the pan, allowing them to warm through in the mixture. Spoon the chimichurri over both the chicken and couscous and serve immediately.

Substitutions:

● **Vegan or vegetarian?** Sub the chicken for tofu, tempeh or your favourite meat-free protein alternative. Swap the chicken stock for vegetable stock. ● **Gluten-free?** Sub the couscous for cooked quinoa.

Future you:

🍲 Cool and place in an airtight container, storing in the fridge for up to 3 days.
❄ Cool and freeze for up to 2 months.
💧 Thaw in the fridge overnight, or at room temperature for a few hours.
🔥 Reheat in the microwave for 2–3 minutes, stirring halfway, until piping hot.

Greek-Inspired Orzo

V

VE/O

DF/O

GF/O

Not a week goes by without an orzo dish coming to my table, and this particular recipe is a repeat hit. Bursting with Mediterranean flavours, it has a richness that not only packs a punch on first bite, but keeps perfectly too (AKA the best leftovers!). If you want to keep this dish meat-free, pile your bowl high and serve as is. However, I usually like to amp up the protein by serving it as a side with something like chicken, salmon or prawns. It makes the meal more hearty and satisfying, but also means more yummy leftovers to tuck into for the rest of the week. Win!

1 red onion, finely diced

3 garlic cloves, minced

100 g/3½ oz/1 cup pitted Kalamata olives

1 x 200-g/7-oz can chickpeas/garbanzo beans, drained

80 g/3 oz/generous ¾ cup sun-dried tomatoes, roughly chopped

1 tsp dried oregano

250 g/9 oz orzo

500 g/1 lb 2 oz passata/strained tomatoes

500 ml/18 fl oz/2 cups vegetable stock

20 g/¾ oz/scant ¼ cup crumbled feta

a handful of roughly chopped dill

a handful of roughly chopped parsley

salt and pepper

olive oil, for cooking

1 Heat 1 tablespoon of olive oil in a deep lidded frying pan/skillet over medium heat. Sweat the onion and garlic for about 3 minutes, then add the olives, chickpeas, sun-dried tomatoes and oregano. Cook for another 3 minutes, stirring often to ensure nothing catches on the bottom of the pan.

2 Tip in the orzo and give everything a good stir to coat the pasta in the mixture. Pour in the passata and stock, season to taste with salt and pepper, and stir once more before bringing to the boil. Once boiling, reduce the heat, cover the pan, and simmer for about 6-10 minutes according to your orzo's packet instructions. Take the lid off to stir occasionally, and if the mixture looks too dry, add a splash of water from the kettle.

3 After the 6-10 minutes of cooking time are up, test a piece of orzo. If it needs more time, re-cover and continue to simmer. You're looking for the orzo to be tender and the liquid mostly absorbed.

4 Once done and ready to serve, crumble the feta over the top and finish with a sprinkling of dill and parsley.

Substitutions:

● **Gluten-free?** Use a gluten-free pasta alternative. ● **Vegan or dairy-free?** Use a dairy-free feta alternative.

Future you:

▣ Cool and place in an airtight container, storing in the fridge for up to 4 days.
❄ Cool and freeze for up to 2 months.
◗ Thaw in the fridge overnight, or on low power in the microwave.
🔥 Reheat in the microwave for 2–3 minutes, stirring halfway through.

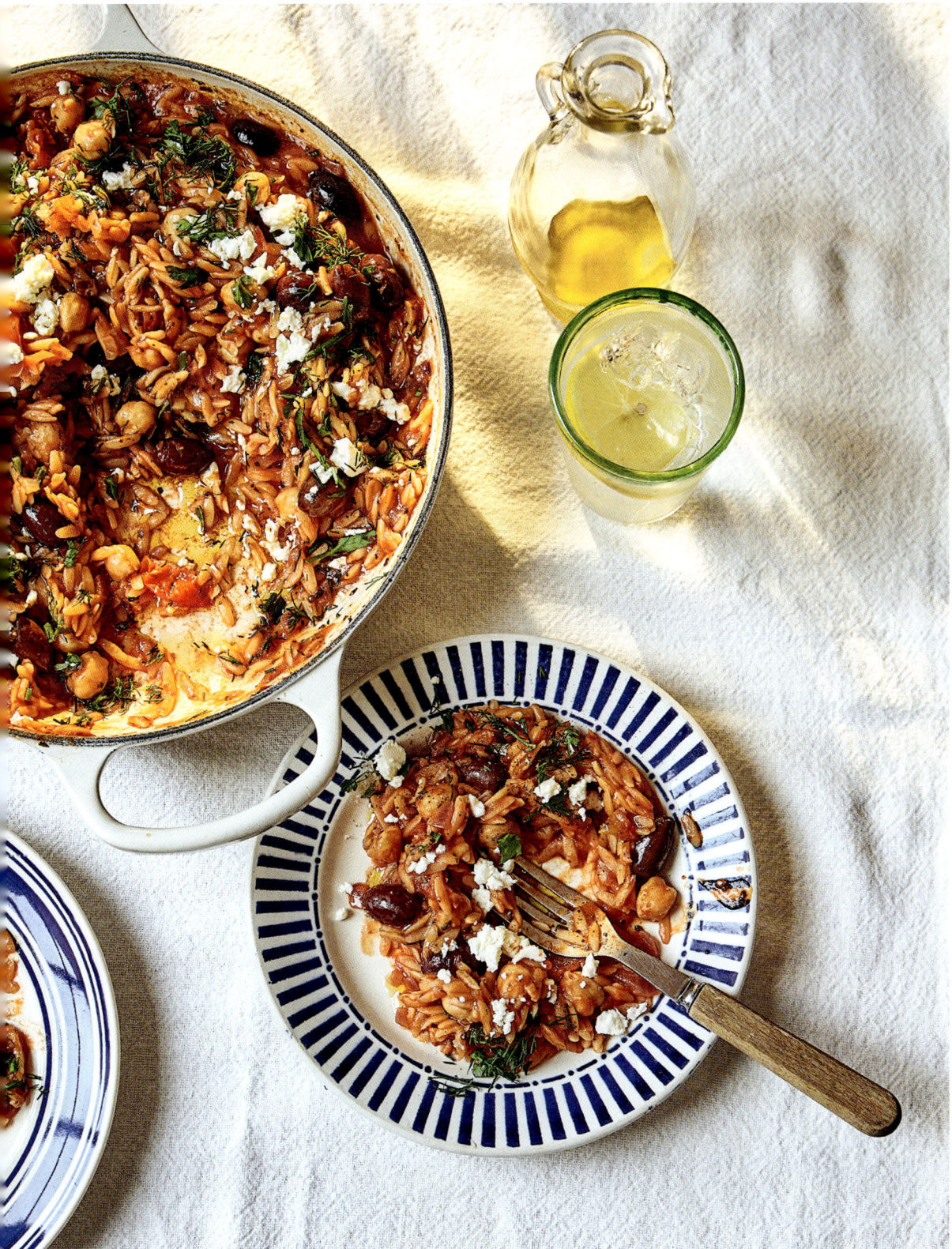

One-Pan Lasagne

(V/O)
(VE/O)
(DF/O)
(GF/O)

Raise your hand if you love eating a rich, cheesy lasagne. Uh-huh, me too. Now, raise your hand if you dread making a lasagne. Same. Endless dirty pans, components and hours spent in the kitchen? Not exactly enticing. Which is why you need this one-pan lasagne in your life. It captures all elements of our beloved lasagne without any of the faff (plus slightly more nutritional value) and it'll be ready to serve in just 35 minutes.

1 onion, finely diced

1 carrot, finely diced

1 courgette/zucchini, finely diced

3 garlic cloves, minced

500 g/1 lb 2 oz turkey thigh mince/ ground turkey thigh

2 tsp dried mixed herbs

3 tbsp tomato purée/paste

300 ml/10 fl oz/1¼ cups chicken stock

1 x 400-g/14-oz can chopped tomatoes

300 g/10½ oz fresh lasagne sheets

100 g/3½ oz/scant ½ cup ricotta

50 g/1¾ oz/scant ½ cup grated mozzarella

20 g/¾ oz/¼ cup grated Italian hard cheese

salt and pepper

olive oil, for cooking

side salad, to serve

1   Heat 1 tablespoon of olive oil in a large, shallow flameproof casserole dish or deep lidded frying pan/skillet over medium heat. Once the oil is hot, add the onion, carrot and courgette and sauté for a few minutes until the vegetables begin to soften. Stir in the garlic and cook for another couple of minutes until fragrant.

2   Add the mince to the pan, breaking it up with a spatula as it cooks. Let it cook for 4–5 minutes until evenly browned, then stir in the mixed herbs and tomato purée. Once everything is well combined, pour in the stock and chopped tomatoes, and season with salt and pepper. Give the mixture a good stir, then bring it to a gentle boil.

3   While the sauce bubbles away, roughly chop the fresh lasagne sheets into thirds and add them to the pan, stirring to evenly coat them in the sauce. Lower the heat to a gentle simmer, cover, and let the pasta cook for 5–10 minutes, stirring occasionally, until it becomes tender and most of the liquid has been absorbed.

4   Finally, the cheesy top. Drop spoonfuls of ricotta across the lasagne, then generously sprinkle mozzarella and hard cheese over the top. Cover the pan and allow the cheese to melt, or, for even better results, place the pan under a hot grill/broiler for a few minutes until the top is golden and bubbling.

5   Serve immediately, accompanied by your favourite side salad.

Future you:

🍲 Cool and place in an airtight container, storing in the fridge for up to 3 days.

❄ Cool and freeze for up to 2 months.

💧 Thaw in the fridge overnight, or at room temperature for a few hours.

🔥 Cover and pop into the microwave for 2–3 minutes, gently stirring halfway through, until piping hot.

Substitutions:

● **Vegetarian?** Swap the turkey mince for 2 x 400-g/14-oz cans cooked lentils. Sub the chicken stock for vegetable stock. ● **Vegan?** Follow the vegetarian and gluten-free advice (using egg-free dried pasta instead of fresh). Use dairy-free cheese alternatives for the topping. ● **Dairy-free?** Use dairy-free cheese alternatives to top. ● **Gluten-free?** Swap the fresh lasagne sheets for gluten-free dried lasagne sheets. You will need to increase the quantity of stock to 800 ml/1¾ pints/3¼ cups and cook the lasagne, covered, for 10–15 minutes, until the pasta is al dente and liquid absorbed, at step 3.

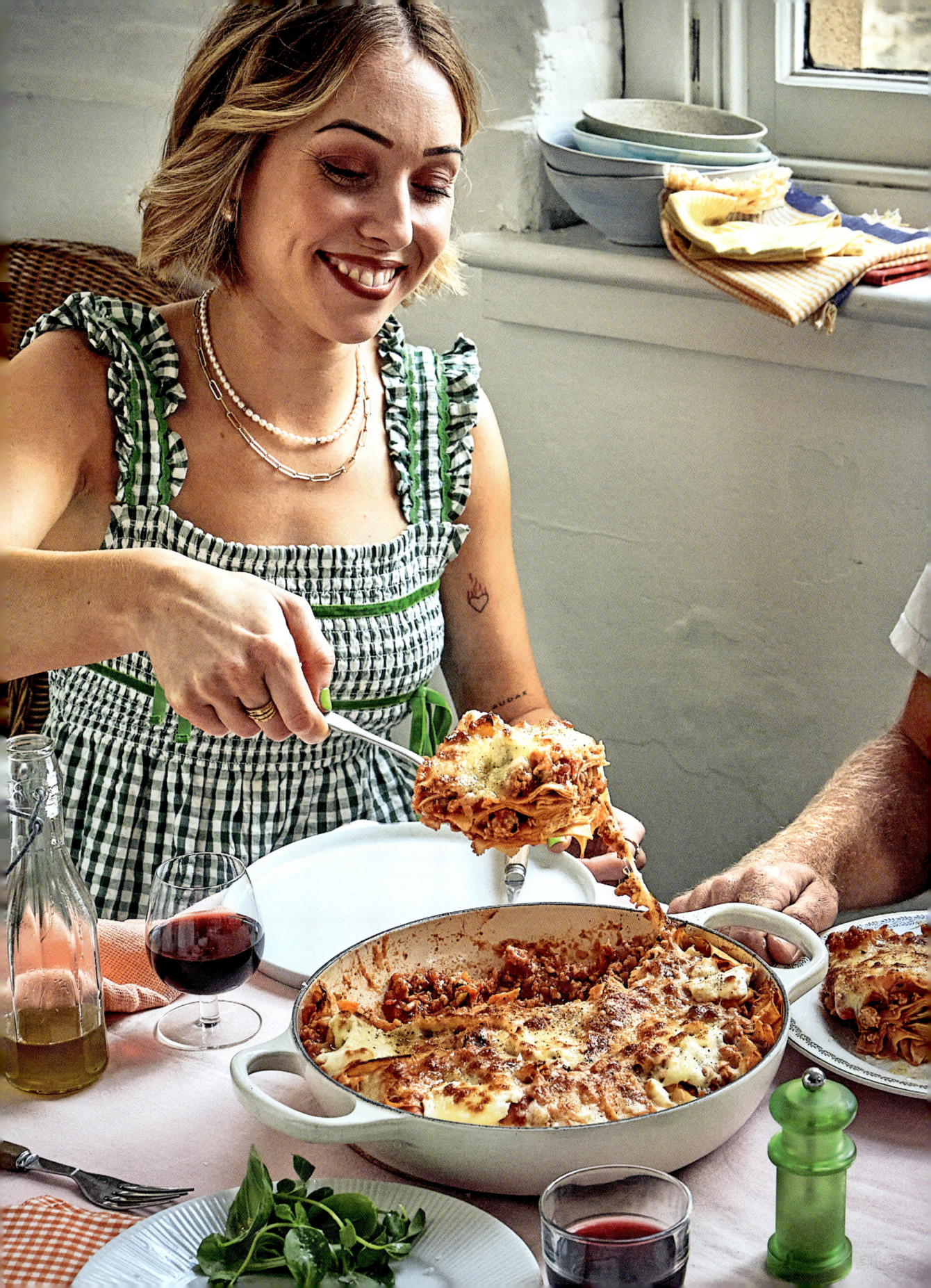

Enchilada Rice + Crumbled Tempeh

V

VE/O

DF/O

GF

This recipe is exactly what I want you to take away from *Healthy-ish*: dishes that are packed with nutritional diversity, protein and flavour, but will never – *ever* – shy away from a glorious, melty cheesy top. It's all about getting the perfect balance between feeling good and nourished, and satisfying our comfort food needs (especially the cheesy ones). One pan, one fork, and one delicious dinner in your belly. You're welcome.

1 tbsp olive oil

1 red onion, finely diced

3 garlic cloves, minced

1 x 200-g/7-oz block tempeh, cut into small cubes

1 red (bell) pepper, finely diced

1 green (bell) pepper, finely diced

2 tsp ground cumin

1 tsp ground coriander

1 tsp smoked paprika

½ tsp cayenne pepper

1 x 400-g/14-oz can black beans, drained

150 g/5½ oz/1 cup sweetcorn/corn

240 g/9 oz/1⅓ cups easy-cook long-grain rice

500 g/1 lb 2 oz passata/strained tomatoes

400 ml/14 fl oz/1¾ cups vegetable stock

60 g/2 oz/½ cup grated cheese (I used cheddar)

a handful of roughly chopped coriander/cilantro

1 spring onion/scallion, thinly sliced

salt and pepper

yogurt, to serve (optional)

1 Heat the olive oil in a large, deep lidded frying pan/skillet over medium heat. Once hot, add the onion and garlic, and cook for 2 minutes until they begin to soften. Toss in the tempeh and peppers and cook for another 4–5 minutes until lightly browned all over. Sprinkle in the spices and give everything a good stir, ensuring everything is well coated with the fragrant mix.

2 Tip the drained beans and sweetcorn into the pan, along with the rice. Stir gently until the rice is coated in the mixture, then pour in the passata and stock, stirring everything to combine. Bring the mixture to a gentle boil, then reduce the heat slightly. Season well with salt and pepper. Cover the pan and let everything simmer for about 10 minutes (note that regular rice will take longer to cook), giving it a stir every so often to prevent the rice from sticking to the bottom of the pan.

3 After 10 minutes, remove the lid and cook uncovered for a further 5 minutes, or until the rice is cooked and the remaining liquid absorbed.

4 Sprinkle the grated cheese over the top straight away, and wait a minute or two for the residual heat to melt it into the dish.

5 Top with the coriander and sliced spring onion and serve with dollops of yogurt, if you like.

Substitutions:

● **No tempeh?** Sub for tofu or chicken instead.

Future you:

🍲 Cool and place in an airtight container, storing in the fridge for up to 3 days.
❄ Cool and freeze for up to 2 months.
💧 Thaw in the fridge overnight.
🔥 Microwave for 3 minutes, stirring halfway through, until piping hot. Cooked rice must only be reheated once.

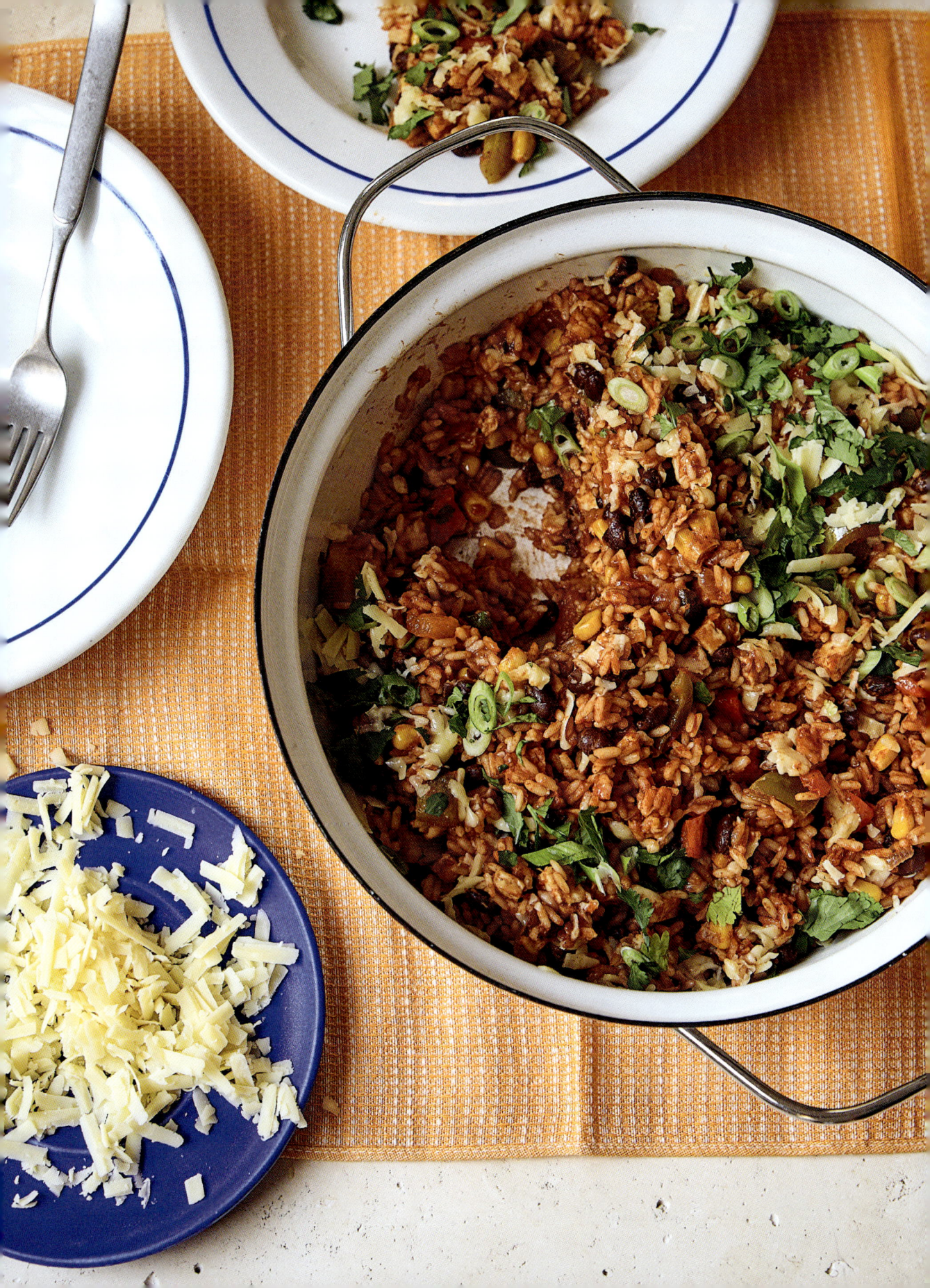

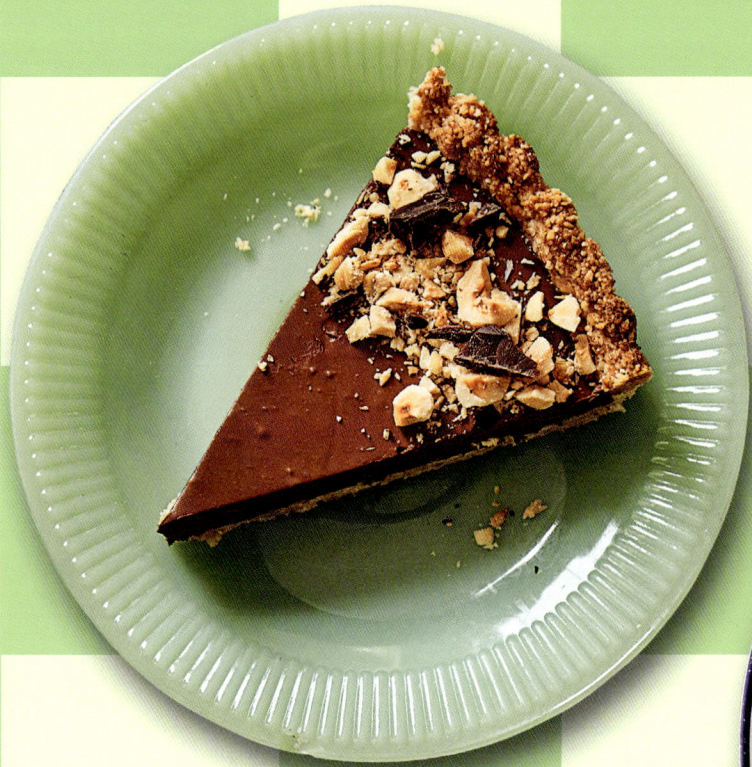

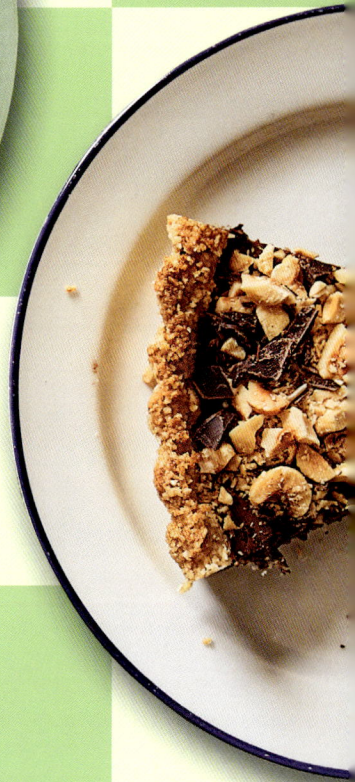

Sweet Treats

Refined Sugar-Free Treats to Satisfy Any Sweet Tooth

For every other sweet tooth out there! From homely bakes and protein-packed snacks to delicious desserts worthy of a dinner party – this chapter has it covered. Without compromising on any flavour or decadence, all of these recipes are free of refined sugars, meaning they use natural sweeteners, such as maple syrup, dates, honey and coconut sugar. Trust me, you will love them all.

Carrot Cake

V

VE/O

DF/O

GF/O

N

My mum was (and still is) an avid baker, and I found it mesmerizing watching her in the kitchen when I was little. On my 6th Christmas, I got a giant A4-sized cookbook, and flipping through its pages now – some pristine, others half rubbed with butter smears – reveals the firm favourite: carrot cake. I'll just never forget how confused little Emma was that something made with vegetables could taste so delicious! This healthier version is every bit as good as the original, so I hope you love it as much as I do. Please also feel free to smear whatever you like on this hopefully well-loved page, just as little Emma did.

2 x 20-cm/8-in cake tins, greased and lined

320 g/11 oz/scant 2½ cups plain/all-purpose flour

300 g/10½ oz carrots, coarsely grated

2 tsp bicarbonate of soda/baking soda

2 tsp ground cinnamon, plus extra to decorate

1 tsp ground ginger

½ tsp fine sea salt

160 g/5½ oz raisins or sultanas/golden raisins

120 g/4 oz/1 cup pecan halves, roughly chopped, plus extra to decorate

4 large/US extra-large eggs

2 tsp vanilla extract

juice of 1 large orange

60 g/2 oz/5 tbsp coconut sugar

60 ml/2 fl oz/¼ cup maple syrup

80 ml/2¾ fl oz/⅓ cup milk

120 g/4 oz/½ cup coconut oil, melted and cooled

For the frosting

200 g/7 oz/scant 1 cup cream cheese

200 g/7 oz/scant 1 cup thick yogurt

3 tbsp maple syrup

1   Preheat the oven to 175°C fan/195°C/375°F/gas mark 5.

2   In a large mixing bowl, combine the flour and grated carrot. Toss them together until every carrot strand is coated in flour – this will ensure an even distribution of carrot throughout the cake. After that, mix in the bicarbonate of soda, cinnamon, ginger, salt, raisins and pecans.

3   In a separate bowl, combine the eggs, vanilla, orange juice, sugar, maple syrup, milk and coconut oil, whisking until well combined.

4   Carefully pour the wet mixture into the bowl of dry ingredients. Using a flat rubber spatula, gently fold the batter together. Mix just until no streaks of flour remain, being careful not to overmix to keep the cake light and fluffy.

5   Divide the batter evenly between the 2 prepared cake tins and smooth the mixture to the edges. Slide the tins onto the middle shelf of the oven and bake for 22–25 minutes, or until a toothpick inserted into the centre of the cakes comes out clean.

6   Once the cakes are done, remove the tins from the oven. Leave the cakes to cool in the tins for 10 minutes, then turn them out onto a wire rack to cool further. Patience is key here (sorry!) – you want them fully cooled before adding the frosting.

7   The frosting is really simple: just stir together the cream cheese, yogurt and maple syrup in a small bowl.

8   Once the cakes are completely cool, it's time to assemble. Place one cake flat-side up on a serving plate and spoon half of the frosting in the middle. Spread it out evenly, but make sure to leave a 2-cm/¾-in border around the edges. Gently place the second cake on top, flat-side down. Spoon the remaining frosting onto the top, spreading it all the way to the edges. For extra decoration points, finish with chopped nuts and a sprinkle of cinnamon.

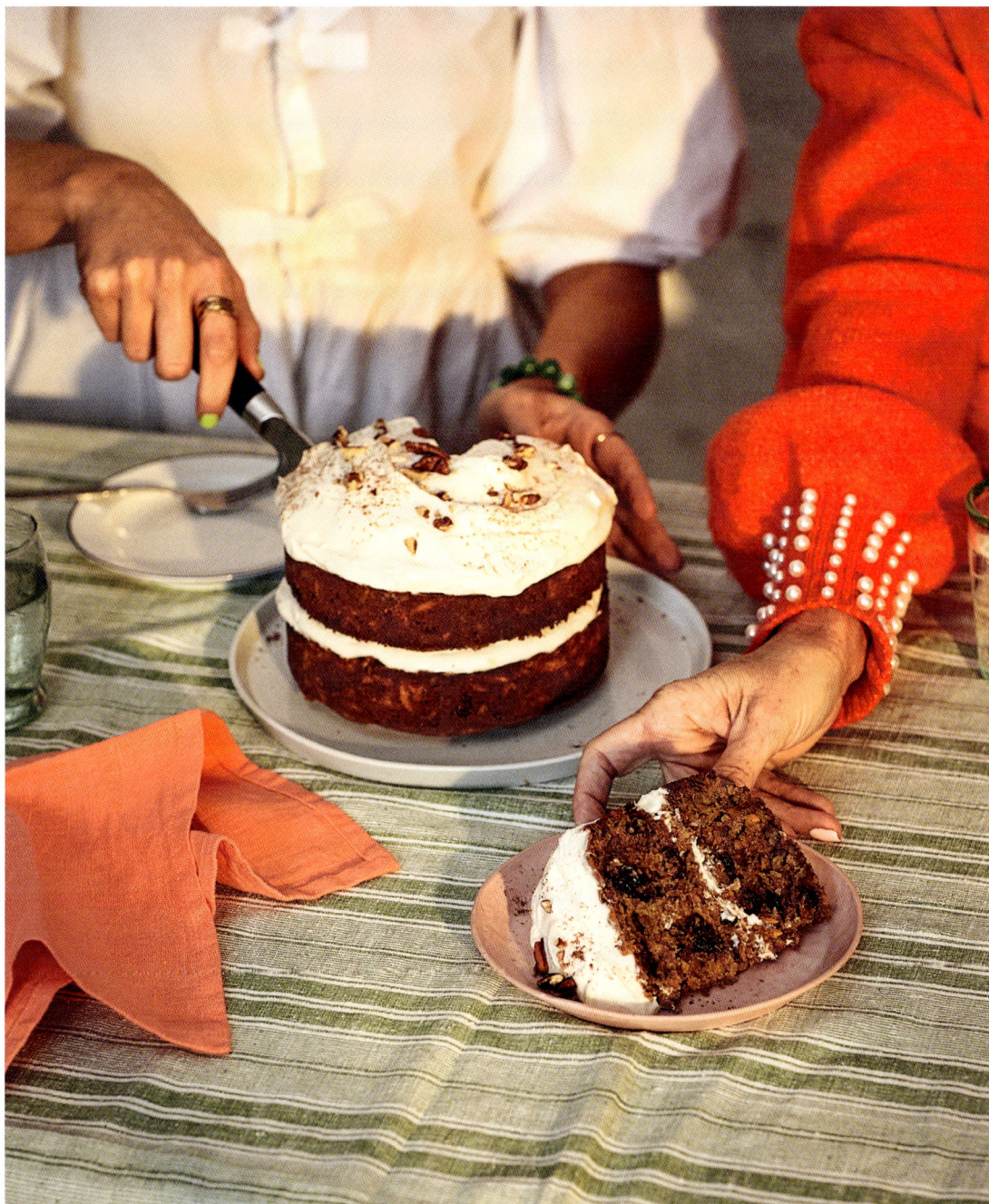

Substitutions:

● **No coconut oil?** Use a neutral oil, such as vegetable oil or mild olive oil instead. ● **Vegan?** Make flaxseed 'eggs' by mixing 2 tbsp milled flaxseed with 5 tbsp water. Use dairy-free alternatives for the cream cheese and yogurt. ● **Gluten-free?** Use gluten-free flour.

Future you:

🍲 Cool and place in an airtight container, storing in the fridge for up to 5 days.

❄ The unfrosted cake can be frozen for up to 2 months.

💧 Thaw in the fridge overnight, or at room temperature for a few hours.

The Best Choc Chunk Banana Bread

(V) (VE) (DF)

Nothing sparks more joy in me than the smell of freshly baked banana bread filling the kitchen, and let me tell you, this is the only banana bread recipe you'll ever need. Not only is it perfectly moist and delicious, but it's totally vegan and the end result is like getting a warm hug from your oven. So, the moment you see freckles invade your bananas, you know where to come. Enjoy it as is, or go all-out with a layer of nut butter on top. Pure comfort-food heaven.

900-g/2-lb loaf tin, lined

2 tbsp milled flaxseed/linseed

3 large ripe bananas

60 ml/2 fl oz/¼ cup maple syrup

1 tsp vanilla extract

55 g/2 oz/scant ½ cup coconut oil, melted and cooled

40 ml/1⅓ fl oz/2½ tbsp unsweetened almond milk

200 g/7 oz/1½ cups plain/all-purpose flour

1 tsp baking powder

½ tsp bicarbonate of soda/baking soda

¼ tsp fine sea salt

1 tsp ground cinnamon

100 g/3½ oz dark/bittersweet chocolate, roughly chopped

1   Preheat the oven to 180°C fan/200°C/400°F/gas mark 6.

2   In a small bowl, mix together the flaxseed and 5 tablespoons of water and set aside for a few minutes to thicken. As there are no eggs in this recipe, this will act as the binder.

3   In a separate large mixing bowl, mash the bananas until smooth, then add the flaxseed mixture, maple syrup, vanilla extract, melted coconut oil and almond milk. Whisk until well combined.

4   After that, add the flour, baking powder, bicarbonate of soda, salt and cinnamon. Using a flat rubber spatula, gently fold the ingredients together until no streaks of flour remain, being careful not to overmix – this will keep the loaf light and fluffy. Tip in most of the chopped chocolate, reserving a generous handful for the topping, and fold it into the batter a few times until evenly distributed.

5   Pour the batter into the prepared loaf tin, using your spatula to smooth the batter into the corners and level the top. Scatter over the remaining chocolate chunks, then pop the tin on the middle shelf of the oven. Bake this for 40–45 minutes, or until a toothpick inserted into the centre comes out clean.

6   Let the loaf cool for 10 minutes in the tin, before transferring to a wire rack and slicing.

Substitutions:

● **No coconut oil?** Use a neutral oil, such as vegetable oil or mild olive oil instead. ● **No maple syrup?** Use honey or agave instead. ● **No flaxseed?** If you are not vegan, substitute for 2 regular eggs and, in turn, reduce the amount of milk to 20 ml/4 tsp.

Future you:

🍱 Cool and place in an airtight container, storing in the fridge for up to 6 days.
❄ Cool and freeze for up to 2 months.
💧 Thaw in the fridge overnight or at room temperature for a few hours.
🔥 Enjoy at room temperature or warm in the microwave for 20 seconds.

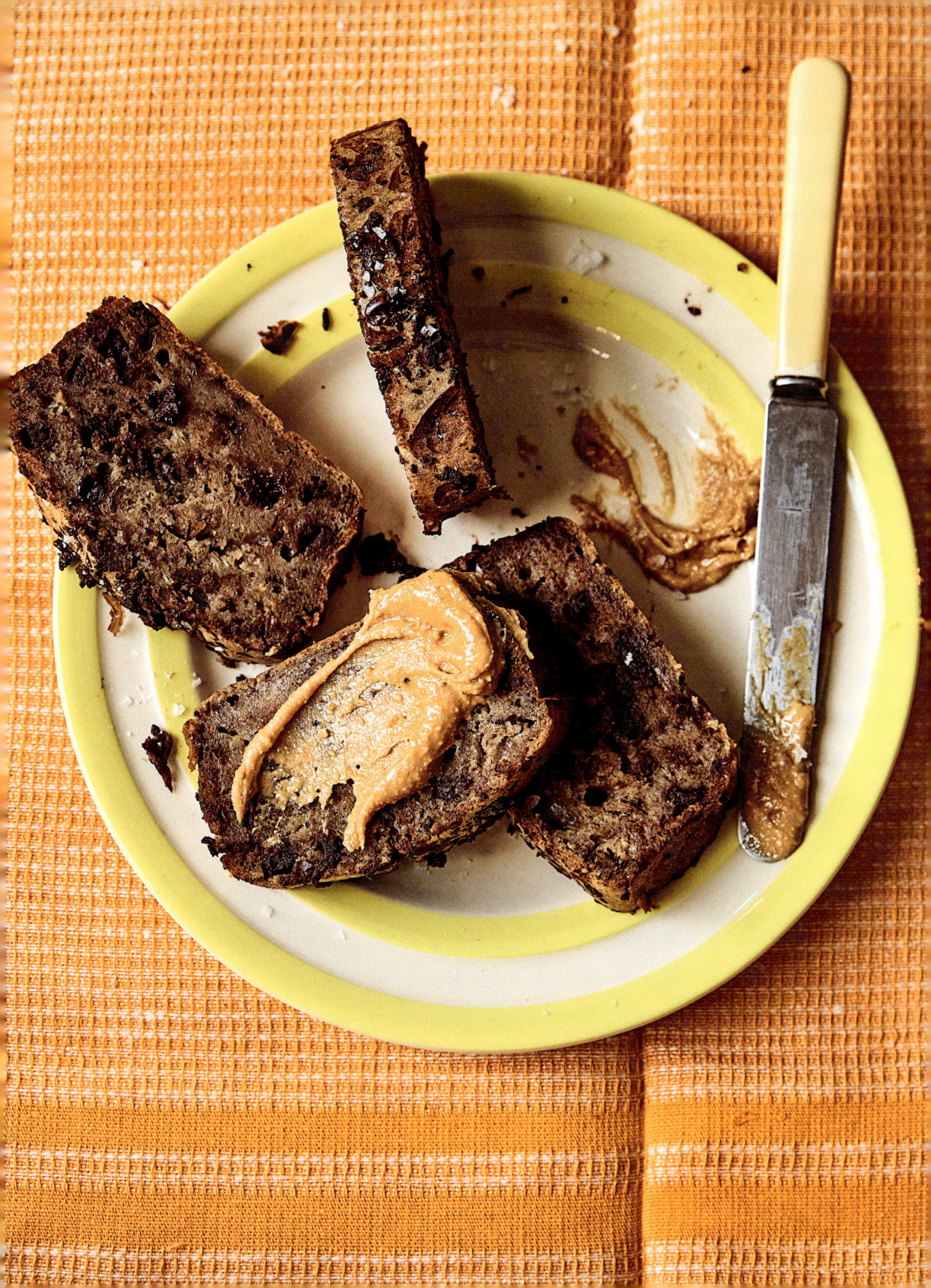

Peach, Ginger + Almond Galette

V

VE/O

DF

Give me any dessert with cooked fruit and pastry, and I'm one happy girl. A galette is essentially the rustic cousin of a pie, but so much easier to make. Naturally, my version is not only healthier than the traditional one but also quicker, thanks to swapping butter for coconut oil, which significantly reduces the chilling time.

large baking sheet, lined

100 g/3½ oz/¾ cup plain/all-purpose flour

70 g/2½ oz/⅔ cup spelt flour

25 g/1 oz/2 tbsp coconut sugar, plus extra for sprinkling

¼ tsp fine sea salt

100 g/3½ oz/6½ tbsp coconut oil, softened but not melted completely

2 tbsp ice-cold water

450 g/1 lb (about 4) ripe peaches, stoned and thinly sliced

2 tbsp honey

1 tsp ground cinnamon

1 tsp ground ginger

1 egg, beaten

20 g/¾ oz/¼ cup flaked/slivered almonds

ice cream, to serve (optional)

1 Preheat the oven to 190°C fan/210°C/400°F/gas mark 6.

2 To make the dough, combine the plain flour, spelt flour, coconut sugar, and salt in a large mixing bowl. Stir to mix, then pour in the coconut oil and cold water. Mix until the dough forms a smooth, cohesive ball.

3 Wrap the dough tightly in cling film/plastic wrap and chill in the fridge for 5–10 minutes. Be cautious not to over-chill; if the coconut oil hardens too much, the dough may crack when rolled. If this happens, let it sit at room temperature until it softens enough to roll out smoothly.

4 While the dough chills, make the fruit filling. In a bowl, combine the peaches, honey, cinnamon and ginger. Mix until the fruit is coated.

5 Remove the dough from the fridge and unwrap it. Remove the parchment paper from the baking sheet and place the dough in the centre. Roll the dough out into a rough 30-cm/12-in circle. Spoon the fruit filling into the middle, arranging it as neatly or as casually as you like, but leaving a 2.5-cm/1-in border around the edges.

6 Fold the edges of the dough over the filling, to create a rustic crust. Brush the crust with the beaten egg, then sprinkle with the flaked almonds and coconut sugar.

7 Carefully transfer the parchment paper with the assembled galette onto the baking sheet. Bake in the preheated oven for 30–35 minutes, or until the crust is golden and the fruit filling is bubbling. Serve while still warm, with a scoop of ice cream, if you like.

Substitutions:

● **No peaches?** Try nectarines, strawberries, blueberries, blackberries, apples or pears – or go savoury! ● **Vegan?** Swap the honey for maple syrup. Use plant-based milk, rather than the egg, to glaze the edges. ● **No spelt flour?** Sub for plain/all-purpose flour.

Future you:

▣ Cool and place in an airtight container, storing in the fridge for up to 4 days.
❄ Cool and freeze for up to 2 months.
◊ Thaw in the fridge overnight, or at room temperature for a few hours.
♨ Reheat in the oven for 10–15 minutes at 140°C fan/160°C/325°F/gas mark 3, or microwave individual portions for 20–30 seconds.

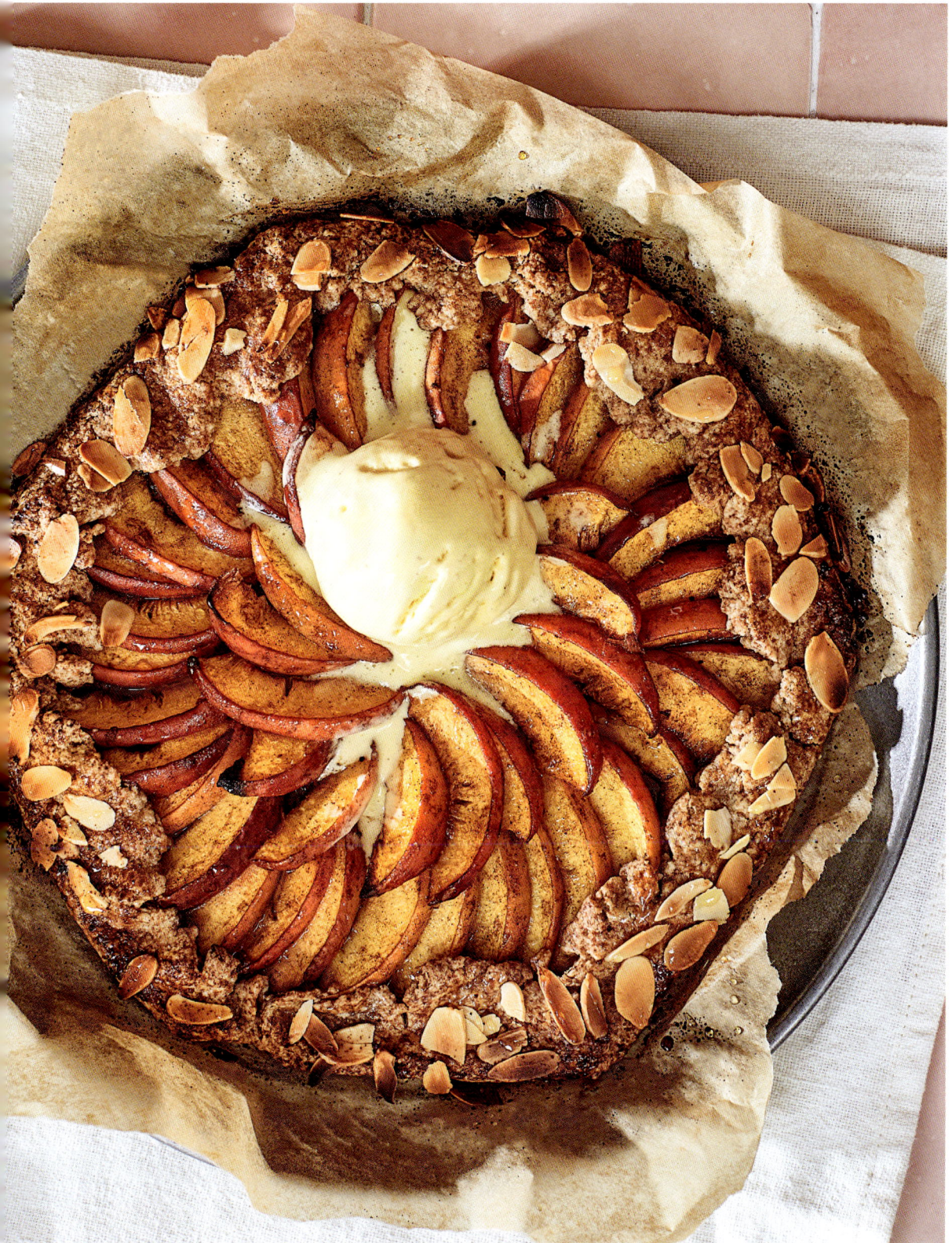

Chocolate Tart

(V)
(VE)
(DF)
(N)

If you didn't know that you can make a rich and decadent chocolate filling using silken tofu and melted chocolate, now's the time to let your mind (and taste buds) be blown. This sneakily high-protein combo creates a velvety smooth texture that's so indulgent, you'd never guess it's dairy-free and healthy(ish!). Normally, I serve the filling mixture alone to make little chocolate pots (which I highly recommend trying too), but in a stroke of genius, I figured it would be absolutely mega in a tart — and let me tell you, the result is exceptional. Such a perfect dinner party or special occasion dessert that can be prepped in advance and can suit almost any dietary restriction around your table.

23-cm/9-in loose-bottom tart or cake tin, lined

200 g/7 oz/2 cups ground almonds/almond meal

50 g/1¾ oz/generous ⅓ cup oat flour

grated zest of 1 orange

½ tsp fine sea salt

70 g/2½ oz/4½ tbsp coconut oil, melted and cooled

3 tbsp maple syrup

grated dark/bittersweet chocolate, to decorate

chopped hazelnuts, to decorate

For the filling

600 g/1 lb 5 oz silken tofu (not firm tofu)

200 g/7 oz 70 per cent dark/bittersweet chocolate, melted

2 tbsp cacao powder

3 tbsp maple syrup

juice of 1 orange

a pinch of flaky sea salt

1 Preheat the oven to 180°C fan/200°C/400°F/gas mark 6.

2 In a bowl, combine the ground almonds, oat flour, orange zest, salt, coconut oil and maple syrup until the ingredients come together into a sticky, fragrant mixture. Tip this mixture into your prepared tin and use your fingers to press it evenly across the bottom and up the sides, forming a smooth and even crust.

3 Using a fork, poke holes all over the bottom and a few along the sides of the crust to stop it from puffing up too much during baking.

4 Place the tin in the oven and bake for about 12 minutes, or until the crust turns a light golden brown. Once baked, remove from the oven and let it cool. While the crust is still warm, use the back of a spoon to gently press down and re-form the edges if needed, creating a neat rim.

5 As the crust cools, prepare the chocolate filling. In a food processor, blend together the tofu, melted chocolate, cacao powder, maple syrup, orange juice and salt. Blend until the mixture is completely smooth and velvety.

6 Once the crust has cooled, pour the chocolate filling into the tart shell, smoothing it out to ensure there are no air bubbles. Place the tart in the fridge to set for at least 3 hours.

7 Just before serving, decorate the tart with grated dark chocolate and chopped hazelnuts.

Substitutions:

● **Not a fan of chocolate orange?** Simply omit the orange juice and zest. ● **Gluten-free?** Ensure your oat flour is gluten-free. ● **Nut-free?** Sub ground almonds for oat flour and omit hazelnuts.

Future you:

▭ Cool and place in an airtight container, storing in the fridge for up to 7 days.
❄ Cool and freeze for up to 2 months.
◖ Thaw in the fridge overnight, or at room temperature for a few hours.

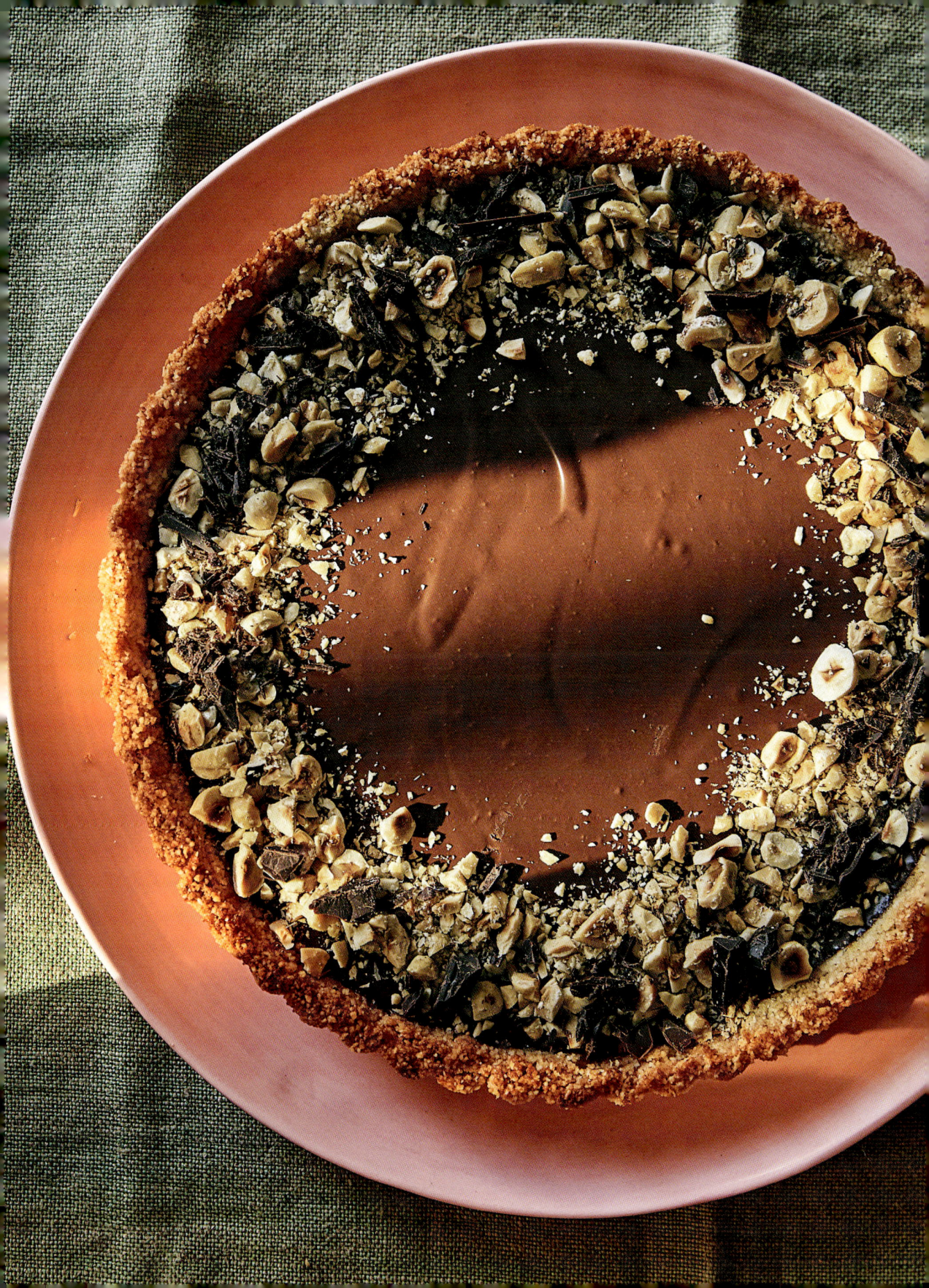

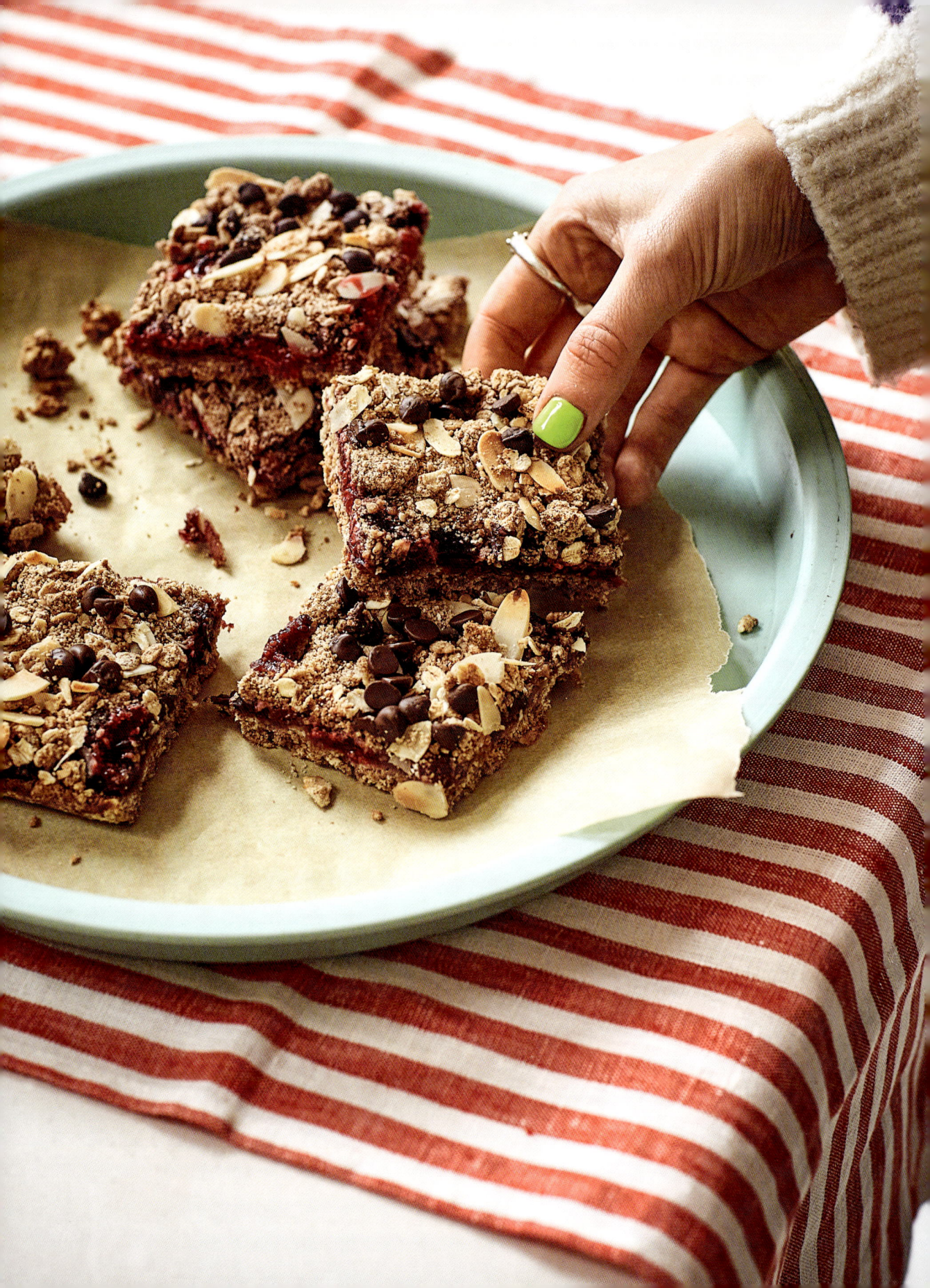

Chocolate Cherry Crumble Bars

V
VE
DF
N

Every time I make these (and I do so often), I'm blown away by how good they are. They'll work with any frozen berries, so feel free to experiment each time you make them, but I'm letting cherries be the star here because the cherry-almond-chocolate combo is quite simply a decadent match made in heaven. Enjoy them as dessert, with yogurt for breakfast, or with a coffee for an ultimate mid-afternoon treat.

20-cm/8-in loose-bottom square tin, lined

200 g/7 oz/1½ cups oat flour

100 g/3½ oz/1 cup rolled/old-fashioned oats

30 g/1 oz/scant ⅓ cup ground almonds/almond meal

40 g/1½ oz/3¼ tbsp coconut sugar

1 tsp baking powder

1 tsp ground cinnamon

¼ tsp fine sea salt

1 tbsp maple syrup

60 g/2 oz/4 tbsp coconut oil, melted and cooled

400 g/14 oz frozen cherries

15 g/½ oz/1 tbsp chia seeds

1 tbsp maple syrup

20 g/¾ oz/¼ cup flaked/slivered almonds

20 g/¾ oz/2 tbsp dark/bittersweet chocolate chips

1   Preheat the oven to 180°C fan/200°C/400°F/gas mark 6.

2   In a large bowl, combine the flour, rolled oats, ground almonds, sugar, baking powder, cinnamon and salt. Add the maple syrup and coconut oil and stir until the mixture is crumbly, but holds when packed.

3   Transfer two-thirds of the mixture into the lined tin and, using your fingers or a flat rubber spatula, pack it down in an even layer.

4   Place the cherries, chia seeds and maple syrup into a microwave-safe bowl. Microwave for 3 minutes on full power, stirring halfway through. Depending on the berries you use (and as is the case for cherries), you may find that some fruits have not broken down very much. If this happens, use the back of a fork or a masher to squash everything together a few times to achieve a jammier consistency.

5   Pour the berry mixture and any residual juices on top of the oaty base layer in the tin.

6   Add the flaked almonds to the remaining crumble mixture left in the bowl. Then, sprinkle the crumble over the top of the berries and scatter the chocolate chips across the top. Place the tin into the oven and bake for 25 minutes.

7   Remove the tin from the oven and allow the mix to cool in the tin for at least 15 minutes before turning out and slicing into bars or squares. This will ensure the base holds itself together when cut.

Substitutions:

● **Gluten-free?** Ensure your oats and oat flour are gluten-free.
● **No coconut oil?** Use a neutral oil, such as vegetable oil or mild olive oil instead. ● **Nut free?** Omit the ground almonds and flaked almonds.

Future you:

🥡 Cool and place in an airtight container, storing in the fridge for up to 6 days.
❄ Cool and freeze for up to 3 months.
💧 Thaw in the fridge overnight.
🔥 Enjoy at room temperature or reheat in an oven or air fryer on a low heat (around 140°C fan/160°C/325°F/gas mark 3) for 5–10 minutes. Only microwave them if you're serving in a bowl with ice cream, as microwaving will further soften them.

Apple Fritter Loaf

V

VE/O

DF/O

This really does taste like an apple fritter in cake form. The syrupy cinnamon apples running throughout are perfectly soft, but still hold a little bite, while the cake itself practically melts in your mouth. Plus, your kitchen will smell so, so incredible.

900-g/2-lb loaf tin, lined

2 tbsp milled flaxseed/linseed

60 ml/2 fl oz/¼ cup maple syrup

60 g/2 oz/¼ cup coconut oil, melted

120 g/4 oz/scant ½ cup unsweetened apple purée/apple sauce

juice of ½ lemon

80 ml/2¾ fl oz/⅓ cup milk

190 g/6¾ oz/scant 1½ cups plain/all-purpose flour

1 tsp bicarbonate of soda/baking soda

1 tsp ground cinnamon

¼ tsp fine sea salt

For the caramelized apples

3 sweet apples, peeled and diced into 1-cm/½-in chunks

2 tbsp maple syrup

1 tsp ground cinnamon

coconut oil, for cooking

For the glaze

3 tbsp runny yogurt

1 tbsp cream cheese

1 tsp maple syrup

1 Preheat the oven to 180°C fan/200°C/400°F/gas mark 6.

2 In a small bowl, combine the flaxseed and 5 tablespoons of water. Set this mixture aside for a few minutes to thicken. As there are no eggs in this recipe, this will act as the binder.

3 For the caramelized apples, toss the apples with maple syrup and cinnamon in a small bowl. Heat 1 teaspoon of coconut oil in a medium frying pan/skillet over medium heat. Cook the apples for 6-8 minutes, stirring occasionally, until caramelized and tender, but still retaining some bite. Remove from the heat and set aside.

4 In a large bowl, whisk the flaxseed mixture, maple syrup, coconut oil, apple purée, lemon juice and milk until smooth. Fold in the flour, bicarbonate of soda, cinnamon and salt with a spatula until just combined – avoid overmixing to keep the loaf light and fluffy.

5 Pour half of the batter into the prepared loaf tin, then layer with half of the caramelized apples. Add the remaining batter on top, and finish by layering the rest of the apples over the surface along with any residual syrupy juices.

6 Place the loaf tin on the middle shelf of the oven and bake for 40–45 minutes, or until a toothpick inserted into the centre comes out clean.

7 Let the loaf cool in the tin for 10 minutes, then transfer to a wire rack.

8 For the glaze, mix the yogurt, cream cheese and maple syrup in a bowl until smooth. Drizzle over the cooled loaf, and serve.

Substitutions:

● **No flaxseed?** If you are not vegan, substitute for 2 regular eggs and, in turn, reduce the amount of milk to 50 ml/1½ fl oz/3½ tbsp. ● **Vegan?** Omit the glaze.

Future you:

🥡 Cool and place in an airtight container, storing in the fridge for up to 7 days.
❄ Cool and freeze the unglazed loaf for up to 2 months.
💧 Thaw in the fridge overnight or at room temperature for a few hours.
🔥 Best enjoyed at room temperature. However, if you would like to warm, microwave a slice for 20 seconds.

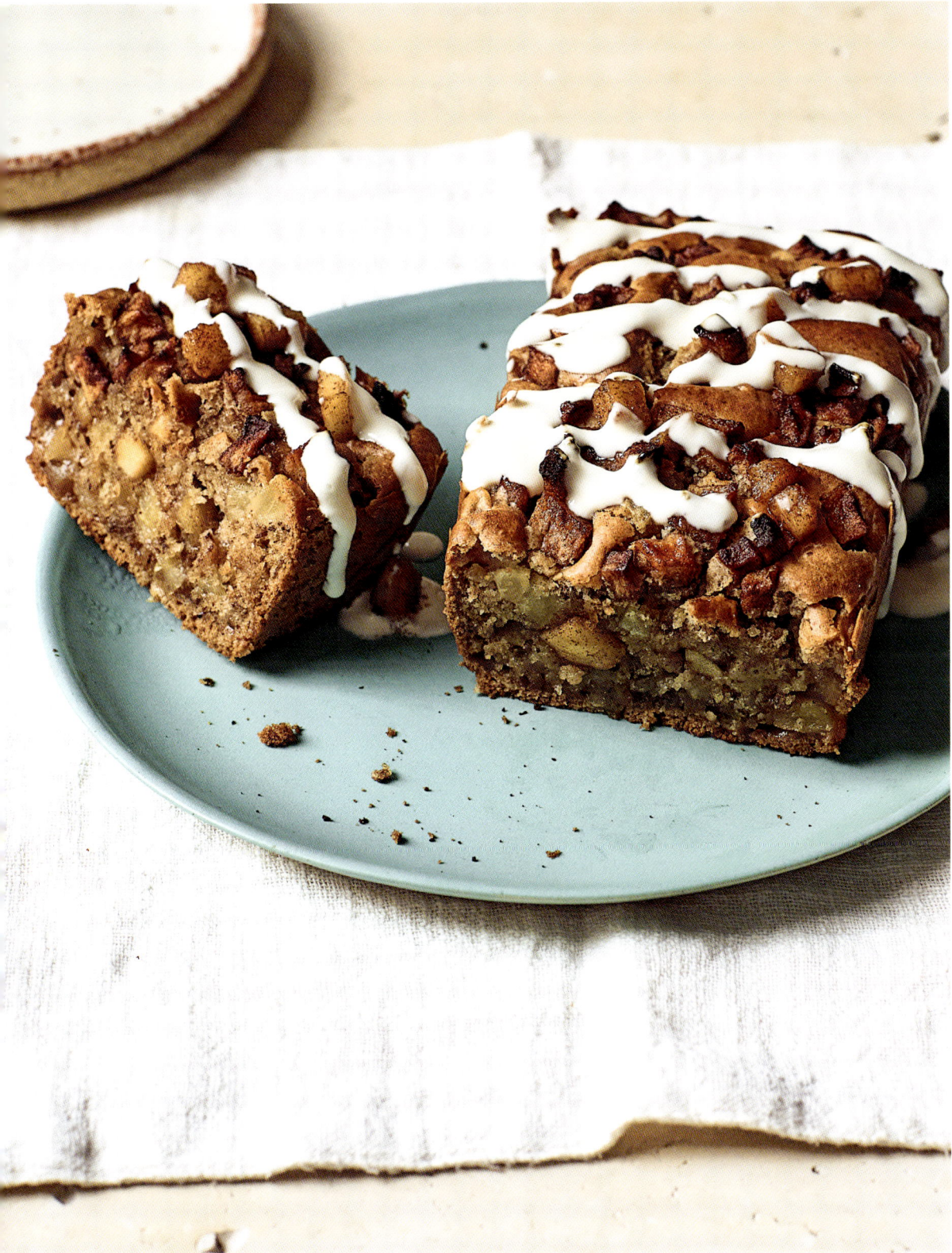

Healthy-ish Fudgy Brownies

(V)
(VE/O)
(DF)

We've all experienced the let-down of a brownie at some point in our lives. Whether you order one for pudding at a restaurant or bake a batch at home, the anticipation of biting into a gorgeously gooey and rich square can sometimes end in dry, cakey regret. That risk is even greater when you venture into 'healthy' brownie territory... So, naturally, here I am, doing just that. But trust me on this one – these brownies rival any butter-laden delight, and no avocados, black beans or sweet potatoes were harmed in the process. For this reason they definitely fall more into the -ish category, but they are so worth it. Utterly delicious, rich and decadent. Are you salivating yet? I am.

18-cm/7-in square brownie tin, lined with excess paper overhanging the sides

140 g/5 oz 70 per cent dark/bittersweet chocolate, broken into pieces

100 g/3½ oz/6½ tbsp coconut oil

3 large/US extra-large eggs, at room temperature

160 g/5½ oz/generous ¾ cup coconut sugar

85 g/3 oz/⅔ cup plain/all-purpose flour

35 g/1 oz/⅓ cup unsweetened cocoa powder

¼ tsp fine sea salt

60 g/2 oz/generous ⅓ cup dark/bittersweet chocolate chips or chunks

a pinch of flaky sea salt

1 Preheat the oven to 160°C fan/180°C/350°F/gas mark 4.

2 Add the chocolate and oil to a microwave-safe bowl. Heat in the microwave, in 20–30 second intervals, stirring between each, until the chocolate is melted, smooth and glossy.

3 In another bowl, use a handheld electric mixer to cream the eggs and sugar together until the mixture is paler, fluffy and at least doubled in volume – expect this to take no less than 4 minutes. After that, pour in the melted chocolate and gently fold it in with a flat rubber spatula until fully incorporated – be patient, this will take some time.

4 Sift the flour, cocoa powder and salt into the chocolate mixture. Using the spatula, gently fold everything together until no traces of flour remain. Tip in the chocolate chunks and fold a few more times to evenly distribute them.

5 Pour the batter into the prepared tin, spreading evenly to the edges and smoothing the top. Slide the tin onto the middle shelf of the preheated oven and bake for 14–18 minutes. The brownies will continue to cook after being removed from the oven, so it's better to err on the side of underbaking to ensure a perfectly gooey texture.

6 Once baked, resist the urge to dig in! Let the brownies cool in the tin for at least 10 minutes before transferring them to a wire rack to cool further. Finish with a sprinkle of flaky sea salt before slicing and serving.

Substitutions:

● **Vegan?** Make flaxseed 'eggs' by mixing 2 tbsp milled flaxseed with 5 tbsp water. You will also need to add ¼ tsp of baking powder with the flour at step 4.

Future you:

🍲 Cool and place in an airtight container, storing in the fridge for up to 10 days.
❄ Cool and freeze for up to 2 months.
💧 Thaw in the fridge overnight, or at room temperature for a few hours.
🔥 Enjoy at room temperature or, to make them extra gooey, warm in the microwave for 10–20 seconds.

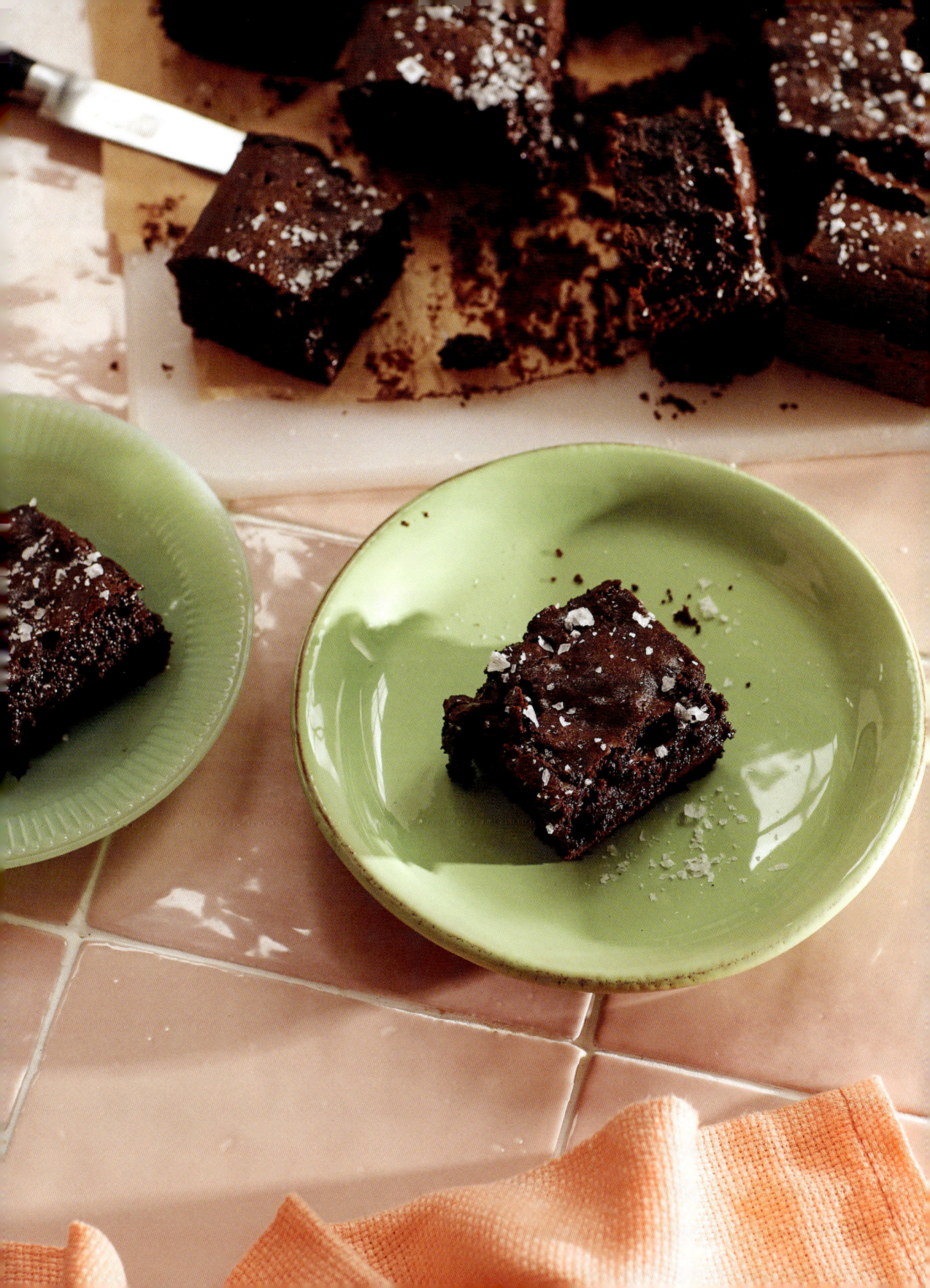

Dark Chocolate Macadamia Cookies

V
VE/O
DF
GF/O
N

Crisp on the outside and soft and chewy in the centre – these nutty delights are everything a good cookie should be. All you need is one bowl and they come together in no time, especially as I developed them with the intention of skipping the usual lengthy dough-chilling step. This makes them a perfect choice for any day you crave something wholesome and want your kitchen to smell like a bakery, without breaking a single sweat.

large baking sheet, lined

160 g/5½ oz/generous ¾ cup coconut sugar

1 large/US extra-large egg, at room temperature

70 ml/2⅓ fl oz/4½ tbsp mild olive oil

1 tsp vanilla extract

140 g/5 oz/1 cup plain/all-purpose flour

1 tsp cornflour/cornstarch

½ tsp bicarbonate of soda/baking soda

¼ tsp fine sea salt

40 g/1½ oz macadamia nuts, roughly chopped

60 g/2 oz dark/bittersweet chocolate, roughly chopped

a pinch of flaky sea salt

1 Preheat the oven to 170°C fan/190°C/375°F/gas mark 5.

2 In a medium mixing bowl, beat together the sugar, egg, oil and vanilla for about a minute until the mixture becomes light and fluffy.

3 Sift in the flour, cornflour, bicarbonate of soda and salt, then gently fold everything together with a flat rubber spatula, stopping just before the flour is fully incorporated. Add the nuts and chocolate, folding until evenly distributed and no streaks of flour remain.

4 Using an ice-cream scoop or a large spoon, divide the dough into 6–8 equal portions, depending on your desired cookie size. Place each portion in a heap on the prepared baking sheet, being careful not to press them down too much. Make sure to leave plenty of space between each one to allow for spreading.

5 Bake the cookies for 10–12 minutes, keeping a close eye on them from the 8-minute mark. You're looking for golden edges and a centre that is just set, as the cookies will continue to cook as they cool.

6 Once baked, tap the baking sheet lightly on the worktop a couple of times to slightly deflate the cookies – this trick helps to achieve a chewy texture. Sprinkle with a pinch of flaky sea salt and let the cookies cool on the baking sheet for at least 15 minutes to ensure they set and hold their shape before serving.

Substitutions:

● **No macadamias?** Sub for any other type of nut – hazelnuts, peanuts, walnuts or almonds would be delicious. ● **Vegan?** Replace the egg with 75 g/6 oz/⅓ cup dairy-free yogurt. ● **Gluten-free?** Use gluten-free flour. ● **Nut free?** Omit the nuts.

Future you:

🍵 Cool and place in an airtight container, storing in the fridge for up to 7 days.
❄ Cool and freeze for up to 2 months.
💧 Thaw in the fridge overnight, or at room temperature for a few hours.
🔥 Enjoy at room temperature, or microwave on full power for 5–10 seconds for a gooier experience!

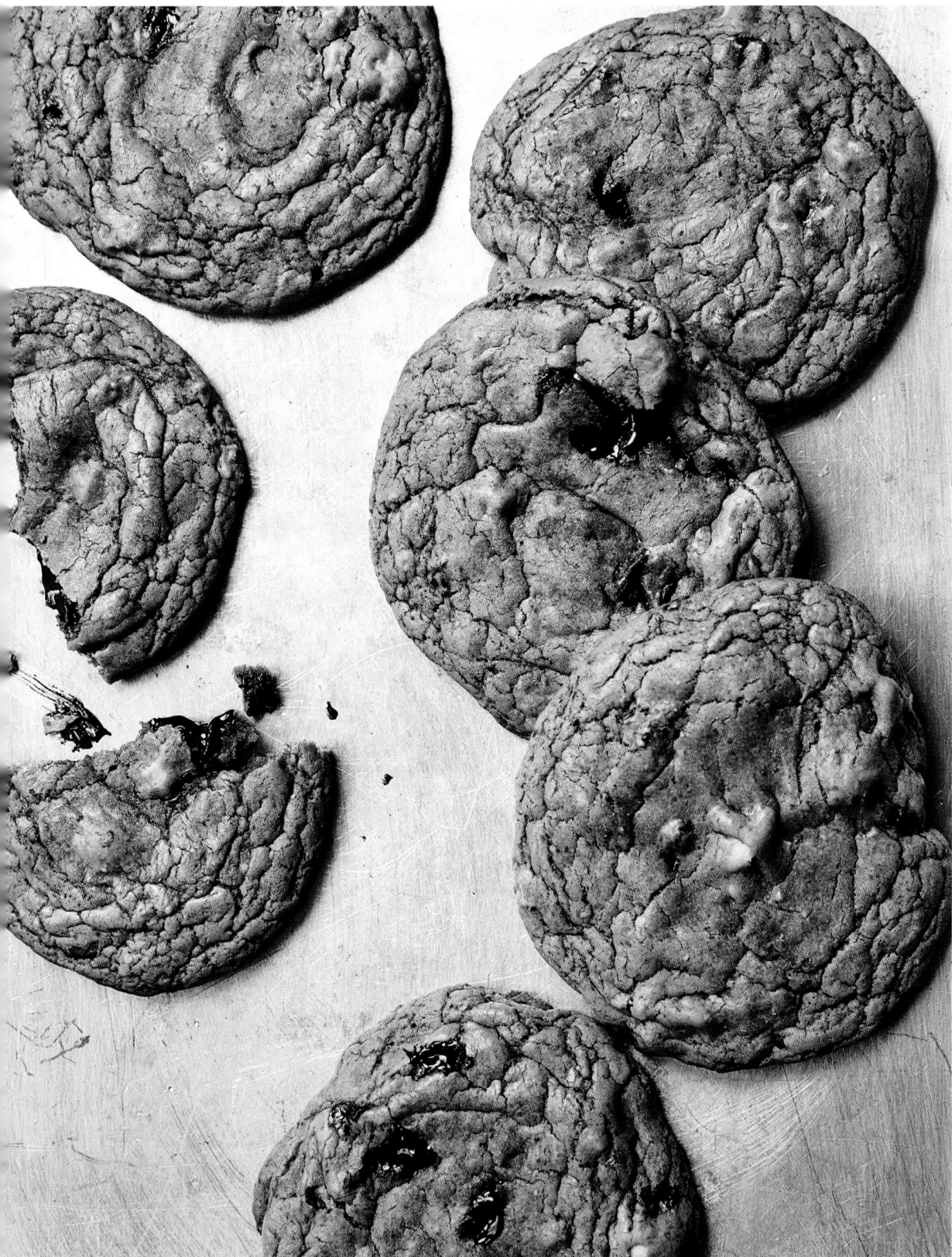

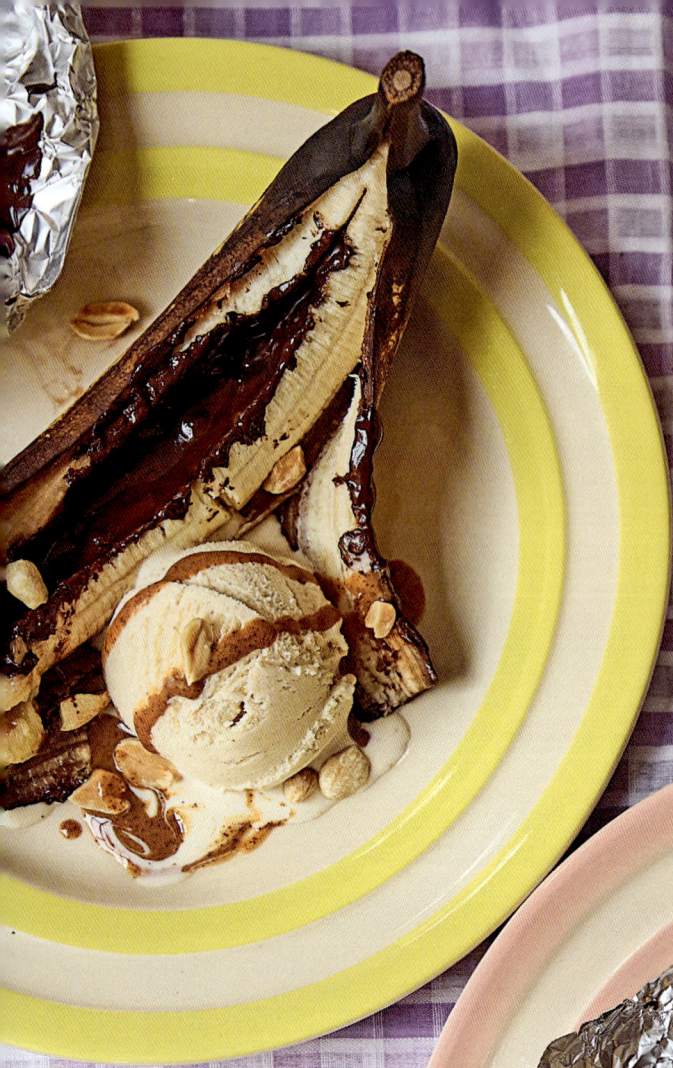

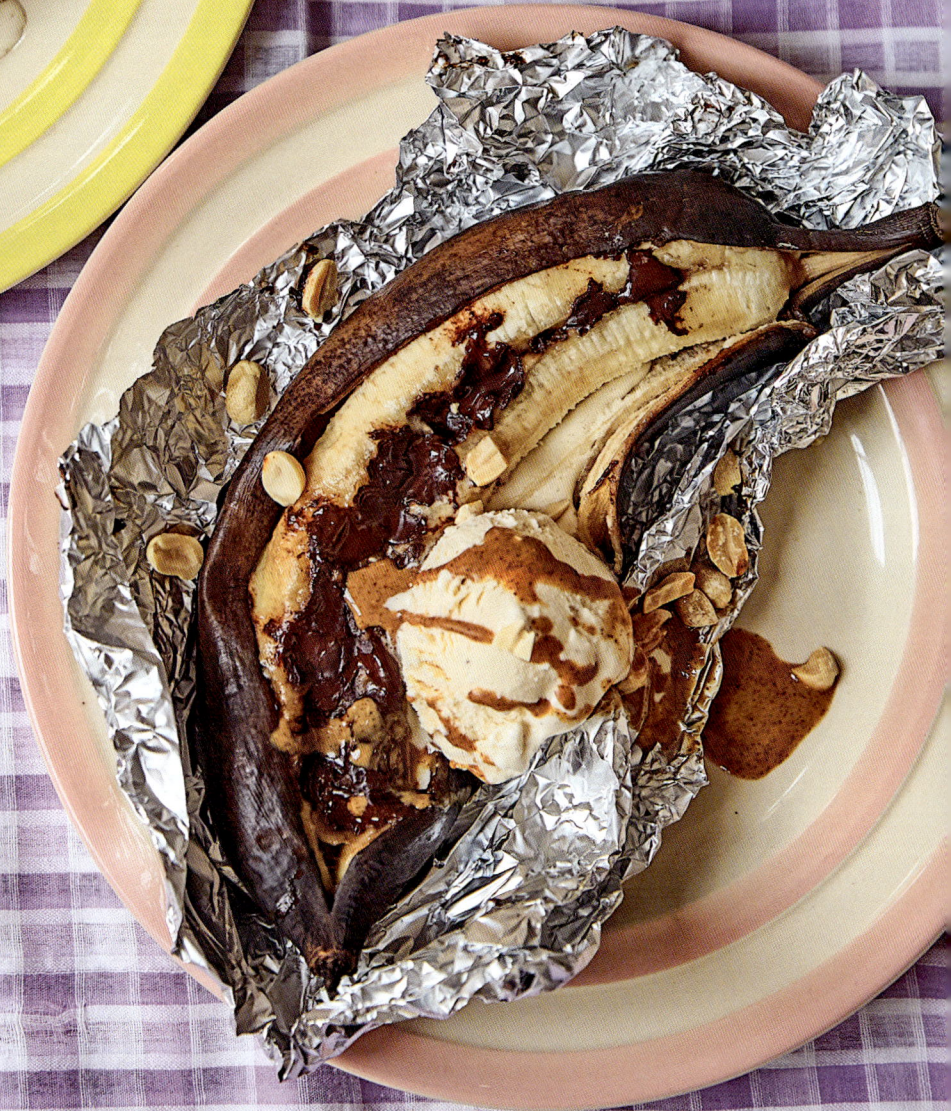

Campfire Bananas

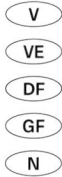

(V) (VE) (DF) (GF) (N)

While I love a beach holiday, camping will always have my heart. Growing up, camping trips were an annual thing, and a campfire feast was the best bit. After a dinner of burgers and hot dogs, the demands for 'foil bananas' would begin. The smell of caramelized bananas mingled with the smoky campfire is just pure bliss. Luckily, I've found that the oven does a surprisingly good job of recreating that nostalgia, so I present you with my grown-up version. It's just as delicious, melty, and gooey, with the added convenience of not needing to build a roaring fire! Simply wrap the bananas in foil, stuff them with your favourite things and bake.

2 ripe bananas

20 g/¾ oz/2 tbsp dark/bittersweet chocolate chips

a pinch of flaky sea salt

1 tsp peanuts, crushed

20 g/¾ oz/4 tsp natural peanut butter

ice cream, to serve (optional)

1 Preheat the air fryer or oven to 210°C fan/230°C/450°F/gas mark 8.

2 Carefully make a deep slice through the peel of each banana from stem to bottom, cutting the banana lengthways without going all the way through to the peel on the back side. Gently open the banana flesh just enough to create a pocket, and tuck in the pieces of chocolate.

3 Wrap each banana snugly in foil and place them into your preheated oven or air fryer. Cook for 15–20 minutes until the chocolate has melted and the banana is soft.

4 Carefully unwrap the hot bananas and plate them up with the peel prised slightly open. Sprinkle with a pinch of flaky sea salt, then top with crushed peanuts and a drizzle of peanut butter. Serve with a generous scoop of ice cream, if using, and dig in straight from the peel with a spoon.

Substitutions:

● **Nut free?** Use tahini in place of the peanut butter and replace the peanuts with another topping of your choice.

Lemon + Pistachio Olive Oil Cake

(V) (VE/O) (DF/O) (N)

Lemon cake lovers, this one's for you. Bright and zesty, with pistachios adding nuttiness to a sponge that's light, moist, and irresistible. Olive oil is the secret here – you can go bold with extra virgin for a real fruity richness (my fave), or keep it subtle with a milder variety, letting the lemon fully steal the show.

20-cm/8-in square tin, lined (allow the paper to overhang the edges)

100 g/3½ oz/¾ cup unsalted pistachio kernels

200 g/7 oz/1½ cups plain/all-purpose flour

¼ tsp fine sea salt

1 tsp bicarbonate of soda/baking soda

½ tsp baking powder

2 large/US extra-large eggs

100 g/3½ oz/scant ½ cup low-fat Greek yogurt

50 ml/1½ fl oz/3½ tbsp olive oil

grated zest and juice of 1 lemon, plus extra grated zest to decorate

1 tsp vanilla extract

150 ml/5 fl oz/⅔ cup honey

For the frosting

130 g/4½ oz/1 cup cream cheese

70 g/2½ oz/⅓ cup thick yogurt

2 tbsp honey

1 tsp freshly squeezed lemon juice

1   Preheat the oven to 180°C fan/200°C/400°F/gas mark 6.

2   In a food processor, blend the pistachios for 1–2 minutes until they have a mostly fine, dusty texture. Set them aside.

3   Grab a bowl and whisk together the flour, salt, bicarbonate of soda and baking powder.

4   In a separate, larger bowl, whisk together the eggs, yogurt, olive oil, lemon zest, lemon juice, vanilla and honey until smooth.

5   Sift the dry ingredients into the wet, add most of the pistachios (reserve some for topping), and gently fold everything together until no streaks of flour remain. Be cautious not to over-mix to keep the cake light and fluffy.

6   Pour the batter into the prepared tin, spreading it evenly to the edges. It may look bubbly; this is fine. Bake on the middle shelf for 17–18 minutes, or until a toothpick inserted in the centre comes out clean.

7   Once baked, allow the cake to cool in the tin for 10 minutes before transferring it to a wire rack to cool completely.

8   For the frosting, whisk together the cream cheese, yogurt, honey and lemon juice until smooth.

9   Once the cake is cool to the touch, spread the frosting evenly over the top, sprinkle across the reserved pistachios, and finish with a little lemon zest. Cut into 9 even portions and serve.

Substitutions:

● **Vegan?** Make flaxseed 'eggs' by mixing 2 tbsp milled flaxseed with 5 tbsp water. Use maple syrup in place of honey. Use dairy-free alternatives for the yogurt and cream cheese.

Future you:

🍱 Cool and place in an airtight container, storing in the fridge for up to 5 days.
❄ Cool and freeze for up to 2 months.
💧 Thaw in the fridge overnight, or at room temperature for a few hours.
🔥 Best enjoyed at room temperature.

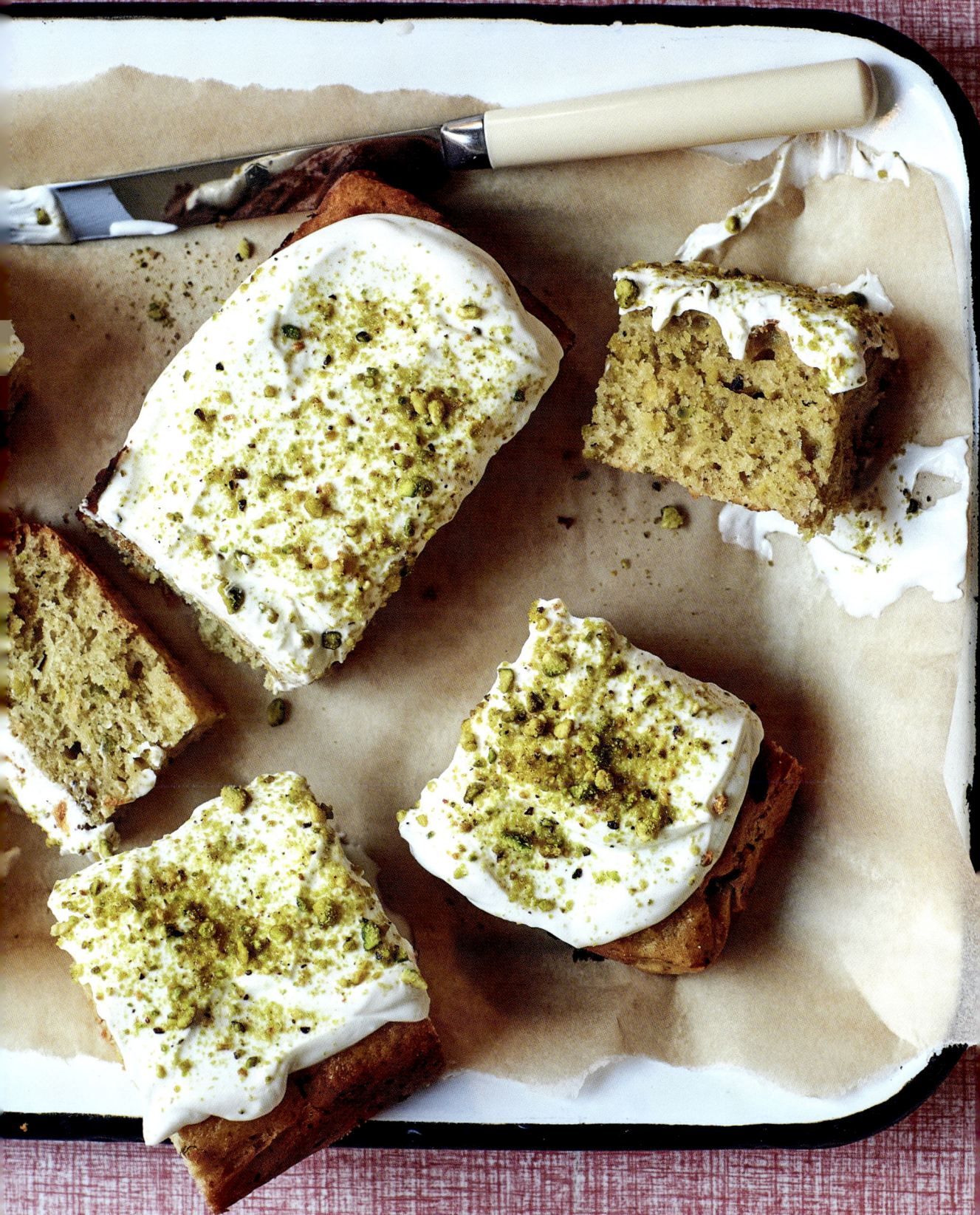

Blueberry Cobbler

V

VE/O

DF/O

N

If you've never met a cobbler before, allow me to introduce you. It's a classic American pud that I've come to adore – partly because it's so simple to throw together, but mostly because it's ridiculously delicious. If you're unfamiliar with how they work, cobblers are typically made up of a juicy fruit filling, topped with mounds of dough that bake up into a glorious scone-like (or biscuit-like, if you're stateside) layer. In other words, pure dessert bliss. You'll notice that ice cream is listed as optional, but I'll be honest – you'll never catch me eating this one without it.

23 x 15-cm/9 x 6-in baking dish

500 g/1 lb 2 oz/4 cups blueberries

2 tbsp agave or maple syrup

juice of ½ lemon

1 tbsp cornflour/cornstarch

ice cream, to serve (optional)

For the cobbler topping

180 g/6 oz/1⅓ cups plain/all-purpose flour

40 g/1½ oz/generous ⅓ cup ground almonds/almond meal

1 tsp baking powder

grated zest of ½ lemon

¼ tsp fine sea salt

50 g/1¾ oz/3½ tbsp coconut oil, melted and cooled

50 ml/1½ fl oz/3½ tbsp agave or maple syrup

1 tsp vanilla extract

100 ml/3½ fl oz/6½ tbsp milk

1 Preheat the oven to 180°C fan/200°C/400°F/gas mark 6.

2 In a mixing bowl, stir together the blueberries, syrup for the filling, lemon juice (be sure to zest the lemon first) and cornflour. Set aside.

3 In a separate bowl, make the cobbler topping. Whisk together the flour, ground almonds, baking powder, lemon zest and salt until combined. Pour in the melted coconut oil, along with the syrup, vanilla and milk. Gently fold with a rubber spatula to combine, stopping as soon as no patches of flour remain. The batter should be just about thick enough to be scooped up with an ice-cream scoop.

4 Pour the blueberries, as well as any syrupy juices left in the bottom of the bowl, into the baking dish and spread them out into an even layer.

5 Grab an ice-cream scoop, or large spoon, and make 6 dollops of the cobbler batter on top of the blueberries, ensuring to leave a few gaps in between. Slide the dish onto the middle shelf of the oven and bake for 30 minutes, or until the topping has turned golden and the blueberries are jammy and bubbling.

6 Serve immediately, with a big scoop of vanilla ice cream on top (if you like).

Substitutions:

● **No blueberries?** This is also delicious with other fruits such as cherries, peaches, apples or strawberries. ● **Nut free?** Replace the ground almonds with 20 g/¾ oz/2 tbsp flour of your choice.

Future you:

☕ Cool and place in an airtight container, storing in the fridge for up to 5 days.
❄ Cool and freeze for up to 2 months.
◗ Thaw in the fridge overnight, or on low power in the microwave.
♦ Warm on a low heat (around 140°C fan/160°C/325°F/gas mark 3) for 10–15 minutes, or microwave, covered, for 90 seconds.

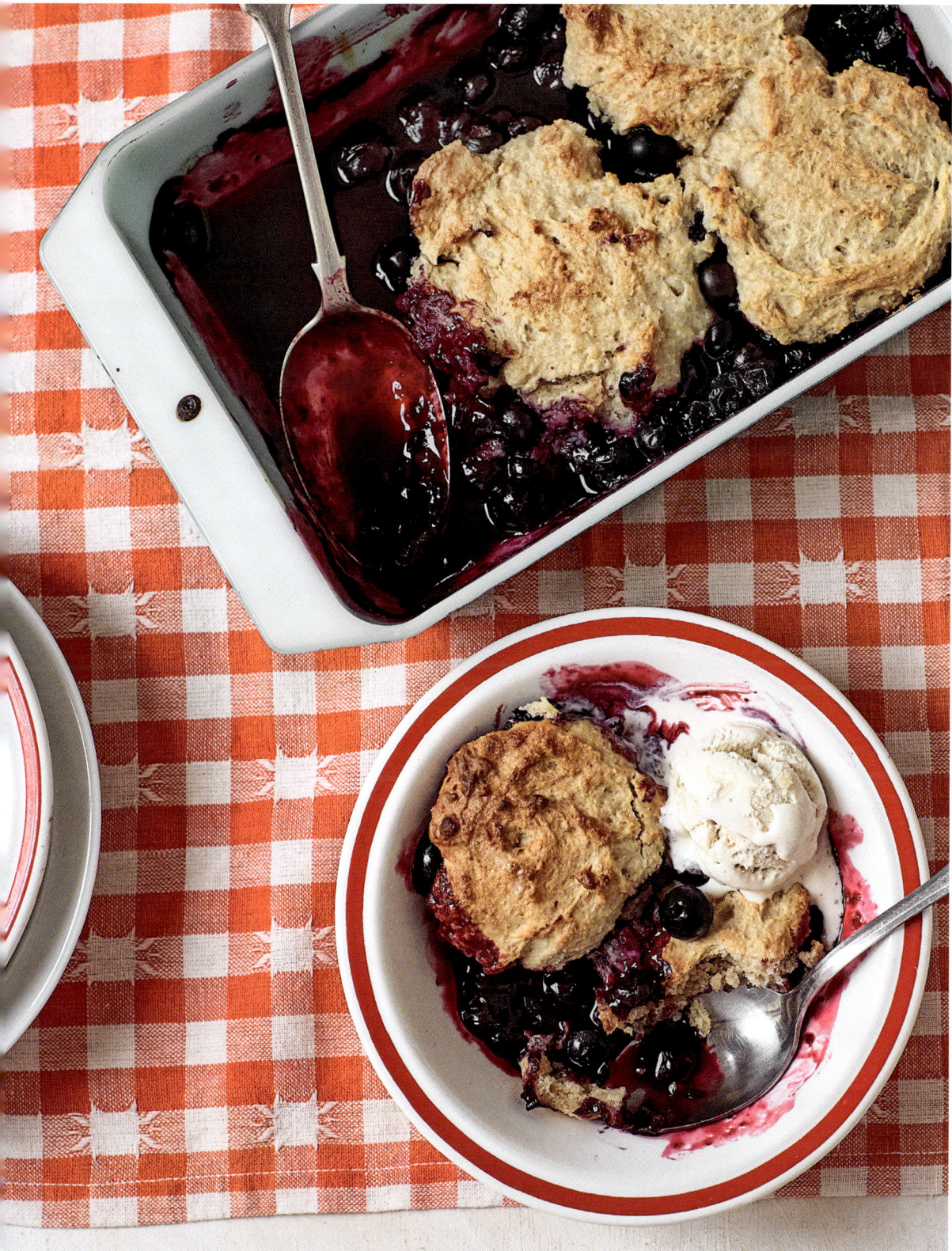

Gooey Chocolate Courgette Loaf Cake

I know what you're thinking. Courgette in a cake?! But hear me out. This cake is so moist it practically melts in your mouth, and every bite oozes with chocolatey goodness. Think: Matilda. That's what I'm promising here. The grated courgette is a secret weapon for adding incredible moisture and no, you can't taste it!

900-g/2-lb loaf tin, lined

2 tbsp milled flaxseed/linseed

1 courgette/zucchini

1 large ripe banana

60 g/2 oz/¼ cup coconut oil, melted

1 tsp vanilla extract

60 g/2 oz/5 tbsp coconut sugar

150 ml/5 fl oz/⅔ cup milk

160 g/5½ oz/scant 1¼ cups plain/all-purpose flour

40 g/1½ oz/generous ⅓ cup unsweetened cocoa powder

1 tsp bicarbonate of soda/baking soda

1 tsp baking powder

¼ tsp fine sea salt

100 g/3½ oz/⅔ cup dark/bittersweet chocolate chips, plus extra to decorate

For the frosting

130 g/4½ oz/scant ⅔ cup thick yogurt

1 tbsp unsweetened cocoa powder

50 g/1¾ oz/3½ tbsp natural peanut butter

2 tbsp maple syrup

1 Preheat the oven to 180°C fan/200°C/400°F/gas mark 6.

2 In a small bowl, combine the flaxseed with 5 tablespoons of water and set aside so it can thicken. As there are no eggs in this recipe, this acts as the binder.

3 Finely grate the courgette using the Parmesan side of a cheese grater and squeeze out as much water as possible using a paper towel. Aim for about half its original weight (140 g/5 oz) to prevent a watery loaf.

4 In a large bowl, mash the banana until smooth, then whisk in the courgette, flaxseed mixture, coconut oil, vanilla, sugar, and milk.

5 Sift the flour, cocoa powder, bicarbonate of soda and salt into the wet ingredients. Fold together gently with a spatula until just combined, then stir in the chocolate chips.

6 Pour the batter into the prepared loaf tin and smooth the top with your spatula. Bake for 40 minutes, or until a toothpick inserted into the centre comes out mostly clean (melted chocolate chips are fine!).

7 Leave the loaf to cool in the tin for about 10 minutes before turning out onto a wire rack to cool completely.

8 While the loaf cools, whip up the frosting. Whisk together the yogurt, cocoa powder, peanut butter and maple syrup until smooth.

9 Once the loaf is completely cool, spoon the frosting on top and spread it into an even layer, or serve the icing in a dollop on the side (the cake will last longer if not frosted).

Substitutions:

● **No flaxseed?** If you are not vegan, substitute for 2 regular eggs and reduce the amount of milk to 100 ml/3½ fl oz/6½ tablespoons.
● **Nut-free?** Use tahini instead of peanut butter.

Future you:

🍱 Cool and place in an airtight container, storing in the fridge for up to 6 days.
❄ The unfrosted cake can be frozen for up to 2 months.
💧 Thaw in the fridge overnight, or at room temperature for a few hours.
🔥 Best enjoyed at room temperature.

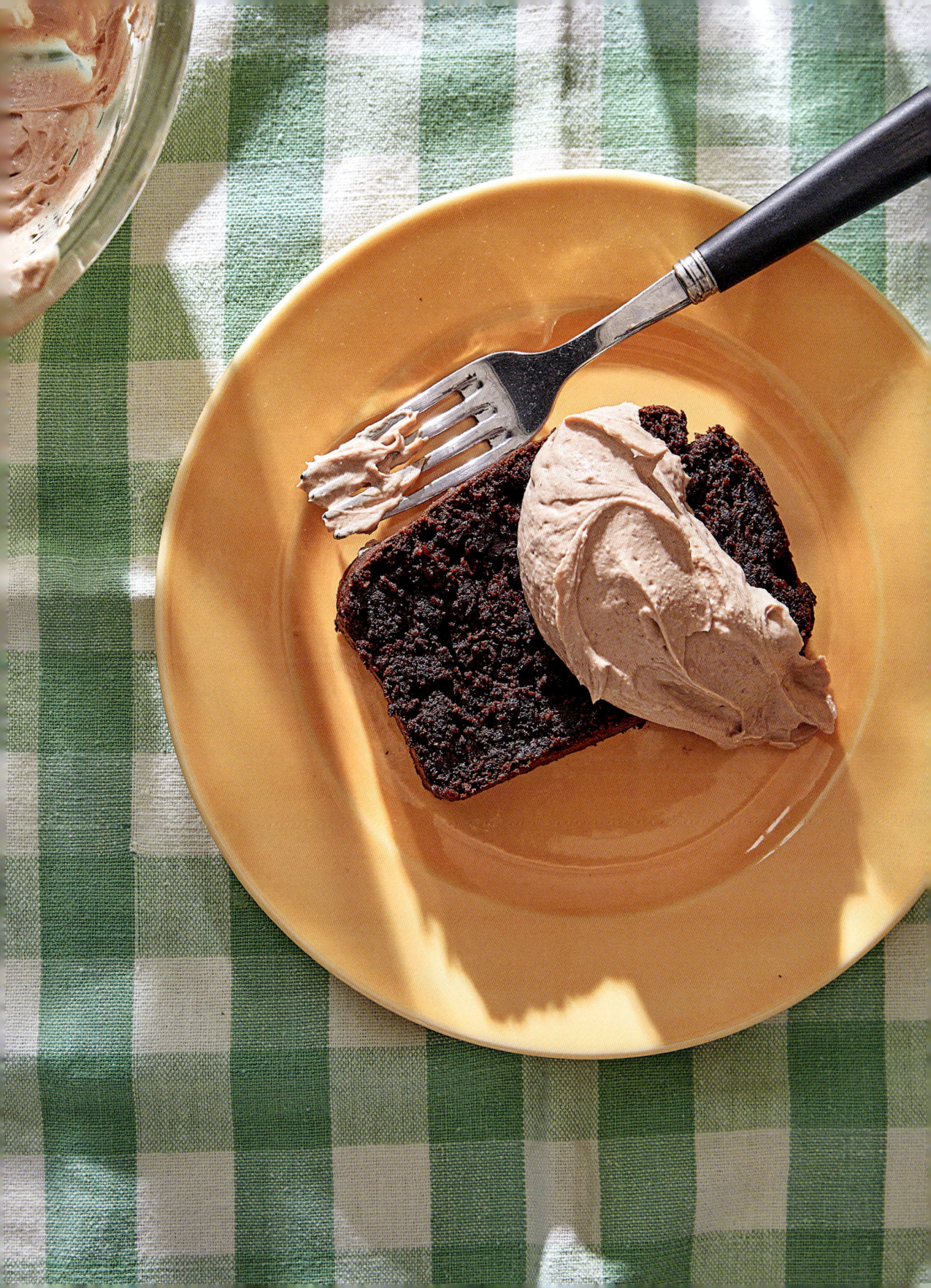

Index

Thank Yous

I still can't quite believe that *Healthy-ish* is here, tangible, real, and being held in your hands!

Just over a year ago, this cookbook was nothing more than an ambitious, and very "Emma-style", bells and whistles PowerPoint that I was nervously ready to pitch to the daunting world of publishing. To my amazement (and immense relief!), Pavilion immediately got the vision for *Healthy-ish*, and from the first meeting we just clicked. Laura, Ellen, Alice, Caroline, Emma, and everyone at Pavilion, I wish I had the word count to gush properly about how grateful I am for each and every one of you. Just look at the beauty of this book! It's quite literally all thanks to you. Thank you for embracing this dream with open arms and boundless talent. I really couldn't have asked for a better team to bring *Healthy-ish* to life.

To the incredible shoot team who made the long days feel like a laugh with friends, this book wouldn't have the life it does without your magic. Lizzie, your gorgeous photography gave every dish its own personality. Flossy, your food styling made every recipe look even more mouthwatering than I could have hoped. Maisie, thank you for giving each recipe the attention it deserved and for constantly reassuring me that my recipes actually work! And Ollie, my number 1 fan! My imposter syndrome was at an all-time high when I walked into the shoot on day 1, so having you hype up how genuinely delicious my food was, without fail, every single day, was the confidence boost you didn't know I needed.

Emily Sweet, my incredible literary agent, thank you for guiding me through this journey with such grace and wisdom. You coined "Healthy-ish" as the title after hearing me use it to describe my food in our very first meeting, and it couldn't be more perfect. To Ellie and Chloe at 84 World, who are so much more than just my managers, thank you for always being by my side, taking things off my plate when I needed it most, and extinguishing my self-doubt whenever it crept in.

And now, most importantly, to my family. Mum, Dad, Tom and the entire Petersen/Bagot crew – where do I even begin?! From the early days of my ever-changing hobbies to the day I dubiously announced that I was leaving my career as a lawyer to chase my dreams in food, you've stood by me with unwavering faith (even though it sometimes required a brief and frank "are you absolutely sure?" chat first!). You're my rocks, my constant support, and my biggest cheerleaders, no matter what path I take. I am beyond grateful for each of you and everything you've done to help me get here.

Thank you to my gorgeous partner, Matt, who took his taste-testing "duties" very seriously! And my best friends and hype girls Ilse and Imo, thank you all for being my calm in the storm and for your belief in me, especially on days when mine wavered.

To my wonderful online community, from those who've been here since the start to the newest faces, thank you. Your messages, comments and constant support fuelled this book, pushed me forward on the hard days, and reminded me why I love doing this so much.

And finally, to you – yes, you holding this book! You're the reason I've poured my heart into every page. I hope this book makes cooking easier, a little bit healthier, and a lot more delicious for you. Thank you for bringing *Healthy-ish* into your kitchen, and I hope you enjoy every bite.

With love, Emma x

Pavilion
An imprint of HarperCollinsPublishers Ltd
1 London Bridge Street
London SE1 9GF

www.harpercollins.co.uk

HarperCollinsPublishers
Macken House
39/40 Mayor Street Upper
Dublin 1
D01 C9W8
Ireland

10 9 8 7 6 5 4 3 2 1

First published in Great Britain by Pavilion
An imprint of HarperCollinsPublishers 2025

ISBN 978-0-00- 8730567

MIX
FSC
www.fsc.org
Paper | Supporting
responsible forestry
FSC™ C007454

This book contains FSC™ certified paper and
other controlled sources to ensure responsible
forest management.

For more information visit:
www.harpercollins.co.uk/green

Publishing Director: Laura Russell
Commissioning Editor: Ellen Simmons
Design Manager: Alice Kennedy-Owen
Designer: Studio Nic&Lou
Production Controller: Grace O'Byrne
Production Assistant: Emma Hatlen
Photographer: Lizzie Mayson
Food Stylist/Prop Stylist: Flossy McAslan
Copyeditor: Kate Reeves-Brown
Proofreader: Laura Nickoll
Indexer: Ruth Ellis
Reproduction: Rival Colour Limited

Printed and bound by GPS Group in Bosnia
and Herzegovina